Fundamental Critical Care Support

Fourth Edition

Printed in the United States of America
Second Printing, November 2007
Society of Critical Care Medicine
Headquarters
500 Midway Drive
Mount Prospect, IL 60056 USA
Phone +1 (847)827-6869
Fax +1 (847)827-6886
www.sccm.org
International Standard Book Number: 978-0-936145-30-3

Fourth Edition Contributors

Editors:

Barbara McLean, MN, CCRN, CCNS, CCNP, FCCM
Atlanta Medical Center
Atlanta, Georgia
Guidelines Consultant: Piedmont Hospital System

Janice L. Zimmerman, MD, FCCM
The Methodist Hospital
Houston, Texas
No disclosures

Associate Editors:

Marie Baldisseri, MD
University of Pittsburgh Medical Center
Pittsburgh, Pennsylvania
No disclosures

J. Christopher Farmer, MD, FCCM
Mayo Foundation
Rochester, Minnesota
No disclosures

R. Phillip Dellinger, MD, FCCM
Cooper University Hospital
Camden, New Jersey
No disclosures

Thomas E. Grissom, MD, FCCM
University of Maryland School of Medicine
Baltimore, Maryland
No disclosures

Contributors:

Prasad E. Abraham, PharmD, BCPS
Grady Health Systems
Atlanta, Georgia
No disclosures

Robert Aranson, MD
Parkview Adventist Medical Center
Freeport, Maine
No disclosures

James A. Barker, MD
Palmetto Richland Hospital
Columbia, South Carolina
No disclosures

Kent D. Blad, MS, ACNP, FNP, FCCM
Brigham Young University
Riverton, Utah
No disclosures

Thomas P. Bleck, MD, FCCM
Evanston Northwestern Healthcare
Evanston, Illinois
No disclosures

Eric L. Bloomfield, MD, FCCM
Mayo Clinic
Rochester, Minnesota
No disclosures

Gregory H. Botz, MD
M.D. Anderson Cancer Center
Houston, Texas
No disclosures

William A. Brock, MD, FCCM
Sentara Healthcare
Chesapeake, Virginia
No disclosures

Ronald G. Caravano, Jr.
Medical Education Technologies, Inc.
Sarasota, Florida
Employee: Medical Education Technologies Inc.

Daniel H. Ceraso, MD, FCCM
Hospital Juan A. Fernandez
Buenos Aires, Argentina
No disclosures

Eric A. Crawley, MD
Tripler Army Medical Center
Kailua, Hawaii
No disclosures

Gavin D. Divertie, MD
Mayo Clinic
Jacksonville, Florida
No disclosures

David J. Dries, MD, FCCM
Regions Hospital
Saint Paul, Minnesota
No disclosures

Brandon Foster, MSN, APRN, CSN
Palmetto Neurosurgery & Spine
Lexington, South Carolina
No disclosures

Ross C. Freebairn, MD
Hawkes Bay Hospital
Hastings, New Zealand
No disclosures

Eugene B. Freid, MD, FCCM
Nemours Children's Clinics
Jacksonville, Florida
Consultant: Medical Education Technologies, Inc.

Andrea Gabrielli, MD, FCCM
University of Florida
Gainesville, Florida
No disclosures

Ahmed I. Ghali, MD
Dar Al-Fouad Hospital
Touristic Zone, Giza, Egypt
No disclosures

Manuel R. Gonzalez-Brito, DO
University of Miami School of Medicine
South Miami, Florida
No disclosures

K. Dean Gubler, DO, FCCM
Legacy Emanuel Trauma
Portland, Oregon
No dislcosures

Steven M. Hollenberg, MD, FCCM
Cooper University Hospital
Camden, New Jersey
No disclosures

Mary Anne House-Fancher, ACNP, CCRN, ARNP
Health-First Heart Institute
Melbourne, Florida
No disclosures

Edgar Jimenez, MD, FCCM
Orlando Regional Medical Center
Orlando, Florida
No disclosures

Maria T. Kinsella, RN, BSN
Exempla Saint Joseph Hospital
Denver, Colorado
No disclosures

Peter K. Linden, MD
University of Pittsburgh Medical Center
Pittsburgh, Pennsylvania
No disclosures

Donald K. Maxwell, DO
Banner Desert Medical Center
Tempe, Arizona
No disclosures

Rodrigo Mejia, MD, FCCM
University of Texas M.D. Anderson Cancer Center
Houston, Texas
No disclosures

William S. Miles, MD, FCCM
Carolinas Medical Center
Charlotte, North Carolina
No disclosures

Nicholas Namias, MD, FACS, FCCM
Miller School of Medicine / University of Miami
Miami, Florida
No disclosures

Jorge A. Neira, MD, FCCM
Sanatoria De La Trinidad
Ciudad De Buenos Aires, Argentina
No disclosures

Scot Nolan, MS, RN, CNS, PHN, CCRN, CNRN, WCC
Scripps Mercy Hospital
San Diego, California
No disclosures

J. Robert Osborne, MD
Atlanta Medical Center
Atlanta Georgia
No disclosures

William B. Owens, MD
University of South Carolina
Columbia, South Carolina
No disclosures

Jose Luis do Pico, MD
Hospital de Necochea
Necochea, Argentina
No disclosures

Ignacio Jose Previgliano, MD
Sociedad Argentina De Terapia Invesiva
Capital Federal, Argentina
No disclosures

Nestor O. Raimondi, MD, FCCM
Hospital Juan A. Fernandez
Buenos Aires, Argentina
No disclosures

Sophia Chu Rogers, MSN, ACNP, FAANP, FCCM
Lovelace Health Systems
Albuquerque, New Mexico
Employee: Lovelace Health Systems

Joan L. Settlemyer, PharmD
Carolinas Medical Center
Charlotte, North Carolina
No disclosures

Khalid Ahmad I. Shukri, MD, MBA, FCCM,
FIPACCM
King Fahad Specialist Hospital
Dammam, Saudi Arabia
No disclosures

Alexander O. Sy, MD, FCCP, FASM
University of Scouth Carolina School of Medicine
Columbia, South Carolina
No disclosures

James E. Szalados, MD, MBA, FCCM, JD
Park Ridge Hospital
Rochester, New York
No disclosures

Robert J. Tiller, MD
Self Regional Healthcare
Greenwood, South Carolina
No disclosures

Johannes G. van der Hoeven, MD, PhD
Radboud University Medical Centre
Mook, Netherlands
No disclosures

Nick Widder, RRT
Carolinas Medical Center
Charlotte, North Carolina
No disclosures

Kenneth E. Wood, DO, FCCM
University of Wisconsin Hospital and Clinics
Madison, Wisconsin
No disclosures

Thomas E. Woodcock, MD, MB, BS
Southampton University Hospital
Southampton, United Kingdom
No disclosures

FUNDAMENTAL CRITICAL CARE SUPPORT
FOURTH EDITION

The Fundamental Critical Care Support (FCCS) program of the Society of Critical Care Medicine (SCCM) has grown enormously since its inception in 1994. It is doubtful that those who conceived this idea would have ever thought that the course would be offered in five languages, at approximately 240 sites annually, in 36 countries, and that this textbook would be in its fourth edition. Most importantly, the overall success of the FCCS program has been the result of many individuals who have volunteered to teach the important concepts and principles...the fundamentals of critical care.

This fourth edition has been developed as a result of the energy and resolve of the SCCM staff, especially Gervaise Nicklas, MS, RN, and Lynn Retford; the diverse and multi-professional individuals who contributed the chapters; the very hard work of the four associate editors who reviewed content and provided feedback; and the perseverance and dedication of our two co-editors: Barbara McLean, MN, CCRN, CCNS, CCNP, FCCM and Janice L. Zimmerman, MD, FCCM.

In hope of increasing the utility of the text, a new format is being introduced. Course participants will find that each chapter opens with a brief scenario that generates a context for the successive discussions. Also, key considerations are highlighted in text boxes throughout each chapter.

The FCCS program has been one of the main cornerstones of the Society's educational foundation and the successful completion of this new edition has been a priority of SCCM leadership. It is hoped that, in the tradition of the FCCS program and the previous versions of this book, many professionals will learn about critical care and, importantly, that many patients will benefit as a consequence of that knowledge.

Frederick P. Ognibene, MD, FCCM
2007 President, Society of Critical Care Medicine

Table of Contents

Table of Contents

Chapter 1

RECOGNITION AND ASSESSMENT OF THE SERIOUSLY ILL PATIENT

✓ Objectives

- Explain the importance of early identification of patients at risk for life-threatening illness or injury and the importance of early intervention.

- Recognize the early signs and symptoms of critical illness.

- Discuss the initial assessment and early treatment of the critically ill or injured patient.

Case Study

A 54-year-old diabetic woman with cholelithiasis and recurrent episodes of pancreatitis undergoes a laparoscopic cholecystectomy. On the third postoperative day, she develops shortness of breath. The surgeon asks you to see the patient.

- What history is important to obtain for this patient?

- Which aspects of the physical examination would you concentrate on initially?

- Which investigations would you order for this patient?

I. INTRODUCTION

As the old adage goes, an ounce of prevention is worth a pound of cure. That principle often applies in the care of critically ill patients. Early identification of patients at risk for life-threatening illness makes it easier to manage them appropriately and prevent further deterioration. Many clinical problems, if recognized early, can be managed with simple measures such as oxygen, respiratory therapy interventions, intravenous fluids, or effective analgesia. The early identification of patients in trouble allows clinicians time to identify the main physiological problem, determine its underlying cause, and begin treatment. The longer the interval between the onset of an acute illness and the appropriate intervention, the more likely it is that the patient's condition will deteriorate, even to cardiopulmonary arrest. Several studies have demonstrated that physiological deterioration precedes many cardiopulmonary arrests by hours, suggesting that early intervention could prevent the need for resuscitation, admission to the intensive care unit (ICU), and other sentinel events. Many hospitals are using medical emergency teams (METs) to identify patients at risk and begin early treatment. (See **Appendix 1** for further information on organization and implementation of medical emergency teams.) The purpose of this chapter is to describe the general principles involved in recognizing and assessing acutely ill patients.

II. RECOGNIZING THE PATIENT AT RISK

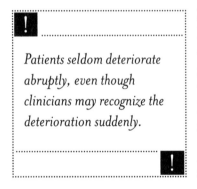

Patients seldom deteriorate abruptly, even though clinicians may recognize the deterioration suddenly.

Recognizing that a patient is seriously ill is usually not difficult. It may be more challenging, however, if the patient is in the very early stages of the process. Young and otherwise fit patients may be much slower to exhibit the signs and symptoms of an acute illness than may elderly patients with impaired cardiopulmonary function. Individuals that are immunosuppressed or debilitated may not mount a vigorous and clinically obvious inflammatory response. Some conditions, such as cardiac arrhythmias, do not evolve with progressively worsening and easily detectable changes in physiology but present as an abrupt change of state. In most circumstances, a balance exists between the patient's reserve and the acute disease. Patients with limited reserve are more likely to be susceptible to severe illness and to experience greater degrees of organ-system impairment. Identifying patients at risk of deterioration therefore requires assessment of their background health, their current disease process, and their current physiological condition.

A. Assessing Severity

"How sick is this patient?" is one of the most important questions a clinician must answer. Determining the response requires the measurement of vital signs and other specific physiological variables (**Appendix 1**). Acute illness typically causes predictable changes in physiology that are associated with a limited range of clinical signs. For example, a patient's physiological response to a bacterial infection may result in fever, delirium, shaking chills, and tachypnea. The most important step is to recognize these signs and initiate physiologic monitoring in order to quantify the severity of disease and take appropriate action. Sick patients may present with confusion, irritability, impaired consciousness, or a sense of impending doom. They may appear short of breath and may demonstrate signs of a sympathetic response, such as pallor, sweating, or cool extremities. Symptoms may be nonspecific, such as nausea and weakness, or, like chest pain, they may identify the involvement of a particular organ system. A high index of suspicion is therefore required when starting the measurement of vital signs: pulse rate, blood pressure, respiratory rate, oxygenation, temperature, and urine output. Clinical monitoring helps to quantify the severity of the disease process, tracks trends and rates of deterioration, and directs attention to those aspects of physiology that most urgently need treatment. The goals at this stage of assessment are to recognize that a problem exists and to maintain physiological stability while pursuing the cause and initiating treatment.

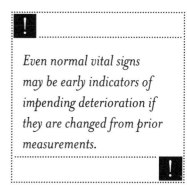

Even normal vital signs may be early indicators of impending deterioration if they are changed from prior measurements.

Tachycardia in response to physiologic abnormalities (ie, fever, low cardiac output) may be increased with pain and anxiety or suppressed in patients with conduction abnormalities or receiving ß-blockade.

B. Making a Diagnosis

Making an accurate diagnosis in the acutely ill patient often must take second place to treating life-threatening physiological abnormalities. It is important to ask the question, "What physiological problem needs to be corrected now to prevent further deterioration of the patient's condition?" Correcting the problem may be as simple as providing oxygen or intravenous fluids. Time for the leisurely pursuit of a differential diagnosis is not likely to be available. However, an accurate diagnosis is essential for refining treatment options once physiological stability is achieved. The general principles of taking an accurate history, performing a brief, directed clinical examination followed by a secondary survey, and organizing laboratory investigations are fundamentally important. Good clinical skills and a disciplined approach in circumstances that may be frightening for inexperienced staff are required to accomplish these tasks.

III. INITIAL ASSESSMENT OF THE CRITICALLY ILL PATIENT

> **!**
>
> *A primary and secondary survey approach is recommended in the assessment of a seriously ill patient.*
>
> **!**

A framework for assessing the acutely ill patient is provided in **Table 1-1** and discussed below. Further information on specific issues and treatments can be found in later chapters of this text.

Table 1-1 Framework for Assessing the Acutely Ill or Injured Patient

	PHASE I **Initial Contact— First Minutes** (Primary Survey) What is the main physiological problem?	**PHASE II** **Subsequent Reviews** (Secondary Survey) What is the underlying cause?
History	**Main features of circumstances and environment** • Witnesses, healthcare personnel, relatives • Main symptoms: pain, dyspnea, altered mental status, weakness • Trauma or no trauma • Operative or nonoperative • Medications and/or toxins	**More detailed information** • Present complaint • Past history, chronic diseases, surgeries • Hospital course (if applicable) • Psychosocial and physical independence • Medications and allergies • Family history • Ethical or legal issues, code status • Systems review
Examination	**Look, listen, feel** • Airway • Breathing and oxygenation • Circulation • Level of consciousness	**Structured examination of organ systems** • Respiratory system • Cardiovascular system • Abdomen and genitourinary tract • Central nervous and musculoskeletal systems • Endocrine and hematological systems
Chart review, documentation	**Essential physiology, vital signs** • Heart rate, rhythm • Blood pressure • Respiratory rate and pulse oximetry • Level of consciousness	**Case records and note keeping** • Examine medical records, if available • Formulate specific diagnosis or differential diagnosis • Document current events
Investigations	• Blood gas analysis (use venous if arterial access is difficult) • Blood glucose	• Laboratory blood tests • Radiology • Electrocardiogram • Microbiology
Treatment	**Proceeds in parallel with the above** • Ensure adequate airway and oxygen • Provide intravenous access ± fluids • Assess response to immediate resuscitation • CALL FOR MORE EXPERIENCED ADVICE AND ASSISTANCE	**Refine treatment, assess responses, review trends** • Provide support for specific organ systems as required • Choose most appropriate site for care • Obtain specialists' advice and assistance

A. History

The patient's history provides the greatest contribution to diagnosis. Often the current history, past medical history, and medication list must be obtained from family members, caregivers, friends, neighbors, or other healthcare providers. The risk of critical illness is increased in patients with the following characteristics:

- Emergency admission (limited information)

- Advanced age (limited reserve)

- Severe coexisting chronic illness (limited reserve, limited options for management)

- Severe physiological abnormalities (limited reserve, refractory to therapy)

- Need for or recently undergone major surgery, especially an emergency procedure

- Severe hemorrhage or need for a massive blood transfusion

- Deterioration or lack of improvement

- Immunodeficiency

- Combination of the preceding problems

A complete history includes the present complaint, treatment history, hospital course to the present (if applicable), past illnesses, past surgeries, current medications, and any medication allergies. A social history, including alcohol, tobacco, or illicit drug use, and a family history, including the degree of physical and psychosocial independence, are essential and often omitted. The history of the present complaint must include a brief review of systems that should be replicated in the examination that follows.

Critical illness is often associated with inadequate cardiac output, respiratory compromise, and a depressed level of consciousness. Specific symptoms will typically be associated with the underlying condition. Patients may complain of nonspecific symptoms such as malaise, fever, lethargy, anorexia, or thirst. Organ-specific symptoms may direct attention to the respiratory, cardiovascular, or gastrointestinal systems. Distinguishing acute from chronic disease is important at this point, as chronic conditions may be difficult to reverse and may act as rate-limiting factors during the recovery phase of critical illness.

B. Examination

Look, listen, and feel. The patient must be fully exposed for a complete examination. The initial examination must be brief, directed, and concentrated on the basic elements: airway, breathing, circulation, and level of consciousness. As the treatment proceeds, a more detailed secondary survey should be conducted to refine the preliminary diagnosis and assess the response to initial treatment. A full examination must be performed at some point and will be guided by the history and other findings. Ongoing deterioration or development of new symptoms warrants a further primary survey.

Remember the ABCs of resuscitation: airway, breathing, circulation. The airway and respiratory system should be assessed first, as summarized in **Table 1-2**. Observe the patient's mouth and chest. There may be obvious signs suggesting airway obstruction as well as vomitus, blood, or a foreign body. The patient's respiratory rate, pattern of breathing, and use of accessory respiratory muscles will help to confirm respiratory distress or airway obstruction (see **Chapter 2**). *Tachypnea is the single most important indicator of critical illness.* Therefore, the respiratory rate must be accurately measured and documented. Although tachypnea may result from pain or anxiety, it may also indicate pulmonary disease, severe metabolic abnormalities, or infection. Look for cyanosis, paradoxical respiration, equality and depth of respiration, use of accessory muscles, and tracheal tug. An increase in the depth of respiration (Kussmaul breathing) may indicate severe metabolic acidosis. Periodic breathing (Cheyne-Stokes respiration) usually indicates severe brainstem injury or cardiac dysfunction. Agitation and confusion may result from hypoxemia, whereas hypercapnia will usually depress the level of consciousness. Low oxygen saturation can be detected with pulse oximetry, but this assessment may be unreliable if the patient is hypovolemic, hypotensive, or hypothermic. Noisy breathing (eg, grunting, stridor, wheezing, gurgling) may indicate partial airway obstruction. Complete airway obstruction will result in silence.

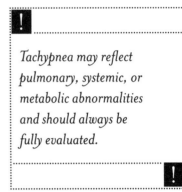

Tachypnea may reflect pulmonary, systemic, or metabolic abnormalities and should always be fully evaluated.

Table 1-2	Assessment of Airway and Breathing
Airway	
Causes of Obstruction	Direct trauma, blood, vomitus, foreign body, central nervous system depression (with soft tissue or tongue blocking airway), infection, inflammation, laryngospasm
LOOK for	Cyanosis, altered respiratory pattern and rate, use of accessory respiratory muscles, tracheal tug, altered level of consciousness
LISTEN for	Noisy breathing (grunting, stridor, wheezing, gurgling); complete obstruction results in silence
FEEL for	Decreased or absent airflow
Breathing	
Causes of Inadequate Breathing or Oxygenation	
Depressed respiratory drive	Central nervous system depression
Decreased respiratory effort	Muscle weakness, nerve/spinal cord damage, debilitation, chest wall abnormalities, pain
Pulmonary disorders	Pneumothorax, hemothorax, aspiration, chronic obstructive pulmonary disease, asthma, pulmonary embolus, lung contusion, acute lung injury, acute respiratory distress syndrome, pulmonary edema, rib fracture, flail chest
LOOK for	Cyanosis, altered level of consciousness, tracheal tug, use of accessory respiratory muscles, altered respiratory pattern, altered respiratory rate, equality and depth of breaths, oxygen saturation
LISTEN for	Dyspnea, inability to talk, noisy breathing, dullness to percussion, auscultation of breath sounds
FEEL for	Symmetry and extent of chest movements, position of trachea, crepitus, abdominal distension

Inadequate circulation may result from primary abnormalities of the cardiovascular system or secondary abnormalities caused by metabolic disturbances, sepsis, hypoxia, or drugs (**Table 1-3**). *A drop in blood pressure may be a late sign of cardiovascular disturbance signaling failure of the compensatory mechanisms.* Central and peripheral pulses should be assessed for rate, regularity, volume, and symmetry. Patients with hypovolemia or low cardiac output will have weak and thready peripheral pulses. A bounding pulse suggests hyperdynamic circulation, and an irregular rhythm usually signifies atrial fibrillation. A ventricular premature beat is often immediately followed by a compensatory pause, and the subsequent beat often has a larger pulse volume. Pulsus paradoxus is a weakening or disappearance of the pulse with deep inspiration and can occur with profound hypovolemia, constrictive pericarditis, cardiac tamponade, asthma, and chronic obstructive pulmonary disease (COPD). The location and character of the left ventricular impulse may suggest left ventricular hypertrophy, congestive heart failure, cardiac enlargement, severe mitral regurgitation, or severe aortic regurgitation. The turbulent flow of blood through a stenotic heart valve or a septal defect may produce a palpable thrill.

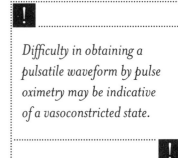

Difficulty in obtaining a pulsatile waveform by pulse oximetry may be indicative of a vasoconstricted state.

Table 1-3.	Assessment of Circulation
	Circulation
Causes of Circulatory Inadequacy	
Primary—directly involving the heart	Ischemia, arrhythmias, valvular disorders, cardiomyopathy, pericardial tamponade
Secondary—pathology originating elsewhere	Drugs, hypoxia, electrolyte disturbances, dehydration, sepsis, acute blood loss, anemia
LOOK for	Reduced peripheral perfusion (pallor, coolness), hemorrhage (obvious or concealed), altered level of consciousness, dyspnea, decreased urine output, jugular venous distension
LISTEN for	Additional or altered heart sounds, carotid bruits
FEEL for	Precordial cardiac pulsation, central and peripheral pulses (assessing rate, quality, regularity, symmetry)

In addition to the ABCs, a quick external examination should look for pallor, cyanosis, diaphoresis, jaundice, erythema, or flushing. The skin may be moist or dry, thin, edematous, or bruised, or may demonstrate a rash (ie, petechia, hives). Fingernails may be clubbed or may show splinter hemorrhages. The eyes may reveal abnormal pupils or jaundice. The conjunctiva may be pale, indicating an anemia. The patient may be alert, agitated, somnolent, asleep, or obtunded.

Palpation of the abdomen is an essential, but often overlooked, part of the examination of the critically ill patient. Areas of abdominal tenderness and palpable masses must be identified. The size of the liver and spleen must be noted as well as any associated tenderness. It is important to assess the abdomen for rigidity, distension, or rebound tenderness. Auscultation may reveal a vascular bruit or the absence of bowel sounds. Intrauterine or ectopic pregnancy must be considered in all women of childbearing age. The flanks and back must be examined, if possible.

The Glasgow Coma Score (GCS) should be recorded during the initial assessment of central nervous system (CNS) function and limb movement (**Chapter 8**). Pupillary size and reaction should be documented, and a more detailed assessment of central and peripheral sensory and motor functions should be undertaken when time permits.

C. Chart Review and Documentation

Critically ill patients have abnormal physiology that must be documented and tracked. Physiological monitoring provides parameters that are useful only when they are accurate and interpreted by trained personnel (**Chapter 6**). The values and trends of this data provide key information for the assessment of the patient's status and guidance for treatment. Data must be charted frequently and accurately to ensure good patient care. Particular attention needs to be paid to the accuracy and reliability of the data. For example, an accurate and reproducible central venous pressure (CVP) measurement depends upon patient position, equipment calibration, and proper zeroing of the instrument, as well as on heart rate and valvular function. The source of the data should also be noted. Is the recorded temperature a rectal measurement or an oral measurement? Was the blood pressure measured with a manual blood pressure cuff or with a pressure transducer in an arterial line? The medication record is an invaluable source of information about prescribed and administered drugs.

Routine monitoring and charting should include heart rate, heart rhythm, respiratory rate, blood pressure, core temperature, fluid balance, and GCS score. The fluid balance should include loss from all tubes and drains. The inspired oxygen concentration should be recorded for any patient receiving oxygen, and oxygen saturation should be charted if measured with pulse oximetry. Patients in the intensive care unit setting may have central venous catheters or pulmonary artery catheters in place. These catheters can measure central venous pressure, various cardiac pressures, cardiac output, and mixed venous saturation. These complex monitoring devices require specific operational expertise. Likewise, the data must be interpreted by someone with clinical experience and expertise in critical care.

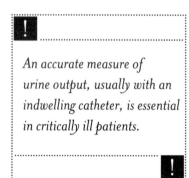

An accurate measure of urine output, usually with an indwelling catheter, is essential in critically ill patients.

D. Investigations

Additional investigative tests should be based on the patient's history and physical examination as well as on previous test results. Standard biochemistry, hematology, microbiology, and radiologic tests should be performed as indicated. *The presence of a metabolic acidosis is one of the most important indicators of critical illness.* When evaluating electrolyte results, decreasing total serum carbon dioxide (CO_2) and/or a widened anion gap are evidence of metabolic acidosis. An arterial blood gas (ABG) analysis is often the most useful test in an acutely ill patient. An ABG will provide information about blood pH, arterial oxygen tension, and arterial carbon dioxide tension. Additional tests such as lactate, blood glucose, serum electrolytes, and renal function can often be obtained from the same blood sample. The presence of lactic acidosis following resuscitation of the cardiorespiratory system is usually an ominous sign that should be closely monitored.

IV. TRANSLATING INFORMATION INTO EFFECTIVE ACTION

The framework in **Table 1-1** lays out a course of action based on first ensuring physiological safety and then proceeding to treatment of the underlying cause. The basic principles are summarized as the ABCs of resuscitating the severely ill patient: airway—ensuring a patent airway; breathing—providing supplemental oxygen and adequate ventilation; and circulation—restoration of circulating volume. These early interventions should proceed regardless of the situation, while the context of the clinical presentation (ie, trauma, postoperative situation, presence of chronic illness, advanced age) directs attention to the differential diagnosis and potential treatments. The clinical history, physical examination, and laboratory tests should aid in clarifying the diagnosis and determining the patient's degree of physiological reserve. Because the external features of critical illness may be more effectively disguised in young and previously fit patients than in elderly or chronically ill ones, an acute deterioration may seem to occur more abruptly in younger individuals. Thus it is particularly important to assess trends in patients' vital signs and physiological parameters as they undergo treatment. These trends can help determine a patient's response to treatment and clarify the diagnosis.

More experienced help must be obtained if a patient's condition is deteriorating and there is uncertainty about the diagnosis or treatment. Transfer to the most appropriate site for care is influenced by resources and local configurations, but transfer to a high-dependency or intensive care unit must be considered.

Key Points

Recognition and Assessment of the Critically Ill Patient

- Early identification of a patient at risk is essential for preventing or minimizing critical illness.

- The clinical manifestations of impending critical illness are often nonspecific. Tachypnea is one of the most important predictors of risk and signals the need for more detailed monitoring and investigation.

- Resuscitation and physiological stabilization will often precede definitive diagnosis and treatment of the underlying cause.

- A detailed history is essential for making an accurate diagnosis, determining a patient's physiological reserve, and establishing a patient's treatment preferences.

- Clinical and laboratory monitoring of a patient's response to treatment is essential.

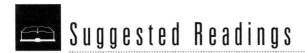

Suggested Readings

1. Buist MD, Moore GE, Bernard SA, Waxman BP, Anderson JN. Effects of a medical emergency team on reduction of incidence of and mortality from unexpected cardiac arrests in hospital: preliminary study. *BMJ*. 2002;324:1.

2. Goldhill DR, White SA, Sumner A. Physiological values and procedures in the 24 h before ICU admission from the ward. *Anaesthesia*. 1999;54:529.

3. Hillman KM, Chey T, Jacques T, Simmons G. Duration of life-threatening antecedents prior to intensive care admission. *Intensive Care Med*. 2002;28:1629.

4. Hodgetts TJ, Kenward G, Vlachonikolis IG, Payne S, Castle N. The identification of risk factors for cardiac arrest and formulation of activation criteria to alert a medical emergency team. *Resuscitation*. 2002;54:125.

5. Subbe DP, Kruger M, Rutherford P, Gemmel L. Validation of a modified early warning score in medical admissions. *QJM*. 2001;94:521.

Chapter 2

Airway Management

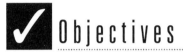

Objectives

- Recognize signs of a threatened airway.

- Describe manual techniques for establishing an airway and for mask ventilation.

- Explain proper application of airway adjuncts.

- Describe preparation for endotracheal intubation, including the recognition of a potentially difficult intubation.

- Describe alternative methods for establishing an airway when endotracheal intubation cannot be accomplished..

Case Study

A 40-year-old, morbidly obese man has arrived in the emergency department with severe respiratory distress. His respiratory rate is 40/min, pulse oximetry is 88% with high-flow oxygen supplementation, and he is actively using his accessory muscles of respiration. He is confused.

- Should this patient be intubated?

- What airway management issues might you anticipate?

- Should you call for help?

I. INTRODUCTION

The focus of this chapter is on ensuring that the airway is open and able to support gas exchange—the *A* in the ABCs of resuscitation. Secondary goals include the preservation of cardiovascular stability and the prevention of aspiration of gastric contents during airway management. Endotracheal intubation will often be required, but establishing and maintaining a patent airway instead of or prior to intubation is equally imperative and often more difficult. Healthcare providers must be skilled in manually supporting the airway and providing the essential processes of oxygenation and ventilation. Securing an artificial airway via orotracheal or nasotracheal intubation, cricothyrotomy, or tracheostomy is an extension of, not a substitute for, the ability to provide that primary response.

II. ASSESSMENT

Assessment of airway patency and spontaneous breathing effort is the crucial first step. The clinician must look, listen, and feel for diminished or absent air movement.

- Observe the patient's level of consciousness and determine if apnea is present. If respiratory efforts are absent and an immediate remedy is not available, proceed to manual support and assisted ventilation while preparing to establish an artificial airway.

- Identify injury to the airway or other conditions (eg, cervical spine fracture) that will affect assessment and manipulation of the airway; see below).

- Observe chest expansion. Ventilation may be adequate with minimal thoracic excursion, but respiratory muscle activity and even vigorous chest movement do not ensure that tidal volume is adequate.

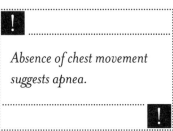

Absence of chest movement suggests apnea.

- Observe for suprasternal, supraclavicular, or intercostal retractions; laryngeal displacement toward the chest during inspiration (a tracheal tug); or nasal flaring. These often represent respiratory distress with or without airway obstruction.

- Auscultate over the neck and chest for breath sounds. Complete airway obstruction is likely when there is visible chest movement but breath sounds are absent. Incomplete obstruction due to soft tissue, liquid, or a foreign body in the airway may be associated with snoring, stridor, gurgling, or noisy breathing.

■ The assessment of protective airway reflexes (ie, cough and gag), although not necessarily associated with obstruction, is part of the initial survey of the airway. However, overly aggressive stimulation of the posterior pharynx while assessing these reflexes may precipitate emesis and aspiration of gastric contents. Absence of protective reflexes generally implies a need for longer term airway support if the cause cannot be immediately reversed.

III. MANUAL METHODS TO ESTABLISH AN AIRWAY

Initial interventions to ensure a patent airway in a spontaneously breathing patient without possible injury to the cervical spine include the triple airway maneuver (**Figure 2-1**):

1. Slight neck extension
2. Elevation of the mandible (jaw thrust maneuver)
3. Opening of the mouth

Figure 2-1 illustrates these steps. If a cervical spine injury is suspected, neck extension is eliminated. After the cervical spine is immobilized, manual elevation of the mandible and opening of the mouth are performed.

Adjunctive devices such as properly sized oropharyngeal or nasopharyngeal airways may be useful. The oropharyngeal airway is intended to hold the base of the tongue forward toward the teeth and away from the glottic opening. The plastic flange should rest against the outer surface of the teeth while the distal end curves around the base of the tongue. If the oropharyngeal airway is too small, it may push the tongue back over the glottic opening; if it is too large, it may stimulate gagging and emesis. Oropharyngeal airways should not be inserted if airway reflexes are intact, as gagging, laryngospasm, and emesis will be provoked. The diameter of a nasopharyngeal airway should be the largest that will easily pass through the nostril into the nasopharynx. Its length should extend to the nasopharynx, but it should not be so long as to obstruct gas flow through the mouth or touch the epiglottis. A nasopharyngeal airway is contraindicated in patients with suspected basilar skull fracture or coagulopathy. The correct size for each airway may be estimated by placing the device against the face in the correct anatomic position.

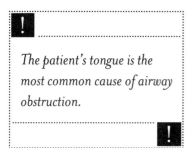

The patient's tongue is the most common cause of airway obstruction.

Figure 2-1. Triple Airway Maneuver

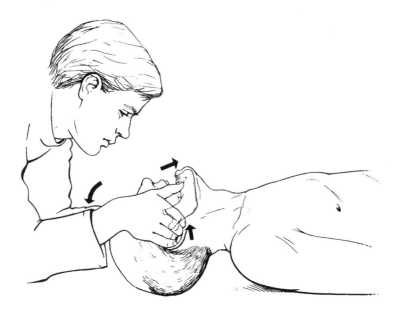

The operator extends the neck and maintains extension with his/her hands on both sides of the mandible. The mandible is elevated with the fingers of both hands to lift the base of the tongue and the thumbs or forefingers are used to open the mouth. Reproduced with permission from Mayo Clinic.

During manual support of the airway, supplemental oxygen should be supplied with a device providing a high concentration of oxygen (100%) at a high flow rate. Such devices include a face mask or a bag-mask resuscitation unit and may include a positive end-expiratory pressure (PEEP) valve.

IV. MANUAL MASK VENTILATION

Manual assisted ventilation by means of a bag-mask resuscitation unit is indicated:

■ If the patient is apneic.

■ If spontaneous tidal volumes are determined by physical examination or ABG analysis to be inadequate.

■ To reduce the work of breathing by assisting the patient during spontaneous inspiration.

■ If hypoxemia is associated with poor spontaneous ventilation.

Successful manual mask ventilation depends upon (1) maintaining an open airway, (2) establishing a seal between the patient's face and the mask, and (3) delivering an adequate minute ventilation from the resuscitation bag to distal lung units. The first 2 elements are combined through the

correct placement of the mask over the patient's nose and mouth (**Figure 2-2**) and completion
of the triple airway maneuver as previously described. It is useful to have masks of different sizes
available in the event that the initial selection does not achieve a good seal between the mask and
face.

Figure 2-2. Application of Face Masks

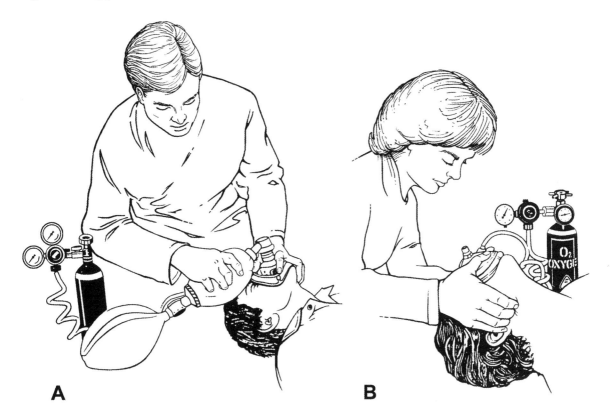

A   **B**

Single-handed (A) and two-handed (B) techniques for placement of a face mask.
Reproduced with permission from Mayo Clinic.

A. When No Cervical Spine Injury Is Suspected

1. If tolerated by the patient, an oropharyngeal airway, or nasopharyngeal airway may
   be placed to maintain a patient airway as needed. A small pad or folded towel may be
   positioned under the occiput.

2. The operator stands above and behind the head of the supine patient. The height of
   the bed should be quickly adjusted for the comfort of the operator.

3. The base of the mask is first placed into the skin crease between the lower lips and the
   chin, and the mouth is gently opened.

4. The apex of the mask is placed over the nose, with care to avoid pressure on the eyes.

5. As most operators are right-handed, the mask is stabilized on the face with the left hand by holding the superior aspect of the mask apex adjacent to its connection to the bag between the thumb and first finger. This position allows gentle downward pressure on the mask over the face.

6. The fifth, fourth, and perhaps third fingers of the left hand are then placed along the mandible on the left side of the patient's jaw. As this placement occurs, it is helpful to gently encircle the left side of the mask with the soft tissues of that cheek to reinforce the seal along the left edge. This position further secures the mask to the patient's face while allowing the mandible to be partially elevated.

7. The operator gently rotates the left wrist to cause slight neck extension and contracts the fingers around the mandible to raise it slightly. The composite motions of the left hand, therefore, produce slight neck extension, mandibular elevation, and gentle downward pressure of the mask on the face.

B. When a Cervical Spine Injury Is Suspected

1. The operator stands in the same position, and an oropharyngeal or nasopharyngeal airway is inserted, if possible.

2. Under unusual circumstances, successful manual ventilation can be accomplished while the neck is stabilized in a cervical collar. Often, however, an assistant is required to stand to the side, facing the patient. The anterior portion of the collar is removed, and the assistant places one hand or arm along each side of the neck to the occiput to limit movement of the neck during manipulation of the airway. Linear traction is not applied.

3. The operator may then proceed with the steps described above, *except no rotation is applied from the left wrist to produce neck extension.* Alternatively, the operator may choose the two-handed method for mask placement, which further assures that no neck movement occurs. This method is discussed below.

C. Alternative 2-Handed Method to Ensure Airway Patency and Mask Application

The alternative 2-handed method is useful if the patient has a large face or a beard, after neck injury, or in any other situation when a mask seal is difficult to secure.

1. The operator stands in the same location at the head of the bed, and adjunctive airway devices are used as previously suggested.

2. The base and apex of the mask are placed in the manner previously described.

3. The operator places the third, fourth, and fifth fingers of both hands along the mandible on each side of the face while the thumbs rest over the apex of the mask and first fingers rest over the base of the mask.

4. Soft tissues of the cheek are brought upward along the side edges of the mask and held in place by each hand to reinforce the mask's seal with the face.

5. In the absence of possible cervical spine injury, the neck is slightly extended as the operator gently elevates the mandible from both sides and provides gentle pressure on the mask over the face.

6. An assistant provides ventilation, as needed, by compressing the resuscitation bag.

D. Compression of the Resuscitation Bag to Provide Assisted Manual Mask Ventilation

The goal of manual mask ventilation is to provide adequate minute ventilation, the product of the tidal volume delivered during each compression of the resuscitation bag and the number of times per minute the bag is compressed. Overzealous compressions of the bag at a rapid rate may produce dangerous hyperventilation and respiratory alkalemia as well as gastric distension.

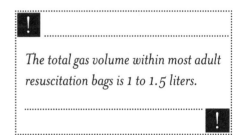

The total gas volume within most adult resuscitation bags is 1 to 1.5 liters.

1. If a single-handed method of mask placement is used, the resuscitation bag is compressed over 1 second by the operator's right hand.

2. The delivered tidal volume must be estimated from the observed initial chest expansion, auscultated breath sounds, and other factors.

3. During bag compression, the operator should listen carefully for any gas leaks around the mask. Similarly, when a good seal is present, the feel of the bag during lung inflation reflects some resistance caused by the normal airway anatomy. If gas is felt to be moving from the bag too easily, a leak is likely to be present.

4. If the patient is apneic but has a pulse, 1-handed compressions of the bag should be delivered 10 to 12 times per minute. If spontaneous breathing is present, bag compression should be synchronized with the patient's inspiratory efforts. If the patient is breathing easily and inhaling adequate tidal volumes frequently enough to produce sufficient minute ventilation, the bag need not be compressed at all.

5. Oxygen (100%) is delivered to the resuscitation bag, usually at a flow rate ≥15 L/min.

6. If the mask-to-face seal is not adequate and a leak is detected, the operator should consider the following interventions:

■ Reposition the mask and hands.

■ Adjust the inflation of the facial cushion of the face mask, if possible, to improve the seal or change to a larger or smaller mask.

■ Apply slightly more downward pressure to the face or displace the mandible in an upward fashion provided cervical spine manipulation is not contraindicated.

■ Convert to the 2-handed technique described above.

■ Reposition an orogastric or nasogastric tube, if present, to a different part of the mask. Leaks are common when such a tube is present, but rarely will it need to be removed.

■ Consider compensating for the leak if it is small by increasing the frequency of bag compressions or the volume of gas delivered per compression.

■ Some resuscitation bags have a pressure-relief (pop-off) valve designed to prevent transmission of high pressures to the lungs. In patients with stiff lungs or high airway resistance, the pop-off valve should be adjusted to ensure adequate tidal volumes.

Manual assisted ventilation should be continued in preparation for intubation or until the cause of inadequate ventilation is reversed, if possible. An assistant should prepare medications, equipment, etc, for intubation while the primary operator maintains ventilation. Pulse oximetry and cardiac monitoring are valuable adjuncts throughout assisted ventilation. The patient should be evaluated continuously for evidence of cyanosis, although this is a late finding in the setting of hypoxemia.

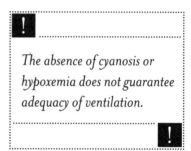

The absence of cyanosis or hypoxemia does not guarantee adequacy of ventilation.

E. Cricoid Pressure

Cricoid pressure (Sellick maneuver) is the application of downward (posterior) pressure on the anterior neck overlying the cricoid cartilage. The downward movement of the cricoid ring will physically occlude the esophagus and may decrease the risk of gastric distension during manual mask ventilation and reduce the risk of passive reflux of gastric contents into the lungs. If the patient lacks protective airway reflexes, cricoid pressure should be applied during mask ventilation and during attempts at tracheal intubation and should be removed only after tracheal intubation has been confirmed. Proper application of cricoid pressure may improve visualization of the vocal cords, similar to the backward, upward, and rightward pressure maneuver (BURP maneuver) described in **Appendix 2**. In the event that a patient vomits, the Sellick maneuver should be discontinued to avoid potential esophageal injury.

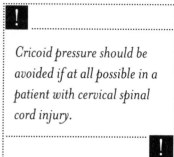

> **!**
>
> *Cricoid pressure should be avoided if at all possible in a patient with cervical spinal cord injury.*
>
> **!**

Guidelines for managing either a known or an unrecognized difficult airway are presented in **Figure 2-3**.

Figure 2-3. Management of the Difficult Airway

Difficult Airway Recognized

Unrecognized Difficult Airway or Emergent Airway

Combative patient
Uncooperative patient

Spontaneous ventilation
– Preparation
– Call for assistance

± Sedation
± Neuromuscular blocker
(with caution)

Expert consultation
– Flexible fiberoptic technique
Awake intubation
– Direct laryngoscopy
– Blind nasal intubation (if spontaneous respirations)
LMA

Manual mask ventilation possible

No → LMA
ET airway device
Needle cricothyrotomy
Call for assistance

Yes

Direct laryngoscopy
Blind nasal intubation (if spontaneous respirations)

Fail →

Succeed   Fail

Expert consultation
– Surgical airway

Succeed   Fail →

Expert consultation
– Flexible fiberoptic technique
– Surgical airway

Abbreviations: LMA, laryngeal mask airway; ET, esophageal-tracheal.

V. AIRWAY ADJUNCTS

In approximately 5% of the general population, manual mask ventilation is difficult or impossible to achieve. Predictors of difficulty are presence of a beard, absence of teeth, history consistent with obstructive sleep apnea, body mass index >26 kg/m², and age >55 years. The presence of 2 of the predictors indicates a high probability of difficulty in manual mask ventilation. Intubation via direct laryngoscopy is difficult in approximately 5% of the general population and impossible in approximately 0.2% to 0.5%. A crisis situation occurs when neither manual mask ventilation nor intubation is possible. The laryngeal mask airway and esophageal-tracheal double-lumen airway device are useful adjuncts to provide an open airway and permit gas exchange in such situations. These devices are blindly inserted, cuffed pharyngeal ventilation devices for use when mask ventilation is difficult or impossible to buy time after failed intubation. The choice of device depends on the experience of the operator and the individual clinical circumstances.

A. Laryngeal Mask Airway

A laryngeal mask airway is an endotracheal tube (ETT) attached to a bowl-shaped cuff that fits in the pharynx behind the tongue. The standard laryngeal mask airway is reusable, but a single-use device is also available. A laryngeal mask airway may be used to ventilate the lungs when mask ventilation is difficult, provided that the patient does not have periglottal pathology. It may also serve as a conduit for intubation when a bronchoscope is used or as a rescue technique after failed intubation. Less sedation is required with a laryngeal mask airway than with direct laryngoscopy because stimulation to the airway (eg, gagging, laryngospasm, sympathetic stimulation) in passing the device is only moderate. It is effective in ventilating patients ranging from neonates to adults, but it does not provide definitive airway protection. For specific details regarding use of a laryngeal mask airway, see **Appendix 3**.

B. Esophageal-Tracheal Double-Lumen Airway Device

Another adjunct for providing an emergency airway is a double-lumen device with 2 inflatable balloon cuffs that is designed primarily for blind intubation during cardiorespiratory arrest. It can provide ventilation if the distal cuffed portion of the tube device is inserted in the esophagus or trachea. When the tube is inserted in the esophagus, the stomach may be suctioned through the tracheal lumen. This double-lumen airway device is contraindicated for patients with central airway obstruction, intact laryngeal or pharyngeal reflexes, known esophageal pathology, or ingestion of caustic substances. Adequate training is required to ensure appropriate use. (For information about inserting an esophageal-tracheal double-lumen airway device, see **Appendix 3**.)

VI. ENDOTRACHEAL INTUBATION

Direct laryngoscopy with orotracheal intubation is the principal method for tracheal intubation because of its speed, success rate, and availability of equipment. Blind nasotracheal intubation may be useful for selected patients. The indications for tracheal intubation are summarized in **Table 2-1**, and the techniques for orotracheal and nasotracheal intubation are discussed and illustrated in **Appendix 2**.

Table 2-1.	Indications for Tracheal Intubation
	Airway protection
	Relief of obstruction
	Provision of mechanical ventilation and oxygen therapy
	Respiratory failure
	Shock
	Hyperventilation for intracranial hypertension
	Reduction of the work of breathing
	Facilitation of suctioning/pulmonary toilet

In preparation for intubation, important issues include:

■ Assessment of airway anatomy and function to estimate degree of difficulty for intubation (see below).

■ Assurance of optimal ventilation and oxygenation. Preoxygenation with 100% oxygen, using a bag-mask resuscitation device, occurs during periods of apnea and intubation attempts.

■ Decompression of the stomach with an existing orogastric or nasogastric tube. In contrast, the insertion of an orogastric or nasogastric tube to decompress the stomach prior to intubation is often counterproductive, as it may elicit emesis and promote passive reflux of gastric contents.

■ Provision of appropriate analgesia, sedation, amnesia, and neuromuscular blockade as required for a safe procedure.

Although emergent intubation leaves little time for evaluation and optimizing of conditions, elective and urgent intubation allows for assessment of factors that promote safe airway management. The patient's clinical situation, intravascular volume status, hemodynamics, and airway evaluation (degree of difficulty) should be assessed as a plan for airway management is formulated. Airway evaluation includes assessment of physical characteristics that together determine if visualization of the vocal cords will be difficult or impossible. This evaluation will suggest whether alternative techniques to direct laryngoscopy (eg, awake intubation, flexible fiberoptic intubation, surgical airway) are likely to be necessary and whether a more experienced individual should be immediately summoned. Keep in mind that many of these physical characteristics also cause difficulty with mask ventilation and the ability to perform an emergent cricothyrotomy. These characteristics are easy to remember if they are considered in the same order as the steps used in oral intubation—that is, head position, mouth opening, displacement of the tongue and jaw, visualization, and insertion of endotracheal tube:

- *Neck mobility*. The presence of possible cervical spine injury, short neck, or limitation of neck mobility by prior surgery or arthritis will restrict the ability to position adequately.

- *External face*. Examine for evidence of micrognathia or presence of surgical scars, facial trauma, small nares, or nasal, oral, or pharyngeal bleeding.

- *Mouth*. Mouth opening may be limited due to temporomandibular joint disease or facial scarring. Mouth opening of less than 3 finger breadths (approximately 6 cm) is associated with an increased risk of difficult intubation.

- *Tongue and pharynx*. Tongue size relative to the posterior pharynx estimates the relative amount of room in the pharynx to visualize glottic structures.

- *Jaw*. Thyromental distance—the distance in finger breadths between the anterior prominence of the thyroid cartilage (Adam's apple) and the tip of the mandible (chin)—estimates the length of the mandible and the available space anterior to the larynx. A distance of less than 3 finger breadths (approximately 6 cm) indicates that the larynx may appear more anterior and be more difficult to visualize and enter during laryngoscopy. A more acute angulation of the stylet in the endotracheal tube may be helpful.

If one or a combination of these physical characteristics indicates the possibility of difficult intubation and if time allows, other options for obtaining a secure airway and calling in someone with additional airway expertise should be considered.

When difficulty in mask ventilation or intubation is anticipated, care is advised before suppressing spontaneous ventilation with neuromuscular blocking drugs or sedatives that cannot be reversed. Options for safe airway management include the following, all of which preserve spontaneous ventilation:

Failed intubation attempts can result in periglottic edema and create subsequent difficulty with mask ventilation, leading to a "can't intubate and can't ventilate" situation.

- Awake intubation by direct laryngoscopy or blind nasotracheal intubation

- Flexible fiberoptic intubation (expert consultation required)

- Awake tracheostomy (expert consultation required)

In the event that visualization of the glottis and mask ventilation are both impossible and there is no spontaneous ventilation, options include:

- Laryngeal mask airway or esophageal-tracheal double-lumen airway device

- Needle cricothyrotomy (expert consultation required)

- Surgical cricothyrotomy/tracheostomy (expert consultation required)

- Percutaneous tracheostomy (expert consultation required)

(Recall that an algorithm for managing a potential or confirmed difficult airway is shown in **Figure 2-3**.)

After tracheal intubation, significant alterations in hemodynamics should be anticipated. Hypertension and tachycardia may result from sympathetic stimulation and may require therapy with antihypertensive medications or sedatives in some patients. Hypotension is common, and decreased cardiac output due to reduced venous return with positive pressure ventilation can precipitate arrhythmias or cardiac arrest. The effects of sedative agents on the vasculature or myocardium, hypovolemia, and a possible postintubation pneumothorax may also contribute to hypotension. Other complications associated with positive pressure ventilation are discussed in **Chapter 5**.

VII. PHARMACOLOGIC PREPARATION FOR INTUBATION

During the process of airway management, both parasympathetic and sympathetic responses are common and may need to be blunted with proper pharmacologic therapy. The pharmacologic goal prior to intubation is to provide the patient with optimal analgesia/anesthesia, amnesia, and sedation without altering cardiorespiratory stability. At times, preservation of spontaneous ventilatory drive is necessary. Obviously, the selection of particular methods or drugs depends upon the clinical circumstances and status of the patient, patient allergies, and the experience and preferences of the operator.

A. Analgesia/Anesthesia

- A variety of topical anesthetic sprays are available, or lidocaine may be delivered via aerosol. Anatomic areas for special emphasis include the base of the tongue, directly on the posterior wall of the pharynx, and bilaterally in the tonsillar fossae. Care should be taken not to exceed 4 mg/kg of lidocaine (maximum dose 300 mg), as it is easily absorbed from the airway mucosa.

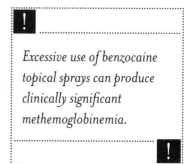

! *Excessive use of benzocaine topical sprays can produce clinically significant methemoglobinemia.* !

■ Administration of nerve blocks and transcricoid membrane lidocaine requires special expertise and is not part of this course.

■ Analgesia is also provided by some agents for sedation.

B. Sedation/Amnesia

Rapid-acting, short-lived, and potentially reversible agents are preferred for sedation. No single agent has every desirable feature, and often more than one agent may be considered to provide a balanced technique. It is important to restate that the status of the patient's intravascular volume and cardiac function must be carefully considered during the selection of an agent and its dosage. Most agents may induce hypotension when heart failure or hypovolemia is present. Examples of commonly used medications are listed in **Table 2-2**.

Table 2-2	Drugs Used to Facilitate Tracheal Intubation		
Agent	**Dosing**	**Benefits**	**Cautions**
Fentanyl	0.5-2 µg /kg IV bolus every several minutes titrated to sedative effect	Rapid onset of action Short acting Reversible with naloxone	Chest wall rigidity with rapid administration Respiratory depression Does not inhibit patient awareness of procedure
Midazolam	0.1-0.2 mg/kg IV bolus titrated to sedative effect every several minutes	Provides amnesia Rapid onset Short acting Reversible with flumazenil	Additive respiratory depression when combined with narcotic Does not provide analgesia
Etomidate	0.3-0.4 mg/kg single IV bolus	Provides sedative effect May be preferred in head injury No adverse cardiovascular effects	May induce myoclonus, including mild trismus (consider premedication with 50 µg fentanyl) No reversal agent Transient adrenal suppression
Lidocaine	1-1.5 mg/kg IV bolus 2-3 minutes before laryngoscopy	Blunts hemodynamic and tracheal response to intubation May reduce elevations of intracranial pressure during laryngoscopy	

C. Neuromuscular Blockers

Often, intubation can be safely and easily performed after topical anesthesia, (ie, an awake intubation) or with sedation alone. Therefore, neuromuscular blockade is not always required prior to endotracheal intubation. Obviously, if the operator cannot intubate the patient after neuromuscular blockers have been given, effective manual mask ventilation must be continued while a more experienced person is sought, an alternative plan to secure the airway is developed, or the agent is metabolized with return of spontaneous ventilation. Hence, a short-acting agent is more advantageous. The following are examples of neuromuscular blockers:

- Succinylcholine, 1 to 1.5 mg/kg intravenous bolus: rapid onset; shortest duration, which provides an element of safety; may cause muscle fasciculations because this agent depolarizes skeletal muscle; emesis may occur if abdominal muscle fasciculations are severe; contraindicated when ocular injury is present; relatively contraindicated when head injury is present or if hyperkalemia is present (potassium release of 0.5-1 mmol/L will occur routinely, and massive potassium release may occur in burn and crush injury, upper motor neuron lesions, or primary muscle disease); may precipitate malignant hyperthermia. Effects are prolonged in patients with atypical cholinesterase or decreased pseudocholinesterase levels.

- Vecuronium, 0.1 to 0.3 mg/kg; rocuronium, 0.6 to 1 mg/kg; or cisatracurium, 0.1 to 0.2 mg/kg intravenous bolus: no fasciculations because these are nondepolarizing agents; slower onset of muscle paralysis; significantly longer duration of effects than with succinylcholine.

D. Rapid Sequence Intubation

Rapid sequence intubation (RSI) is the simultaneous administration of a sedative agent and a neuromuscular blocker along with cricoid pressure, designed to facilitate intubation and reduce the risk of gastric aspiration. It is the technique of choice when there is an increased risk of aspiration (eg, full stomach, pain, gastroesophageal reflux) and examination does not suggest a difficult intubation. Patients for whom intubation is likely to be difficult should not have RSI. The emergency methods described above will be necessary if the patient cannot be intubated and is impossible to ventilate, since the ability to mask ventilate is not tested prior to administration of the neuromuscular blocker.

Airway Management

■ Assessment of the patient's level of consciousness, airway protective reflexes, respiratory drive, obstruction(s) to gas flow into the airway, and work of breathing will determine the steps necessary to ensure appropriate respiratory support.

■ Every primary care provider must be skilled in manual methods to secure and maintain a patent airway.

■ Manual assisted ventilation performed with a bag-mask resuscitation unit is a skill expected of every healthcare provider. The goal is to optimize oxygenation and CO_2 removal prior to, or in lieu of, intubation of the patient.

■ Proper application of cricoid pressure may reduce the risk of gastric distension and passive aspiration.

■ The laryngeal mask airway and the esophageal-tracheal double-lumen airway device are useful airway adjuncts when expertise in intubation is lacking or intubation is unsuccessful.

■ Before intubation, further patient evaluation is necessary to assess the degree of intubation difficulty and determine the appropriateness of analgesia, sedation, amnesia, and possible neuromuscular blockade.

■ A plan for managing a potentially difficult intubation includes maintenance of spontaneous ventilation, alternatives to endotracheal intubation, and requests for expert assistance. When manual mask ventilation is impossible after failed intubation, proper use of adjunct devices, cricothyrotomy, or percutaneous tracheostomy may be lifesaving.

 Suggested Readings

1. Agro F, Frass M, Benumof J, et al. The esophageal tracheal Combitube as a noninvasive alternative to endotracheal intubation: a review. *Minerva Anestesiologica.* 2001;67:863.

2. American Society of Anesthesiologists Task Force on Management of the Difficult Airway. Practice guidelines for management of the difficult airway: an updated report by the American Society of Anesthesiologists Task Force on Management of the Difficult Airway [published correction appears in Anesthesiology. 2004;101:565]. *Anesthesiology.* 2003;98(5):1269. Available online at http://www.guideline.gov/summary/summary. aspx?ss=15&doc_id=7256&nbr=4318.

3. Danks RR, Danks B. Laryngeal mask airway: review of indications and use. *J Emerg Nurs.* 2004;30:30.

4. Dunham CM, Barraco RD, Clark DE, et al; for the EAST Practice Management Guidelines Work Group. Guidelines for emergency tracheal intubation immediately after traumatic injury. *J Trauma*. 2003;55:162. Available online at http://www.east.org/tpg/intubation.pdf.

5. Henderson JJ, Popat MT, Latto IP, Pearce AC. Difficult Airway Society guidelines for management of unanticipated difficult intubation. *Anaesthesia*. 2004;59:675.

6. Langeron O, Masso E, Huraux C, et al. Prediction of difficult mask ventilation. *Anesthesiology*. 2000;92:1229.

7. Rosenblatt WH. Preoperative planning of airway management in critical care patients. *Crit Care Med*. 2004;32:S186.

8. Society of Critical Care Medicine. Clinical practice guidelines for sustained neuromuscular blockade in the critically ill adult patient. *Crit Care Med*. 2002;30(1):142. Available online at http://www.sccm.org/professional_resources/guidelines/table_of_contents/Documents/NeuromuscularBlockade.pdf.

9. Society of Critical Care Medicine. Clinical practice guidelines for the sustained use of sedatives and analgesics in the critically ill adult. *Crit Care Med*. 2002;30(1):117. Available online at http://www.sccm.org/professional_resources/guidelines/table_of_contents/Documents/Sedatives.pdf.

10. Walz JM, Zayaruzny M, Heard SO. Airway management in critical illness. *Chest*. 2007;131:608.

Chapter 3:

Cardiopulmonary/Cerebral Resuscitation

✓ Objectives

- Identify patients who are likely to benefit from cardiopulmonary resuscitation.

- Propose a process for delegating responsibilities during a resuscitation process.

- Discuss important treatment issues in cardiopulmonary arrest.

- Emphasize goals and interventions for brain protection and recovery, including use of hypothermia.

- Review specific cardiorespiratory events that occur in critically ill, ventilated patients.

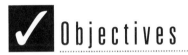 Case Study

The hospital paging operator announces the cardiac arrest of a 54-year-old man on the general floor. On arrival at the scene, you note that one nurse is applying an oxygen mask and another nurse is attempting to measure the patient's blood pressure.

- Assuming the patient should be resuscitated, what are your immediate actions?

- What are the next steps if you are the team leader?

- What tasks are delegated to team members during the resuscitation?

I. INTRODUCTION

The immediate response to an in-hospital cardiac arrest is frequently the responsibility of primary care providers, nurses, housestaff, and other members of the healthcare team. The Society of Critical Care Medicine (SCCM) and the Fundamental Critical Care Support (FCCS) program recognize the valuable training provided by the American Heart Association's Basic Life Support (BLS), Advanced Cardiovascular Life Support (ACLS), and Pediatric Advanced Life Support (PALS) curricula. All healthcare practitioners are encouraged to successfully complete the appropriate course in that series. Algorithms recommended by the American Heart Association from the 2005 International Consensus Conference are reproduced in **Appendix 4**.

II. ETHICAL ISSUES

A. Who Should Be Resuscitated?

The purpose of cardiopulmonary resuscitation (CPR) and advanced life support (ALS) in the critical care setting is to reverse sudden, unexpected death resulting from reversible disease processes or iatrogenic complications. If possible, resuscitation status should always be discussed with the patient, the patient's family, or the surrogate decision maker (**Chapter 15**). Resuscitation

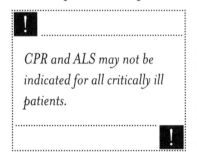

CPR and ALS may not be indicated for all critically ill patients.

is unlikely to benefit patients experiencing cardiac arrest despite maximal medical therapy for progressive cardiogenic or septic shock. Out-of-hospital arrest can carry a very high mortality in conjunction with prolonged CPR. Several other underlying conditions (eg, pneumonia, congestive heart failure, renal failure, and sepsis) make survival from cardiac arrest exceedingly unlikely but not unprecedented. No set of variables is sensitive enough to accurately predict a poor outcome.

B. Level of Therapeutic Support

Cardiopulmonary resuscitation is instituted based on implied consent, without a physician's order, whereas limitation of resuscitation requires an order. "Do not attempt resuscitation" (DNAR) orders should be written on the chart along with an explanation of the rationale. Such orders do not and should not indicate that the patient is not to be treated. Patients and their families should not be emotionally abandoned because of such orders. "No resuscitation" does not mean "no care." Intermediate resuscitative plans suited to a patient's particular wishes and condition should be clearly delineated on the chart by the attending physician and should be respected by the hospital staff. Slow codes that give the illusion of resuscitation are not appropriate.

C. Documentation

Documentation of the level of therapeutic support should be in the patient's chart so that the staff knows exactly how to proceed should an arrest occur unexpectedly. If level of therapeutic support were addressed only in the sickest patients, no instructions would exist for many patients who experience arrest. The staff should follow valid DNAR orders. Information about advance directives, living wills, durable powers of attorney, and related forms should also be well documented in the medical record and should be respected.

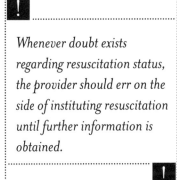

Whenever doubt exists regarding resuscitation status, the provider should err on the side of instituting resuscitation until further information is obtained.

III. PRIMARY RESPONSE

Responders will usually have resuscitation resources available for cardiorespiratory arrests that occur within the hospital. Often, however, the most important aspects of initiating and continuing a successful resuscitation relate to the interactions, knowledge, and skills of the responders and the ability to delegate and accept responsibility for parts of the resuscitation effort. A suggested approach to resuscitation is outlined below and further information is presented in **Appendix 4**.

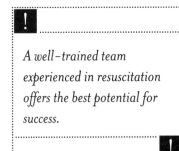

A well-trained team experienced in resuscitation offers the best potential for success.

A. Assessment of the Immediate Situation

Has an appropriate individual assumed the leadership role?

■ If so, how can you assist? Identify yourself and offer help. Be ready to accept a delegated role and to focus your efforts upon that role while remaining aware of other evolving resuscitation activities.

■ If not, you may be required to assume the leadership role until a more qualified individual or the designated team member arrives.

B. The Leader's Role

Proceed with primary assessment and intervention, and delegate appropriate activities to others.

1. Evaluation

■ Assess patient responsiveness.

■ If the patient is unresponsive, assess respiratory effort, pulse, cough, or any body movement that is evidence of circulation. If there is no spontaneous breathing, the initial step should be to open the airway and deliver 2 breaths (with the maximum oxygen concentration available) over 1 second, each with sufficient volume to see the chest rise. In the absence of a pulse, chest compressions at a rate of 100/min are immediately initiated until the cardiac rhythm can be determined.

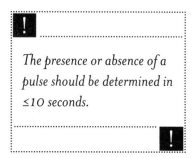

The presence or absence of a pulse should be determined in ≤10 seconds.

■ Defibrillation should proceed as soon as possible after pulselessness is confirmed if monitoring (quick-look paddles, etc) indicates ventricular fibrillation or pulseless ventricular tachycardia (**Appendix 5**). A single shock should be delivered at the energy level appropriate for the defibrillator (360 joules with a monophasic defibrillator and manufacturer's recommended energy level if known, or 200 joules with a biphasic defibrillator). Chest compressions should be resumed immediately after the shock is delivered without checking the pulse or rhythm. Rhythm analysis should usually occur after 2 minutes of compressions, but this sequence may be modified in the hospital setting with continuous electrocardiographic monitoring.

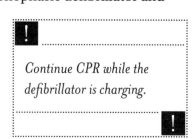

Continue CPR while the defibrillator is charging.

■ If intubated and connected to a mechanical ventilator, the patient must be disconnected and changed to manual bag-mask ventilation.

2. Delegation

■ Delegate tasks to the most appropriate personnel available. Delegation is important, whenever possible, so that the resuscitation leader can maintain an overall perspective, monitor cardiac rhythm, direct assessments and interventions, and prescribe medications. The leader may need to perform some of these tasks or reassign them to another person, if the primary designee is unsuccessful. Obviously, if the number of responders is not sufficient, team members must establish priorities as enumerated below for performance. Delegated duties should include the following:

a. Manage the airway (**Chapter 2**). Establish a patent airway, provide manual bag-mask ventilation, utilize available airway adjuncts, and/or perform endotracheal intubation. Ventilations should not exceed the recommended 8 to 10 breaths/min in order to optimize coronary artery perfusion pressure by decreasing the percentage of time with positive intrathoracic pressure.

b. Perform chest compressions. The resuscitation leader should also designate a second person for relief and instruct the rescuers to exchange responsibilities every 2 minutes. Evidence shows that a compression rate of 100/min results in maximal blood flow for the victim. The ratio of compression to ventilation is 30:2 when the airway is not secured, and the depth of compressions for adults is 1.5 to 2 inches (4-5 cm). The chest should recoil completely between compressions. If the patient is securely intubated, compressions are continuous, and asynchronous ventilation is provided at a rate of 8 to 10 breaths/min. The person on relief should monitor the effectiveness of compressions by checking the carotid or femoral pulse. Although the results of such checks do not correlate highly with intravascular flow, they constitute a minimal monitoring method. Chest compressions are interrupted only for shock delivery and rhythm checks once the airway is secured. Pulse checks are performed only if an organized rhythm is noted.

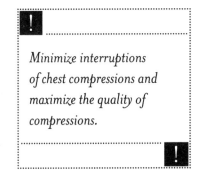

Minimize interruptions of chest compressions and maximize the quality of compressions.

c. Attach ECG monitor/machine.

d. Obtain intravenous access and assume primary responsibility for administering medications. Peripheral venous access with a large catheter is preferred, because it does not require interruption of chest compressions. The intraosseous route can be used as a temporary measure when other vascular sites are not immediately available in children or adults (**Appendix 6**).

e. Provide medications as requested (eg, to manage the code cart, defibrillator/pacer, and so forth).

f. Maintain documentation record of resuscitation interventions and patient assessments.

g. Obtain medical record and/or provide pertinent patient information.

h. Notify the patient's personal attending physician of the cardiopulmonary event and obtain further guidance. Discuss the patient's status, medical history, existence of advance directives, and related topics.

i. Remove furniture, unnecessary equipment, and extra personnel from the resuscitation area.

IV. CONTINUING RESUSCITATION

Once the primary response and assigned tasks have been successfully initiated, each team member continues an appropriate role as the resuscitation interventions are implemented.

■ Critical laboratory data should be obtained to assist with decisions during the resuscitation and, perhaps, to reveal a cause for the cardiac arrest. Important data include levels of glucose, arterial blood gases, potassium, ionized calcium, and magnesium. Suspected abnormalities or those documented from recent laboratory values may be treated empirically. Repetitive blood testing must be expedited by a team member, and the laboratory must be notified of the ongoing resuscitation.

■ Review the patient's chart for history and any possible medication reaction that could lead to arrest, arrhythmia, or decreased ventilatory drive. Notify the primary physician immediately.

■ It is appropriate to assume that the initial code would not have been called if a DNAR or similar directive had been ordered by a physician. However, this should be confirmed as other primary patient information and data are obtained. Whenever doubt exists about a code status, full resuscitative measures should be initiated and continued until clarified with the patient's attending physician and/or family.

■ The point at which family members are notified of the cardiopulmonary arrest will vary. If family is present, a team member should provide information periodically during the resuscitation. The presence of family during resuscitation should be carefully considered and planned for if this practice is accepted by the institution and the resuscitation team.

■ Arrangements for patient transfer to an ICU should be considered early, usually by a nursing supervisor. A transport cart, emergency drugs, external pacer (see **Appendix 7**), portable monitors, oxygen, and other crucial supplies should be available as the patient stabilizes to facilitate immediate transfer. The ICU will need to prepare; therefore, additional patient needs (eg, arterial or central line transducer setups, ECG, chest radiograph, mechanical ventilator) should be communicated.

V. OTHER CONSIDERATIONS IN CARDIOPULMONARY/ CEREBRAL RESUSCITATION

■ The method that best produces blood flow to the coronary arteries, brain, and other organs during a cardiopulmonary arrest has not yet been determined. At present, however, closed-chest compressions remain the standard technique for circulatory support. Interposed abdominal-compression CPR and active compression-decompression CPR (device not available in the United States) may be considered acceptable alternatives whenever personnel trained in the techniques are available. The invasive alternative of open-chest cardiac massage requires a team with special expertise and early institution for optimal outcome. Immediate cardiopulmonary bypass may be effective in improving the success of resuscitation but is not available in most hospitals.

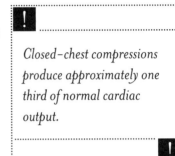

Closed–chest compressions produce approximately one third of normal cardiac output.

■ Early restoration of perfusion to the brain and other organs offers the best chance for recovery of function. Patients who are mildly hypothermic after cardiac arrest should not be actively warmed, because warming increases oxygen demand and alters vascular tone. Mild induced hypothermia (89.6°F-93.2°F [32°C-34°C]) for 12 to 24 hours is recommended to improve neurologic outcome and reduce mortality in comatose patients after initial resuscitation from cardiac arrest due to ventricular fibrillation. Febrile patients should be treated to reach a normal temperature as soon as possible. Seizures must be aggressively treated to avoid further brain injury. Hyperglycemia should be avoided since it has been correlated with a worsened neurologic outcome. Other strategies to protect the brain during and after no-flow states and in conjunction with CPR are under investigation.

VI. RESPIRATORY ARREST

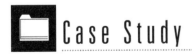 Case Study

You are asked to evaluate a patient with difficulty breathing. The patient is intubated and transferred to the ICU, where mechanical ventilation is instituted. One hour later, the patient's O_2 saturation decreases and the heart rate decreases to 40/min with loss of pulse.

  – What are possible etiologies for the patient's deterioration?

  – What steps should you take to optimize the patient's respiratory status?

A. Respiratory Arrest in the Nonintubated Patient

1. Immediate Concerns

One of the most common catastrophic events in nonintubated patients is respiratory arrest. These patients are typically found in asystole or pulseless electrical activity (PEA) but may be in ventricular fibrillation. Immediate basic life support, including ventilation, should be instituted by the first responders. Early endotracheal intubation allows for the most effective ventilation and oxygenation. Manual bag-mask ventilation with 100% oxygen until a provider experienced in endotracheal intubation arrives is preferable to prolonged, unsuccessful attempts at intubation.

2. Patient Assessment

In many instances, careful assessment of vital signs (including pulse oximetry), air movement, and work of breathing will indicate that respiratory impairment is present. Tachypnea progressing to bradypnea, paradoxical abdominal breathing, and progressively decreasing alertness may herald imminent respiratory arrest. Noninvasive respiratory monitoring may identify patients who are decompensating. Normal arterial blood gases do not rule out the need for mechanical ventilatory support since decompensation can occur precipitously once respiratory muscle fatigue becomes manifest.

B. Special Management Issues

1. Respiratory Arrest in Patients Receiving Mechanical Ventilation

If a patient arrests while receiving mechanical ventilation, some mishap related to mechanical ventilation must be suspected, especially if the initial cardiac rhythm is bradycardia or asystole. Etiologic possibilities include barotrauma (tension pneumothorax), ventilator failure or disconnect, or displacement or obstruction of the endotracheal tube. Patients should be immediately disconnected from the ventilator, and manual ventilation and 100% oxygen should be initiated while further assessment is undertaken. If high resistance to airflow is present, the endotracheal tube should be unsecured and checked for kinks, and attempts should be made to pass a suction catheter. Verification of tube placement with expired CO_2 monitoring is recommended as an adjunct to physical assessment. If tube position or patency is in question, the tube should be removed and the patient reintubated after being adequately oxygenated and ventilated by means of a bag-mask device. Tension pneumothorax should also be considered as a cause of high airway resistance.

2. Tension Pneumothorax

Patients with tension pneumothorax typically have hypotension and/or PEA with narrow complex tachycardia. Physical assessment may reveal jugular venous distension and ipsilateral tympanitic percussion as well as ipsilateral decreased breath sounds. In mechanically ventilated patients, airway pressures for normal tidal volume values will be high, and the ventilator pressure alarm limit may be exceeded. Resistance to bag-mask ventilation would increase as well. For patients with PEA and findings consistent with tension pneumothorax, treatment should be instituted at once, without waiting for radiologic confirmation. Needle thoracostomy can be accomplished on the affected side by sterile placement of a 16- or 18-gauge catheter (a 23-gauge butterfly needle may be used in infants) through the anterior chest wall in the second intercostal space, midclavicular line (**Appendix 8**). Successful decompression is associated with a rush of air, restoration of pulses, and a decrease in airway pressures in response to bag-mask or mechanical ventilation. Successful needle thoracostomy should be followed by standard tube thoracostomy. Endotracheal tube obstruction (from a patient biting the tube or secretions obstructing the tube) can mimic some of the findings described above but does not usually cause severe hypotension or PEA.

VII. ADVANCED LIFE SUPPORT IN THE CRITICAL CARE UNIT

A. General Issues

To be prepared for critical events such as cardiorespiratory arrest, it is important for professionals to know the clinical background and status of patients in the critical care unit. Professionals working in the ICU should review each patient's record during checkout rounds for signs of potential problems, such as electrolyte abnormalities. In addition, the clinical history and course may give clues to the etiology of a potential mishap. For instance, a ventilated patient who is known to have a large emphysematous bulla and who suddenly develops PEA would have a high likelihood of developing a tension pneumothorax secondary to rupture. Making rounds at the beginning of each tour of duty also gives the staff an opportunity to clarify the code status of each patient.

B. Principal Concerns

Airway management and oxygenation/ventilation are important issues in the initial approach to acute decompensation of an ICU patient. Adequate oxygenation/ventilation should be evaluated by physical assessment as well as expired CO_2 monitoring (if intubation is performed). Patients who are mechanically ventilated at the time of their arrest should be immediately disconnected from the ventilator and should receive 100% oxygen by bag-mask ventilation. Patients who are not intubated should have early endotracheal intubation; tube placement should be verified by physical assessment and expired CO_2 detection. Pulselessness can be verified by observing the arterial waveform if a functioning arterial line is in place or by carotid or femoral pulse checks. Chest compressions should be performed and early defibrillation for ventricular fibrillation should be undertaken as recommended by ACLS guidelines.

Cardiopulmonary/Cerebral Resuscitation

Key Points

- ■ The resuscitation status of a patient should be in accordance with that patient's directives.

- ■ Familiarity with recommendations for cardiopulmonary resuscitation (**Appendix 4**) is encouraged for all members of the resuscitation team.

- ■ The person assuming the leadership role during resuscitation must effectively delegate specific duties and supervise the process of resuscitation.

- ■ Resuscitation team members must accept delegation and remain focused upon those duties.

- ■ Chest compressions should be optimized by ensuring a rate of 100/min, changing compressors every 2 minutes, continuing compressions before and after shock delivery, and minimizing interruptions.

- ■ Some mishap related to mechanical ventilation should be suspected in patients who arrest while receiving mechanical ventilation, especially if the arrest is bradyasystolic.

- ■ In patients with hypotension and/or PEA and findings consistent with tension pneumothorax, needle thoracostomy should be instituted without delay.

- ■ Critically ill patients, or patients at risk of becoming critically ill, should be monitored for early signs of physiologic deterioration, and appropriate intervention should be instituted to avoid cardiopulmonary arrest.

 ## Suggested Readings

1. Abella BS, Alvarado JP, Myklebust H, et al. Quality of cardiopulmonary resuscitation during in-hospital cardiac arrest. *JAMA*. 2005;293:305.

2. American Heart Association. 2005 AHA Guidelines for CPR and ECC. *Circulation*. 2005;112(suppl 4):S1.

3. Bernard SA, Gray TW, Buist MD, et al. Treatment of comatose survivors of out-of-hospital cardiac arrest with induced hypothermia. *N Engl J Med*. 2002;346:557.

4. European Resuscitation Council. European Resuscitation Council Guidelines for Resuscitation 2005. *Resuscitation.* 2005;67(suppl):S1.

5. Hypothermia After Cardiac Arrest Study Group. Mild therapeutic hypothermia to improve the neurologic outcome after cardiac arrest. *N Engl J Med.* 2002;346:549.

6. Nadkarni VM, Larkin GL, Peberdy MA, et al. First documented rhythm and clinical outcome from in-hospital cardiac arrest among children and adults. *JAMA.* 2006;295:50.

Web Sites

1. American Heart Association. http://www.americanheart.org. This Web site allows access to the 2005 AHA Guidelines for CPR and ECC and provides other information on resuscitation and cardiac issues.

2. Circulation. http://www.circulationaha.org. This Web site allows access to the 2005 AHA Guidelines for CPR and ECC and provides guidelines for cardiac conditions.

3. European Resuscitation Council. http://www.erc.edu. This Web site provides the ERC Guidelines for Resuscitation 2005 and other educational information and material

Chapter 4

DIAGNOSIS AND MANAGEMENT OF ACUTE RESPIRATORY FAILURE

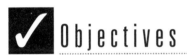 Objectives

- Define and classify acute respiratory failure.

- Describe the pathophysiology and manifestations of acute respiratory failure.

- Review oxygen supplementation strategies in acute respiratory failure.

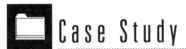 Case Study

A 75-year-old male with a long history of smoking, chronic lung disease, and treatment noncompliance is brought to the emergency department by his daughter, who says that he complained of progressive dyspnea overnight. The patient is awake, alert, and in moderate respiratory distress, with evident use of accessory muscles during inspiration and expiration and a respiratory rate of 30/min. There are audible expiratory wheezes. You are called to assess the patient and initiate treatment.

– What tests would be useful to evaluate the severity of the patient's condition?

– Which oxygen supplementation device should be used?

– What pharmacologic treatment should be initiated?

I. INTRODUCTION

Acute respiratory failure (ARF) is one of the most common disorders leading to ICU admission. Acute respiratory failure is present when the pulmonary system is no longer able to meet the metabolic demands of the individual. The pulmonary system is involved in 2 crucial metabolic roles: elimination of CO_2 and oxygenation of the blood. There are 3 forms of respiratory failure: hypoxemic, hypercapnic, and mixed. Hypoxemic respiratory failure is defined by a room air PaO_2 of ≤50 to 60 mm Hg (≤6.7-8 kPa) or an abnormal ratio of PaO_2 to fraction of inspired oxygen (PaO_2: FiO_2, or P:F ratio; see Section III below). Hypercapnic respiratory failure is defined by a $PaCO_2$ ≥50 mm Hg (≥6.7 kPa), with an accompanying acidosis (pH <7.36). Mixed respiratory failure, with both hypercapnia and hypoxemia, is a common form of respiratory failure in critically ill patients. Respiratory failure may be acute or chronic, depending on the duration and the nature of the compensation. Acute respiratory failure may occur in a person without previous lung disease or may be superimposed on chronic respiratory insufficiency.

II. CAUSES OF ACUTE RESPIRATORY FAILURE

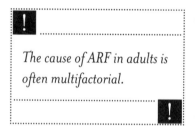

The cause of ARF in adults is often multifactorial.

Acute respiratory failure develops in a variety of clinical settings. Respiratory failure may result from primary pulmonary insults and from other systemic nonpulmonary disorders, as summarized in **Table 4-1**. Abnormalities of the central nervous system, neuromuscular system, upper and lower airways, pulmonary parenchyma, and cardiovascular system may all give rise to ARF.

Hypoxemic respiratory failure is often seen in patients with severe pneumonia, acute lung injury, or acute pulmonary edema. These disorders interfere primarily with the pulmonary system's ability to adequately oxygenate the blood as it circulates through the alveolar capillaries. Hypercapnic respiratory failure is seen in patients with severe airflow obstruction, central respiratory failure, or neuromuscular respiratory failure.

The following are common causes of ARF:

■ Exacerbations of chronic obstructive pulmonary disease (COPD) are characterized by thick mucopurulent secretions as well as bronchospasm. Exacerbations of COPD are often associated with both hypoxemic and hypercapnic acute respiratory failure (ie, mixed ARF).

■ Pneumonia is most commonly associated with hypoxemic respiratory failure, although it can also be associated with hypercapnic respiratory failure, especially in the setting of other diseases such as COPD.

■ Acute respiratory distress syndrome (ARDS) is a manifestation of a systemic inflammatory response caused by pulmonary or nonpulmonary injury or disease. The predominantly hypoxemic respiratory failure is caused primarily by an increased shunt fraction due to alveolar filling.

| Table 4-1 | Causes of Respiratory Failure |

DISORDERS ASSOCIATED WITH ABNORMAL OXYGEN ONLOADING
(HYPOXEMIC RESPIRATORY FAILURE)
Lower Airway and Parenchyma

NEOPLASM	TRAUMA	Acute respiratory distress syndrome
INFECTIONS	Pulmonary contusion	Interstitial lung disease
Viral	Pulmonary laceration	Pulmonary emboli
Bacterial	OTHER	Atelectasis
Fungal	Bronchospasm	Cystic fibrosis
Mycoplasma	Heart failure	
Other		

DISORDERS ASSOCIATED WITH INADEQUATE CARBON DIOXIDE OFFLOADING
(HYPERCAPNIC RESPIRATORY FAILURE)
Brain

DRUGS	METABOLIC	INFECTION
Opioids	Hyponatremia	Meningitis
Benzodiazepines	Hypocalcemia	Encephalitis
Propofol	Hypercapnia (excess carbohydrate)	Abscess
Barbiturates	Alkalosis	Polio
General anesthetics	Hyperglycemia	INCREASED INTRACRANIAL
Poisons	Myxedema	PRESSURE
Others	NEOPLASM	OTHER
		Central alveolar hypoventilation
		Obstructive sleep apnea

Nerves and Muscles

TRAUMA	METABOLIC	OTHER
Spinal cord injury	Hypokalemia, hyperkalemia	Motor neuron disease
Diaphragmatic injury	Hypophosphatemia	Myasthenia gravis
DRUGS/POISONS	Hypomagnesemia	Multiple sclerosis
Neuromuscular blocking	NEOPLASM	Muscular dystrophy
agents	INFECTIONS	Guillain-Barré syndrome
Aminoglycoside antibiotics	Polio (or postpolio syndrome)	
Arsenic	Tetanus	
Strychnine		

Upper Airway

TISSUE ENLARGEMENT	INFECTIONS	OTHER
Tonsil and adenoid	Epiglottitis	Bilateral vocal-cord paralysis
hyperplasia	Laryngotracheitis	Laryngeal edema
Malignant neoplasm	TRAUMA	Tracheomalacia
Polyps		Cricoarytenoid arthritis
Goiter		

Chest Bellows

TRAUMA	OTHER CONTRIBUTING FACTORS	Fibrothorax
Rib fractures	Kyphoscoliosis	Supine position
Flail chest	Scleroderma	Obesity
Burn eschar	Spondylitis	Pain
	Pneumothorax	Ascites
	Pleural effusion	

■ Traumatic brain injury is associated with predominantly hypercapnic respiratory failure, although it can be complicated by hypoxemic respiratory failure in the setting of concurrent aspiration or chronic pulmonary disease.

■ Decompensated congestive heart failure is associated with predominantly hypoxemic failure (secondary to alveolar filling and increased shunt); however, hypercapnic respiratory failure may also occur in severe exacerbations or in the presence of pulmonary disease.

III. PATHOPHYSIOLOGY OF ACUTE RESPIRATORY FAILURE

A. Hypoxemia

The underlying physiologic abnormality in hypoxemic respiratory failure is usually the result of a mismatch of alveolar ventilation ($\dot{V}$) and pulmonary perfusion ($\dot{Q}$), as illustrated in **Figure 4-1**. This mismatch of ventilation and perfusion wherein ventilation is decreased relative to perfusion is called low $\dot{V}/\dot{Q}$. The physiologic effect of this type of $\dot{V}/\dot{Q}$ mismatch is hypoxemia. Disease processes that cause progressive obstruction or atelectasis (eg, pneumonia, aspiration, pulmonary edema) result in a decrease in the amount of oxygen available in distal airways for pulmonary capillary uptake. Although blood flow to such abnormal lung units declines, it usually does not decrease as much as oxygen availability decreases, allowing a greater proportion of unoxygenated blood to return to the left heart. Admixture of poorly oxygenated blood circulating by abnormal alveoli dilutes oxygenated blood from more normal lung units, causing systemic hypoxemia. Treatment of hypoxemia due to $\dot{V}/\dot{Q}$ mismatch should be directed toward treating infections, reversing airway

Figure 4-1. Ventilation and Perfusion Matching in the Lung

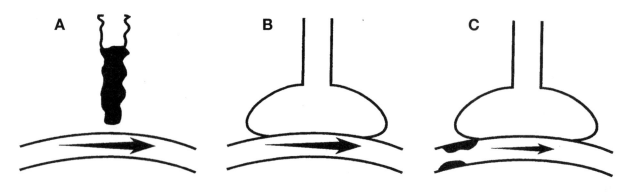

(A) At one end of the pathologic continuum, areas of limited ventilation relative to perfusion produce shunt effect and hypoxemia. (C) At the opposite end of the continuum, areas of better ventilation than perfusion produce dead-space effect. (B) Ventilation and perfusion are matched in the normal lung.

obstruction, reopening (recruiting) atelectatic lung zones, and preventing closure (derecruitment) of the affected lung units.

Other, less common causes of hypoxemia include:

- Decreased diffusion of oxygen across the alveolocapillary membrane complex because of interstitial edema, inflammation, fibrosis, etc

- Alveolar hypoventilation

- High altitude with low inspired oxygen pressure

Therapy for diffusion abnormalities includes treatment of the cause of interstitial pathology (ie, diuretics for cardiogenic pulmonary edema, corticosteroids for inflammatory disorders). Ensuring adequate ventilation will correct hypoxemia that is due to hypercapnia; high altitude is rarely a cause of acute hypoxemia in patients. As a compensatory strategy, increasing oxygen supplementation, that is, FiO_2, while the cause of the hypoxemia is sought and corrected may improve oxygenation.

The gradient between the partial pressure of oxygen in the alveolus (PAO_2) and in the circulation (PaO_2), the $P(A-a)O_2$ gradient, can be used to determine whether hypoxemia is caused only by hypercapnia. The PaO_2 is obtained from an arterial blood gas analysis while the patient breathes room air. The PAO_2 is estimated from the modified alveolar air equation:

$$PAO_2 = [FiO_2 \times (PB - 47)] - (1.25 \times PaCO_2)$$

where FiO_2 is expressed as a fraction (not a percentage), PB is barometric pressure, and $PaCO_2$ is obtained from the same blood gas measurement.

The $P(A-a)O_2$ gradient should be <10 mm Hg (<1.3 kPa) in young adults and <20 mm Hg (<2.7 kPa) in all patients. A normal gradient suggests the hypoxemia is likely due to hypercapnia, whereas an increased gradient suggests that parenchymal changes ($\dot{V}/\dot{Q}$ mismatch, etc) are causing the hypoxemia. The usefulness of this assessment is limited because supplemental oxygen greatly distorts its interpretation. As most hypoxic patients should not be stressed by breathing room air, measurements would usually be done while the patient receives oxygen. Therefore, the $P(A-a)O_2$ gradient has significant limitations.

Numerous methods for quantifying hypoxemia have been proposed to provide a means of following the degree of hypoxemia and to communicate this information to other providers. The P:F ratio is commonly used for quantifying the degree of patient hypoxemia. It requires accurate assessment of FiO_2, which is difficult in the nonintubated patient. The lower the P:F ratio, the worse the patient's hypoxemia.

> **!** *The P:F ratio can be helpful for following trends in a patient's condition and evaluating ventilation strategies.* **!**

B. Hypercapnia

Hypercapnic respiratory failure is caused by 1 or more factors described in the equation for alveolar minute ventilation:

$$V_A = (V_T - V_D)f$$

where V_A is minute alveolar ventilation, V_T is tidal volume, V_D is dead space, and f is respiratory frequency.

Hypercapnia may result from decreased V_T or f, as occurs with drug ingestion, anesthesia, changes in the medullary center for respiration, fatigue, etc. An elevated $PaCO_2$ normally increases ventilatory drive. Therefore, hypercapnic respiratory failure implies that the patient is unable to sustain minute ventilation (respiratory rate [f] × tidal volume [V_T]).

> !
>
> *The more rapidly the negative inspiratory pressure and FVC deteriorate, the lower the threshold for intubation and mechanical ventilation.*
>
> !

Treatment of decreased V_T or respiratory rate may require reversal of sedation or other drugs, intubation/mechanical ventilation to rest fatigued muscles, nutrition, respiratory stimulants, and, as always, treatment of other possible primary causes. Measures of ventilatory mechanics, such as peak negative inspiratory pressure and forced vital capacity (FVC), monitor a patient's course and may signal when endotracheal intubation and mechanical ventilation are warranted. A single measurement is less useful than measurements made over time. Negative inspiratory pressure <-20 to 25 cm H_2O or an FVC <10 mL/kg, or both, should raise concern that a patient's ventilatory mechanics may be sufficiently impaired to warrant tracheal intubation and mechanical ventilation.

Increased physiologic dead space (V_D) may also produce hypercapnia and is another type of mismatch illustrated in **Figure 4-1**. When gas flow to and from airways remains adequate but blood flow is absolutely or relatively diminished, CO_2 does not have the opportunity to diffuse from the pulmonary circulation, and CO_2-rich blood is returned to the left atrium. Increased dead-space ventilation may occur in hypovolemia, pulmonary embolus, poor cardiac output, or when the regional airway pressure is relatively higher than the regional perfusion pressure produced by the pulmonary blood flow in that area.

Therapy of increased dead space may require reduction in peak or mean airway pressures if the patient is receiving mechanical ventilation, augmentation of intravascular volume and/or cardiac output, or treatment of other limitations to pulmonary blood flow. It may be possible to compensate for the symptoms of hypercapnia due to high V_D by modifying parameters to increase minute ventilation during mechanical ventilation while the cause of hypercapnia is sought and corrected. Because of the high solubility of CO_2, a diffusion barrier for CO_2 rarely ever occurs. Increased CO_2 production may contribute to hypercapnia if excessive carbohydrate nutritional calories are given or in extreme hypercatabolic conditions (eg, burns, hyperthyroidism, persistent fever).

C. Mixed Respiratory Failure

It is common for patients to demonstrate characteristics of both pathophysiologic categories of ARF during the course of illness. An understanding of the underlying pathophysiology of each, therefore, is necessary for planning therapeutic support. Several related disease processes often combine and act in concert or synergistically to compound respiratory failure. For example, the patient with chronic pulmonary disease and a large dead space often has associated heart failure, which increases $\dot{V}/\dot{Q}$ mismatching and worsens hypoxemia.

IV. MANIFESTATIONS OF ACUTE RESPIRATORY FAILURE

A. Clinical Presentation of Respiratory Distress

Clinical manifestations of respiratory distress commonly include signs and symptoms of hypoxemia, hypercapnia, or both. These include:

- Altered mental status, ranging from agitation to somnolence

- Evidence of increased work of breathing, such as nasal flaring in infants, use of accessory respiratory muscles, intercostal/suprasternal/supraclavicular muscle retraction, tachypnea, hyperpnea, or a paradoxical or dysynchronous breathing pattern (**Figure 4-2**)

- Bradypnea

- Cyanosis of mucosal membranes (eg, tongue, mouth) or nail beds

- Diaphoresis, tachycardia, hypertension, and other signs of catecholamine release

Figure 4-2. Normal Versus Abnormal Respiration

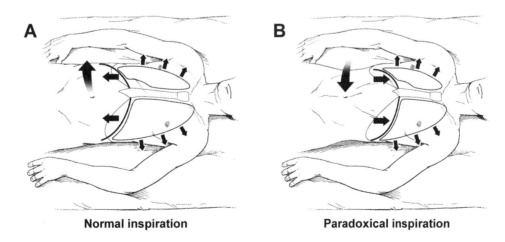

Normal inspiration   **Paradoxical inspiration**

A, The abdominal wall moves outward as the diaphragm moves downward in normal inspiration. B, With respiratory muscle fatigue, the diaphragm becomes flaccid and moves upward during inspiration resulting in inward movement of the abdominal wall. Reproduced with permission from Mayo Clinic.

B. Diagnostic Tests

Pulse oximetry can be used to rapidly evaluate oxygenation in a patient with respiratory distress by estimating the arterial oxyhemoglobin saturation (**Chapter 6**). However, pulse oximetry provides no assessment for hypercapnia. Arterial blood gas analysis is commonly used in severely ill patients to determine the 2 primary measures of respiratory failure, the PaO_2 and $PaCO_2$, as well as pH. Additional tests such as electrolytes, hematocrit, and drug levels may provide clues to the underlying etiology of ARF. A chest radiograph is invaluable in suggesting the underlying pathophysiology. Pulmonary alveolar infiltrates suggest a hypoxemic component for ARF, and clear lung fields suggest possible hypercapnic ARF, although considerable overlap exists.

V. MANAGEMENT CONSIDERATIONS

A. Oxygen Supplementation

Most patients with ARF require supplemental oxygen. Oxygen transfer from alveolar gas to capillary blood occurs by diffusion across the alveolar-capillary membrane and is driven by the oxygen partial-pressure gradient between the PAO_2 and the PO_2 of the pulmonary capillary blood. In most cases of ARF, the PAO_2 can be substantially increased by use of supplemental oxygen, thus increasing the gradient across the membrane and improving the PaO_2.

Supplemental oxygen can be provided by a variety of devices (see **Figure 4-3**). The effectiveness of each is determined by the capacity of the device to deliver sufficient oxygen at a high enough flow rate to match the patient's spontaneous inspiratory flow rate. Matching between the flow capacity of the oxygen device and the patient's inspiratory flow demand determines how much room air the nonintubated patient breathing in an open system may entrain. Any entrained room air ($FIO_2 = 0.21$) will dilute (decrease) the FIO_2 of the delivered gas in such a way that the tracheal FIO_2, and hence PAO_2, may be considerably lower than the FIO_2 delivered from the oxygen source. Therefore, oxygen-supplement systems are usually classified as high oxygen (capable of delivering up to 100% oxygen), controlled oxygen (set oxygen percentage), or low oxygen. Similarly, the devices are also categorized as either high flow, moderate flow, or low flow, reflecting the flow-delivery capacity of the gas at the preset FIO_2 level.

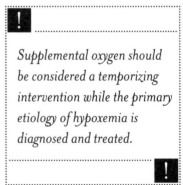

Supplemental oxygen should be considered a temporizing intervention while the primary etiology of hypoxemia is diagnosed and treated.

For example, a tachypneic and hyperpneic patient will have a high inspiratory flow rate during each breath. In such cases, hypoxemia is not likely to respond well to oxygen supplementation by nasal cannula because it is a low-oxygen, low-flow system and cannot match the patient's high inspiratory flow rate. Room air will be entrained during inspiration, and the tracheal FIO_2 will be reduced. A high-oxygen, high-flow system should be selected for this type of patient.

Figure 4-3. Oxygen Supplementation Devices

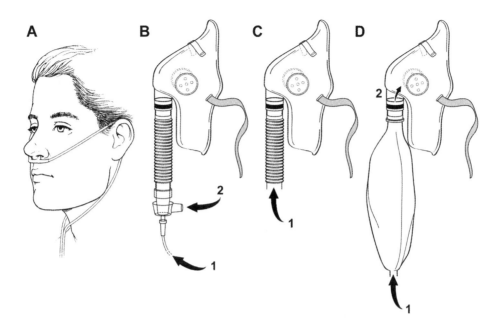

A, Nasal cannula. B, Air-entrainment face mask with 100% oxygen source gas (1) and a changeable nozzle (2), which controls entrainment of room air through an opening. C, Aerosol face mask with blended preset FiO_2 (1) from a nebulizer. D, Reservoir face mask with 100% oxygen (1) supplied to a reservoir, where 1-way valve (2) direct inhaled and exhaled gas. Reproduced with permission from Mayo Clinic.

1. Nasal Cannula

Short prongs of the nasal cannula are inserted into the nares. Oxygen (100%) is delivered through the cannula, but at a low flow rate between 0.5 and 5 L/min. The resulting FiO_2 depends on the patient's minute ventilation and cannot therefore be precisely controlled, but the maximal tracheal FiO_2 is not likely to exceed 0.4 to 0.5 (40% to 50%). Higher flow rates do not result in much higher FiO_2 levels and have a drying and irritating effect on nasal mucosa. The nasal cannula is comfortable and well tolerated by many patients with ARF in whom precise control of FiO_2 is not necessary. It is a low-flow, low-oxygen device.

2. Air-Entrainment Face Mask

Air-entrainment masks (also called Venturi masks) deliver 100% oxygen through a jet-mixing device that increases the velocity of oxygen and causes a controlled entrainment of air. The FiO_2 can be more precisely controlled from 0.24 to 0.5 (24% to 50%) at high flow rates simply by exchanging the interchangeable jet nozzle and adjusting the oxygen flow rate. These masks are most useful in patients with chronic obstructive lung disease who require a degree of hypoxemia to sustain the respiratory drive. Careful titration of FiO_2 is, therefore, required to improve oxygenation without suppressing minute ventilation. It is a high-flow, controlled-oxygen device.

3. Aerosol Face Mask

The commonly used aerosol face mask combines a variable oxygen setting and moderate flows. The mask, which has large side holes, is attached by large-bore tubing to a nebulizer that blends 100% oxygen and room air to deliver gas at a preset FiO_2 level. Flow matching can be evaluated by observing the patient during spontaneous breathing. If the entire aerosol mist disappears from the mask during inhalation, the patient's inspiratory-flow demands are probably exceeding the capacity of the nebulizer and room air is being entrained. The aerosol face mask is a variable-oxygen, moderate-flow device.

4. Reservoir Face Mask

The reservoir face mask incorporates a reservoir bag with the mask from which the patient breathes. The reservoir bag is filled from a supply source of 100% oxygen. The flow rate of oxygen is adjusted so that the bag remains completely or partially distended throughout the respiratory cycle. When the mask is properly applied, oxygen delivery to the nonintubated patient can be maximized but rarely exceeds an FiO_2 of 0.6 to 0.9. The reservoir face mask is a high-oxygen, high-flow device.

> [!]
>
> *A reservoir mask is frequently used for improving oxygenation in patients with severe hypoxemia until further evaluation and treatments are accomplished.* [!]

5. Resuscitation Bag-Mask Unit

Although not commonly considered an oxygen-supplement device, bag-mask units are usually included with other emergency equipment and, therefore, are readily accessible. When the mask is held firmly over the patient's face, room air entrainment is largely excluded. If the oxygen flow to the bag is kept high ($\geq$15 L/min), a high oxygen supply is provided at sufficient flow. The resuscitation bag need not be compressed to supply oxygen. It is a high-oxygen, high-flow device.

B. Pharmacologic Adjuncts

Many diseases that cause ARF produce similar anatomic and physiologic derangements, including bronchial inflammation, mucosal edema, smooth muscle contraction, and increased mucus production and viscosity. Each of these processes may contribute to obstruction of airway gas flow, increased airway resistance, mismatch, and elevated V_D. Some pharmacologic agents may be helpful in the care of such patients and may directly alter shunt or dead-space effects.

1. β_2-Agonists

Inhaled β_2-agonists are important therapy in patients with ARF secondary to many causes. Stimulation of β_2-adrenergic receptors causes bronchial and vascular smooth-muscle relaxation. These agents are typically administered by metered-dose inhaler (MDI) or by intermittent or continuous nebulization (**Table 4-2**). On rare occasions, in very critically ill patients with obstructive airway disease, β_2-agonists are administered by both inhalation and subcutaneous injection. Long-acting inhaled β_2-agonists do not have a role in the management of patients with acute respiratory deterioration. Racemic epinephrine aerosol is an established therapy for upper-airway obstruction in children with croup and is also used for laryngeal edema in adults.

| Table 4-2 | Pharmacologic Agents for Obstructive Airway Disease | | |

Drug	Preparation	Route of Administration	Dosage
Albuterol	0.5% solution	Inhaled (aerosol)	*Adult:* 2.5–5 mg q 2–4 h[a]
			Pediatric: 0.05–0.15 mg/kg q 4–6 h[a]
	MDI (90 µg/puff)	Inhaled	*Adult:* 1–2 puffs q 2–4 h[a]
			Pediatric: 1–2 puffs q 4–6 h[a]
Levalbuterol	0.31, 0.63, or 1.25 mg/unit dose solution	Inhaled (aerosol)	*Adult and children* ≥12 y: 0.63–1.25 mg q 6–8 h
			Pediatric (6–11 y): 0.31–0.63 mg q 6–8 h; more aggressive dosing may be used in acute exacerbations
	MDI (45 µg/puff)	Inhaled	*Adult:* 1–2 puffs q 4–6 h
			Pediatric: (age ≥4 y):1–2 puffs q 4–6 h
Metaproterenol Sulfate	5% solution	Inhaled (aerosol)	*Adult:* 0.3 mL q 2–4 h[a]
			Pediatric: 0.25–0.5 mg/kg q 2–4 h[a]
	MDI (0.65 µg/puff)	Inhaled	*Adult:* 2–3 puffs q 4–6 h[a]
			Pediatric: 1–3 puffs q 4–6 h[a]
Terbutaline	MDI (0.2 µg/puff)	Inhaled	*Adult:* 1–2 puffs q 4–6 h[a]
			Pediatric: 1–2 puffs q 4–6 h[a]
	0.1% solution	Subcutaneous	*Adult:* 0.2–0.4 mL; repeat in 15–30 min
			Pediatric: 0.2 mg/kg; maximum 6 mg
Epinephrine	1 mg/mL (1:1000)	Subcutaneous	*Adult:* 0.1–0.5 mg; repeat in 20–30 min
			Pediatric: 0.01 mg/kg
Racemic Epinephrine	2.25% solution	Inhaled	*Adult:* 0.3–1 mL
			Pediatric: 0.05 mL/kg/dose; maximum 0.5 mL/dose diluted to 3 mL with NS
Ipratropium	0.025% solution	Inhaled (aerosol)	*Adult:* 500 µg q 6–8 h
			Pediatric: Infant and child: 250 µg q 6–8 h
			>12 y: 250–500 µg q 6–8 h
	MDI (18 µg/puff)	Inhaled	*Adult:* 2–4 puffs q 6 h
			Pediatric: 1–2 puffs q 8 h

Abbreviations: MDI, metered-dose inhaler; NS, normal saline
[a]In patients with severe asthma, frequency of administration of inhaled β-agonists should be guided by response to therapy and risk for side effects. Therapy is routinely initiated with 3 treatments every 20 minutes. Further therapy adjustments are then based on response. Continuous nebulization may also be employed. Caution should be exercised when considering use of continuous nebulized β_2-agonists, particularly in older patients and those with underlying cardiac disease.

2. Anticholinergic Agents

Ipratropium bromide competes with acetylcholine at the bronchial receptor site, resulting in bronchial smooth-muscle relaxation. This agent is delivered by MDI or nebulization (**Table 4-2**). Ipratropium has a more delayed onset of action than β_2-agonists and has more consistent bronchodilatory effects in COPD than in asthma. The addition of ipratropium to albuterol appears to have an additive benefit in approximately 30% of asthma patients. Tiotropium is a long-acting anticholinergic bronchodilator that has sustained bronchodilator effects in COPD patients, but its use in acute exacerbations is not recommended.

3. Corticosteroids

The central role of inflammation in obstructive airway disease is established, and the benefit from aggressive corticosteroid use in the asthmatic patient with ARF is well documented. In addition, corticosteroids may decrease β-receptor tachyphylaxis. Limited consensus exists on dosing schedules in asthma. Doses of methylprednisolone of 80 mg/24 h have been as effective as >360 mg/24 h. Some clinicians use doses equivalent to those given for asthma when treating COPD, whereas others begin with doses equivalent to 1 mg/kg/24 h, adjusting as patient response dictates. The intravenous and oral routes are equally effective. Careful monitoring of corticosteroid side effects is warranted. Acute myopathies have been described after moderate to high dosages of corticosteroids in patients with COPD and/or asthma. After the acute exacerbation, inhaled corticosteroids are often useful adjuncts to therapy and may allow reduction in systemic corticosteroid dosage. However, routine use of inhalational agents is not recommended in the setting of acute severe bronchospasm.

4. Antibiotics

Bacterial infection (bronchitis/pneumonia) frequently precipitates ARF. Antibiotics should be used when there is clinical suspicion that bacterial pulmonary infection is present (eg, change in sputum characteristics, pulmonary infiltrates on the chest radiograph, fever, leukocytosis) and should be chosen to effectively treat usual pathogens (see **Chapter 11**). Therapy may be focused subsequently, when culture and sensitivity data become available.

E. Miscellaneous Agents and Treatments

Agents to hydrate or otherwise alter the composition, elasticity, or viscosity of mucus have been used, although their efficacy has not been demonstrated except in selected patient groups (eg, patients with cystic fibrosis) or in severe alterations in mucus composition. These include mucolytics such as acetylcysteine or propylene glycol, bronchorrheic agents such as saturated solution of potassium iodide (SSKI) or glycerol guaiacolate, and alkalinizing agents such as aerosolized sodium bicarbonate.

Postural drainage, chest physical therapy, nasotracheal suctioning, incentive spirometry, intermittent positive-pressure breathing (IPPB), and cough/deep-breathing exercises have long histories of use. Also available are newer measures such as positive expiratory pressure (PEP) therapy, vest device (high-frequency chest oscillator), and even bed percussion modules. Many of these modalities may be applied to treat specific symptoms of ARF or the cause of respiratory failure. The effectiveness and positive impact of the bedside nurse's or the respiratory care practitioner's contributions to care and the avoidance of intubation/mechanical ventilation should not be underestimated.

Diagnosis and Management of Acute Respiratory Failure

Key Points

■ Acute respiratory failure is classified as hypoxemic, hypercapnic, or mixed. Arterial blood gas measurements are the primary assessment tool for determining this classification.

■ The most common pathophysiologic mechanism for hypoxemic acute respiratory failure is ventilation/perfusion mismatch.

■ Hypercapnic acute respiratory failure is primarily the result of a change in 1 or more determinants of the alveolar minute ventilation equation: tidal volume, respiratory frequency, and physiologic dead space.

■ Oxygen supplementation is commonly used to treat hypoxemia. The oxygen supply device that is chosen must be capable of matching the oxygen and respiratory flow demands of the patient.

■ Pharmacologic and therapeutic adjuncts should be considered when treating patients with acute respiratory failure.

Suggested Readings

1. Dolovich MB, Ahrens RC, Hess DR, et al. Device selection and outcomes of aerosolized therapy: evidence-based guidelines. *Chest.* 2005;127:335.

2. Manser R, Reid D, Abramson M. Corticosteroids for acute severe asthma in hospitalised patients. *Cochrane Database Syst Rev.* 2007;(2):CD001740. doi:10.1002/14651858. CD001740.

Chapter 5

MECHANICAL VENTILATION

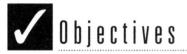

Objectives

■ Discuss the indications and techniques for noninvasive positive-pressure ventilation.

■ Describe the characteristics of different types of breaths and modes of mechanical ventilation.

■ Outline ventilator settings and monitoring needs for the initiation of mechanical ventilation.

■ Describe interactions between ventilatory parameters and modifications needed to avoid harmful effects of mechanical ventilation.

■ Review the guidelines for initial ventilator management that apply to specific clinical situations.

Case Study

A 65-year-old woman with an exacerbation of chronic obstructive pulmonary disease is admitted to the hospital. She is receiving oxygen at 3 L/min by nasal cannula. She continues to have significant respiratory distress after receiving 2 bronchodilator nebulizer treatments. Her vital signs are blood pressure 160/110 mm Hg, heart rate 110/min, respirations 30/min, and temperature 99.0°F (37.2°C). Physical examination is remarkable for use of accessory muscles of respiration and diffuse wheezing bilaterally. An arterial blood gas analysis shows pH 7.24, PCO_2 60 mm Hg (8 kPa), and PO_2 65 mm Hg (8.7 kPa).

– What type of respiratory support should be initiated?

– What settings should be selected for respiratory support?

– What are the goals of respiratory support?

I. INTRODUCTION

When hypoxic or hypercapnic respiratory failure cannot be treated by other means, as discussed in **Chapter 4,** more advanced support with positive pressure ventilation may be needed. Positive pressure ventilation can be delivered noninvasively via a mask or helmet or invasively via an endotracheal tube. Generally accepted indications for initiating positive pressure ventilatory support are summarized in **Table 5-1.**

Table 5-1. Indications for Positive Pressure Ventilatory Support	
Ventilation abnormalities	Respiratory muscle dysfunction
	• Respiratory muscle fatigue
	• Chest wall abnormalities
	• Neuromuscular disease
	Decreased ventilatory drive
	Increased airway resistance and/or obstruction
Oxygenation abnormalities	Refractory hypoxemia
	Need for positive end-expiratory pressure
	Excessive work of breathing
Need for sedation and/or neuromuscular blockade	
Need to decrease systemic or myocardial oxygen consumption	
Use of hyperventilation to reduce intracranial pressure	
Facilitation of alveolar recruitment and prevention of atelectasis	

The choice of noninvasive or invasive positive-pressure ventilation will depend on patient characteristics, the type and severity of the respiratory and/or systemic condition, availability of resources, and experience and training of the clinician and healthcare team.

II. NONINVASIVE POSITIVE-PRESSURE VENTILATION

Noninvasive positive-pressure ventilation (NPPV) is a form of mechanical ventilation that provides respiratory assistance without an invasive artificial airway. The potential beneficial effects of NPPV are similar to those of invasive mechanical ventilation and include decreased work of breathing, improved oxygenation, and improved gas exchange. In addition, this type of ventilation avoids many of the complications associated with intubation and invasive mechanical ventilation. Potential advantages and disadvantages of NPPV are listed in **Table 5-2.**

Table 5-2.	Advantages and Disadvantages of NPPV

Advantages	Disadvantages
• Reduced need for sedation	• Claustrophobia
• Preservation of airway-protective reflexes	• Increased workload for respiratory practitioner
• Avoidance of upper airway trauma	• Facial/nasal pressure lesions
• Decreased incidence of nosocomial sinusitis and pneumonia	• Unprotected airway
• Improved patient comfort	• Inability to suction deep airway
• Shorter length of ICU and hospital stay	• Gastric distension with use of face mask or helmet
• Improved survival	• Possible upper-extremity edema, axillary vein thrombosis, tympanic dysfunction, and intrahelmet noise with use of helmet
	• Delay in intubation

NPPV utilizes 2 levels of positive airway pressure that essentially combines the modalities of pressure support ventilation (PSV) and continuous positive airway pressure (CPAP) (see next section). By convention, the PSV modality is referred to as IPAP (inspiratory positive airway pressure), and the CPAP modality is referred to as EPAP (expiratory positive airway pressure). CPAP alone can also be delivered noninvasively but does not provide support of ventilation. CPAP allows spontaneous breathing from a gas source at an elevated baseline system pressure (higher than atmospheric pressure) and is functionally equivalent to positive end-expiratory pressure (PEEP).

Both ventilators designed for noninvasive ventilation and standard ventilators can be used for NPPV. Alarm setups may need to be altered on standard ventilators because the alarms are typically triggered by exhalation, and noninvasive ventilation inherently has more volume loss in comparison to ventilation via an endotracheal tube. Ventilators specifically designed to provide noninvasive patient-triggered pressure support or patient-triggered volume cycled breaths are optimal. The ventilator connects to a tightly fitted face or nasal mask or helmet (**Figure 5-1**). The

Figure 5-1. Devices for Delivery of NPPV

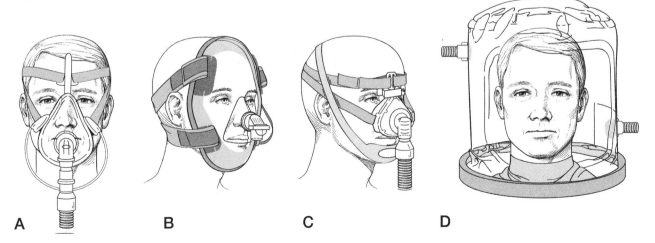

A   B   C   D

Examples of NPPV delivery devices: A, face mask; B, total face mask; C, nasal mask with chin strap; and D, helmet. Reproduced with permission from Mayo Clinic.

nasal mask is better tolerated than the face mask but is less effective in mouth breathers and edentulous patients. Some leakage of gas is anticipated with both masks and can be compensated for by increasing pressure settings or increasing the set tidal volume (VT) level. To reduce the leakage of gas from the mouth when a nasal mask is used, the patient's mouth should be kept closed or chin straps should be secured.

Noninvasive positive-pressure ventilation is best utilized in the alert, cooperative patient whose respiratory condition is expected to improve in 48 to 72 hours. Potential candidates should be hemodynamically stable, able to control airway secretions, and able to coordinate with the ventilator. Patient characteristics that may contraindicate use of NPPV are listed in **Table 5-3.** Noninvasive positive pressure ventilation has been used successfully in both types of acute respiratory failure (ARF), but it may not be desirable when ventilatory requirements and/or the severity of illness are high. Before noninvasive ventilation is initiated, patient characteristics and NPPV's potential for successfully treating the underlying respiratory condition should be evaluated. **Table 5-4** lists

Table 5-3.	Contraindications to Use of NPPV

- Cardiac or respiratory arrest
- Hemodynamic instability
- Myocardial ischemia or arrhythmias
- Patient who is unable to cooperate
- Inability to protect the airway
- High risk for aspiration
- Active upper GI hemorrhage
- Severe hypoxemia
- Severe encephalopathy
- Facial trauma, recent surgery, and/or burns
- Significant agitation

Table 5-4.	Respiratory Conditions Likely to Respond to NPPV

Hypoxemic respiratory failure

- Cardiogenic pulmonary edema without hemodynamic instability
- Respiratory failure in patients with Pneumocystis pneumonia
- Patients who are not candidates for intubation
- Respiratory failure in immunocompromised patients (especially in hematologic malignancies and transplant patients)

Hypercapnic respiratory failure

- Acute exacerbation of COPD
- Acute exacerbation of asthma
- Respiratory failure in patients with cystic fibrosis
- Patients who are not candidates for intubation

respiratory conditions that are likely to benefit from use of NPPV. If a provider skilled in the application of NPPV is not available, if the patient is too sick for this type of support, or if NPPV has failed to benefit the patient, it is critical to move quickly to intubation and mechanical ventilation. The approach to initiating NPPV after appropriate patient evaluation is outlined in **Table 5-5.** Patients receiving NPPV must be monitored closely in a proper setting, and continuous pulse oximetry and cardiac monitoring are suggested.

Table 5-5. Initiation of NPPV

- Do not delay intubation if needed and keep in mind the patient's resuscitation status.
- Arterial blood gas (ABG) analysis should be considered prior to initiation.
- Explain the procedure to the patient.
- Keep head of bed at ≥45°.
- Ensure appropriate mask or helmet size.
- Assess the patient's tolerance of the mask by applying it by hand before securing the harness.
- Use the following initial ventilator settings:
  - Mode: Spontaneous
  - Trigger: Maximum sensitivity
  - FiO_2: 1.00
  - EPAP: 4-5 cm H_2O (higher levels are poorly tolerated initially)
  - IPAP: 10-15 cm H_2O
  - Backup rate: Start at 6/min
- Adjust the difference between EPAP and IPAP to achieve an effective tidal volume and CO_2 clearance. Adjust EPAP for alveolar recruitment in increments of 2 cm H_2O/step to improve oxygenation. Depending on the ventilator, a similar increase in the IPAP may be required to maintain the same V_T.
- If assist-control volume ventilation is used, begin with a V_T of 6 to 8 mL/kg (depending on the underlying pulmonary condition).
- Titrate pressures, volume, and FiO_2 to achieve appropriate PaO_2 and $PaCO_2$ levels. Ventilator changes can be made every 15 to 30 minutes.
- Follow vital signs, pulse oximetry, mental status, clinical appearance, and ABG (if indicated).
- Goals of NPPV may include a respiratory rate <30/min, V_T >7 mL/kg of predicted body weight, improved gas exchange, and patient comfort.

Sedation should be used cautiously and with adequate monitoring as NPPV is initiated. Additional measures that may be considered include application of a protective nose patch when using a nasal mask and gastric decompression if a face mask or helmet is used. Oral intake should be restricted until the patient has stabilized and potential intubation is no longer a consideration. Intubation is usually required when the patient shows clinical worsening, when a follow-up ABG at 1 to 2 hours does not show improvement, or when therapeutic goals cannot be reached within the first 4 to 6 hours. An algorithm for assessing NPPV is presented in **Figure 5-2.**

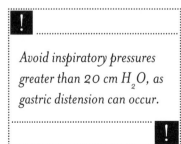

Avoid inspiratory pressures greater than 20 cm H_2O, as gastric distension can occur.

Figure 5-2. Assessment of NPPV

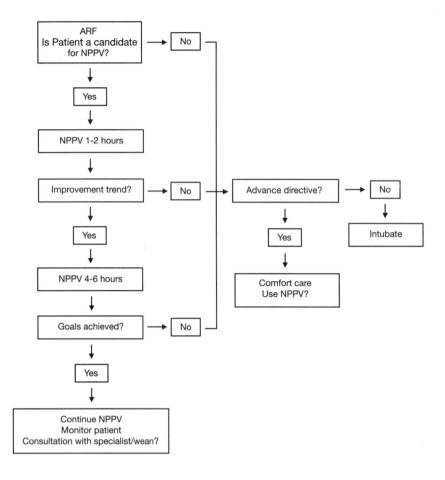

Abbreviations: NPPV, noninvasive positive pressure ventilation; ARF, acute respiratory failure.

III. INVASIVE MECHANICAL VENTILATION

Mechanical ventilation via an endotracheal tube is commonly used to support critically ill patients. It is the definitive intervention to ensure adequate oxygenation and ventilation.

Each mechanical ventilation respiratory cycle can be divided into 2 phases: inspiration and expiration (**Figure 5-3**). Inspiration is the point at which the exhalation valve closes and fresh gas under pressure from the ventilator enters the chest. The amount of gas delivered during inspiration is limited by 3 parameters that can be set on the ventilator: volume, pressure, and/or flow. Cycling is the changeover from the end of inspiration to the second phase, expiration. Cycling can occur in response to elapsed time, delivered volume, or a decrease in flow rate. Expiration begins when the gas flow coming from the ventilator is stopped and the exhalation circuit is opened to allow gas to escape from the lungs. Expiration continues until the next inspiration begins. Triggering is the changeover from expiration to inspiration. All mechanical ventilators require some signal from the patient (except when the patient does not interact with the ventilator) to determine when inspiration should begin. When the patient initiates a breath, it is called an assisted breath, and a triggering signal results when the patient's inspiratory effort produces a drop in airway pressure or a diversion of constant gas flow in the ventilator circuitry. In the absence of patient interaction with the ventilator, breaths are delivered based on elapsed time. This is called an unassisted or mandatory breath. Using these definitions, two ventilator breath types are possible: full ventilator control (mandatory or unassisted) and partial ventilator control (assisted). The most common ventilator breaths are further described below.

Figure 5-3. The Respiratory Cycle During Mechanical Ventilation

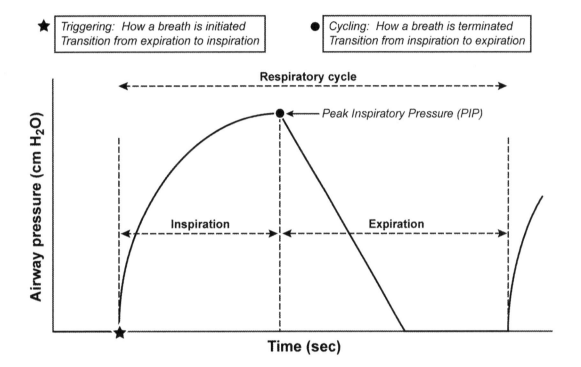

The respiratory cycle is the time from the initiation of one breath until the initiation of the next breath. Triggering (★) signals the transition from expiration to inspiration; Cycling (●) indicates the transition from inspiration to expiration. Reproduced with permission from Mayo Clinic.

A. Volume-Cycled Breath

A volume-cycled breath, often called volume breath, ensures the delivery of a preset tidal volume (unless the peak pressure limit is exceeded). On some ventilators, the setting of peak inspiratory flow rate and the choice of inspiratory flow waveform (square, sine, or decelerating) determine the length of inspiration. As lung resistance and compliance change, some ventilators adjust inspiratory flow to maintain not only the preset tidal volume but also a preset inspiratory time. With volume-cycled breaths, worsening airway resistance or lung/chest-wall compliance results in increases in peak inspiratory pressure with continued delivery of the set tidal volume (unless the peak pressure limit is exceeded).

B. Time-Cycled Breath

A time-cycled breath, often called pressure control breath, applies a constant pressure for a preset time. The constant pressure throughout inspiration produces a square pressure-over-time waveform during inspiration and a decelerating inspiratory flow waveform as the pressure gradient falls between the ventilator (pressure remains constant) and the patient (pressure rises as the lung fills). With this type of breath, changes in airway resistance or lung/chest-wall compliance will alter tidal volume (ie, worsening of airway resistance or lung compliance results in a decrease in tidal volume). This disadvantage of time-cycled (pressure control) breaths may be overcome by delivering pressure-regulated volume-control (PRVC) breaths, in which the ventilator adjusts the pressure up or down in response to a fall or rise of the tidal volume. Each delivered breath is similar to a set tidal-volume breath but is delivered as a time-cycled breath.

C. Flow-Cycled Breath

A flow-cycled breath, usually called a pressure support breath, is very similar to a time-cycled breath in that a constant pressure is applied throughout inspiration and the inspiratory flow waveform is decelerating. However, pressure support breaths are terminated when the flow rate decreases to a predetermined percentage of the initial flow rate (typically 25%). Termination of the patient's inspiratory effort decreases flow, which markedly influences the end of inspiration. Pressure support augments spontaneous breaths.

IV. MODES OF MECHANICAL VENTILATION

The mode of ventilation describes how 1 or more types of ventilator breaths interface with the patient to provide ventilatory support. When mechanical ventilation is initiated, the optimum ventilatory support for a given clinical circumstance and the specific needs of the patient must be determined. A trial of noninvasive positive pressure ventilation (NPPV) may be considered in some circumstances. Although not a mode of mechanical ventilation because positive pressure is not applied during inspiration, continuous positive airway pressure (CPAP) may also be used in a spontaneously breathing patient who is intubated. The respiratory rate and V_T are dependent on the patient's inspiratory effort as the patient inspires against the resistance of the endotracheal tube (ETT). The application of positive end-expiratory pressure using CPAP is seldom used as initial support for acute respiratory conditions in an intubated patient.

Commonly used modes of ventilation include assist-control (AC) ventilation, synchronized intermittent mandatory ventilation (SIMV), and pressure support ventilation (PSV). Many manufacturers have replaced the term "assist-control ventilation" (AC ventilation) with "continuous mandatory ventilation" (CMV). The various modes are achieved by using some combination of the 3 types of ventilator breaths described above. They may be combined with the application of positive end-expiratory pressure (PEEP). Airway pressure and flow tracings of spontaneous respiration, CPAP, and the different modes of mechanical ventilation are illustrated in **Figure 5-4.** Each has advantages and disadvantages, as summarized in **Table 5-6.** In choosing a mode of ventilation, it is important to consider specific goals. The most important goals of mechanical ventilation are adequacy of ventilation and oxygenation, a reduction of the work of breathing, and the assurance of patient comfort and synchrony with the ventilator.

Figure 5-4. Airway Pressure and Flow Tracings

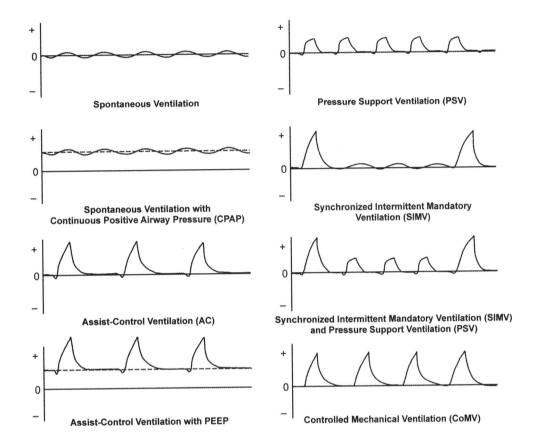

Airway pressure and flow tracings for spontaneous breathing, for CPAP, and for commonly used modes of mechanical ventilation. Time is represented on the horizontal axis and pressure on the vertical axis. The zero line reflects atmospheric pressure. Reproduced with permission from Mayo Clinic.

Table 5-6.	Potential Advantages and Disadvantages of Selected Modes of Mechanical Ventilation

Mode	Advantages	Disadvantages
Assist-control (AC) ventilation (may be called continuous mandatory ventilation [CMV])	Patient can increase ventilatory support; reduced work of breathing compared with spontaneous breathing	Adverse hemodynamic effects; inappropriate hyperventilation; increased work of breathing if V_T and/or flow do not meet patient demands
AC volume ventilation	Guarantees delivery of set V_T (unless peak pressure limit is exceeded)	Excessive inspiratory pressures
AC pressure control ventilation	Limitation of peak inspiratory pressures; variable flow rates accommodate to patient demands	Tidal volume decreases or increases with lung resistance/compliance changes
Pressure support ventilation (PSV)	Patient comfort; improved patient-ventilator interaction; decreased work of breathing	Apnea alarm may not trigger backup ventilation mode; variable patient tolerance
Synchronized intermittent mandatory ventilation (SIMV)	Less interference with normal cardiovascular function	Increased work of breathing compared with AC
Controlled mechanical ventilation (CoMV)	Rests muscles of respiration completely	Requires use of sedation/neuromuscular blockade; adverse hemodynamic effects

A. Assist-Control Ventilation

Assist-control ventilation (also called continuous mandatory ventilation [CMV]) is typically delivered with either volume-cycled or time-cycled (pressure control) breaths. A preset V_T or a preset applied pressure and inspiratory time (pressure control ventilation) is delivered at a preset minimum rate. The patient receives a minimum number of ventilator breaths (backup rate) synchronized to spontaneous effort (if present), and the number of breaths can be increased beyond the preset rate with additional inspiratory efforts. This mode of ventilation is commonly used when mechanical ventilation is initiated in patients with acute respiratory failure.

With proper use of assist-control, the work of breathing may be significantly decreased. However, if the ventilator and the patient are not in synchrony, or if the ventilator inspiratory flow rates are not matched with patient demand, this mode of ventilatory support may lead to a significant amount of patient work.

B. Pressure Support Ventilation

Pressure support ventilation provides a preset level of inspiratory pressure assist with each spontaneous breath. This inspiratory assist is selected to overcome the increased work of breathing imposed by the disease process, the endotracheal tube, the inspiratory valves, and other mechanical aspects of ventilatory support. The set amount of pressure support that is applied augments each patient-generated breath. All breaths are flow cycled. With PSV, the patient controls the respiratory rate and exerts a strong influence on the duration of inspiration, inspiratory flow rate, and V_T. In addition, the delivered V_T is influenced by pulmonary compliance and resistance. Rapid changes in these parameters will, therefore, potentially alter the minute ventilation and work of breathing. Pressure support ventilation may also be coupled with SIMV, primarily as a means to diminish work of breathing during spontaneous breaths (see the section on SIMV below).

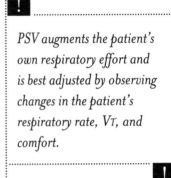

PSV augments the patient's own respiratory effort and is best adjusted by observing changes in the patient's respiratory rate, V_T, and comfort.

The amount of pressure support set during mechanical ventilation is titrated according to the V_T exhaled by the patient. Suggested parameters include a pressure-support setting that achieves one or more of the following goals:

- A V_T of 6 to 10 mL/kg, depending on patient needs

- A slowing of spontaneous breathing rate to an acceptable range

- The desired minute ventilation

Appropriate apnea alarms and a backup ventilation setting are essential. Potential benefits of PSV include the comfort and tolerance this ventilatory mode may offer some patients. In addition, PSV may reduce the work of breathing by enhancing patient-ventilator interaction. Typically, as pressure support is increased in patients with lung disease, the patient's work of breathing and respiratory rate decrease and V_T increases. With PSV, the presence of a bronchopleural fistula or an endotracheal tube cuff leak may interfere with appropriate cycling since flow may never drop to the preset threshold for cycling (typically 25% of the peak flow rate).

C. Synchronized Intermittent Mandatory Ventilation

Synchronized intermittent mandatory ventilation delivers either volume-cycled or time-cycled breaths at a preset mandatory rate. Volume cycling is most commonly used. When the number of inspiratory efforts by the patient exceeds the preset mandatory rate, the additional patient efforts access fresh gas for spontaneous breathing. Typically, SIMV is initially set to deliver full ventilatory support, and support is then decreased as the patient tolerates spontaneous breathing. Synchronization allows for enhanced patient-ventilator interaction by delivering the preset machine breaths in conjunction with the patient's inspiratory effort. When no effort is sensed, the ventilator delivers the preset V_T at the set rate. Synchronized intermittent mandatory ventilation is almost always combined with pressure support ventilation to augment the spontaneous breaths. At a minimum, the pressure support should be set at a level to offset endotracheal tube resistance (usually 5-8 cm H_2O).

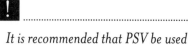

> *It is recommended that PSV be used in conjunction with SIMV to decrease the patient's work of breathing during spontaneous breaths.*

The SIMV mode allows patients to contribute to and determine a portion of their ventilatory requirement. The negative inspiratory pressure generated by spontaneous breathing may lead to increased venous return to the right side of the heart, which may improve cardiac output and cardiovascular function.

D. Controlled Mechanical Ventilation

Controlled mechanical ventilation delivers unassisted ventilator breaths at a preset rate. All breaths are mandatory and are either volume cycled or time cycled (pressure control); no spontaneous breaths are allowed. The patient is not able to initiate any additional ventilator breaths between the set number of controlled breaths. With current ventilators, there is no direct setting of controlled mechanical ventilation, and this mode can be achieved only in patients who are not capable of spontaneous respiratory effort (ie, those who are heavily sedated or receiving neuromuscular blockade). Therefore, AC or SIMV resembles controlled mechanical ventilation during heavy sedation/neuromuscular blockade if the patient does not initiate spontaneous breaths.

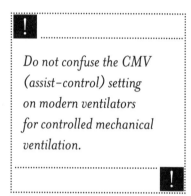

> *Do not confuse the CMV (assist-control) setting on modern ventilators for controlled mechanical ventilation.*

V. INITIAL VENTILATOR SETTINGS

When initiating ventilatory support in adults, an FiO_2 of 1.0 is used to ensure maximal amounts of available oxygen during the patient's adjustment to the ventilator and during the initial attempts to stabilize the patient's condition. In addition, the high level of oxygen offers support for complications that may have occurred before and during intubation. The usual recommended V_T level is 8 to 10 mL/kg and should be calculated by using predicted body weight (PBW). Higher V_T levels should be avoided to reduce the possibility of pulmonary barotrauma or volutrauma. An appropriate respiratory rate should be set to achieve the desired minute ventilation. Normal minute ventilation (V_T × respiratory rate) is approximately 7 to 8 L/min. Minute

> *To Estimate Predicted Body Weight*
> *Males:*
> $50 + 2.3$ *(Height in inches − 60)*
> $50 + 0.91$ *(Height in cm − 152.4)*
> *Females:*
> $45.5 + 2.3$ *(Height in Inches − 60)*
> $45.5 + 0.91$ *(Height in cm − 152.4)*

ventilation should be adjusted to produce the $PaCO_2$ level that allows the appropriate acid/base (pH) status for the patient's clinical condition. As a general rule FiO_2, mean airway pressure, and positive end-expiratory pressure (PEEP) affect the PaO_2, whereas the respiratory rate, dead space (V_D), and V_T affect alveolar minute ventilation and $PaCO_2$. Guidelines for the initiation of mechanical ventilation are listed in **Table 5-7.**

Table 5-7. Guidelines for the Initiation of Mechanical Ventilation

1. Choose the ventilator mode with which you are most familiar. The primary goals of ventilatory support are adequate oxygenation/ventilation, reduced work of breathing, synchrony between patient and ventilator, and avoidance of high end-inspiration alveolar pressures.

2. The initial FiO_2 should be 1.0. The FiO_2 thereafter can be titrated downward to maintain the oxygenation as measured by pulse oximetry (SpO_2) at 92% to 94%. In severe acute respiratory distress syndrome, an $SpO_2 \geq 88\%$ may be acceptable to minimize complications of mechanical ventilation.

3. Initial V_T = 8 to 10 mL/kg in patients with relatively normal lung compliance. In patients with poor lung compliance (eg, ARDS), a target V_T of 6 mL/kg by PBW is recommended to avoid overdistension and to maintain an inspiratory plateau pressure ≤ 30 cm H_2O. (See Section VIII below for more information.)

4. Choose a respiratory rate and minute ventilation appropriate for the particular clinical requirements. Target pH, not $PaCO_2$.

5. Use PEEP in diffuse lung injury to maintain open alveoli at end expiration. If volume is held constant, PEEP may increase peak inspiratory plateau pressure, a potentially undesirable effect in ARDS. PEEP levels >15 cm H_2O are rarely necessary.

6. Set the trigger sensitivity to allow minimal patient effort to initiate inspiration. Beware of autocycling if the trigger setting is too sensitive.

7. In patients at risk of obstructive airways disease, avoid choosing ventilator settings that limit expiratory time and cause or worsen auto-PEEP (see "Relation of Inspiratory Time to Expiratory Time and Auto-PEEP" below).

8. Call the critical care consultant or other appropriate consultant for assistance.

Abbreviations: FiO_2, fraction of inspired oxygen; SpO_2, oxyhemoglobin saturation as measured by pulse oximetry; V_T, tidal volume; ARDS, acute respiratory distress syndrome; PBW, predicted body weight; PEEP, positive end-expiratory pressure.

VI. CONTINUING CARE DURING MECHANICAL VENTILATION

After mechanical ventilation has been initiated, the parameters discussed below should be assessed and titrated to achieve the desired goals. Many important interrelationships exist among ventilator settings, and the consequences of making any change must be appreciated. This interdependency of parameters may lead to beneficial or harmful effects in the respiratory and/or cardiovascular systems. Critical care consultation should be obtained for complex patients.

A. Inspiratory Pressures

During positive-pressure volume-control ventilation, airway pressure rises progressively to a peak inspiratory pressure (Ppeak; **Figure 5-3**), which is reached at end inspiration. Ppeak is the sum of the pressure required to overcome airway resistance and the pressure required to overcome elastic properties of the lung and chest wall. Peak inspiratory pressure is sometimes referred to as PIP or peak airway pressure. When an inspiratory hold is applied at the end of inspiration, gas flow ceases and the pressure drops to a measurement called the inspiratory plateau pressure (Pplat). The Pplat reflects the pressure required to overcome elastic recoil in the lung and chest wall. The Pplat is the best estimate of peak alveolar pressure, which is an important indicator of alveolar distension. Accurate measurement of Pplat requires the absence of any patient effort, which is usually achievable with an inspiratory hold as short as 0.5 second.

Potential adverse effects from high inspiratory pressure include barotrauma, volutrauma, and reduced cardiac output. Barotrauma (pneumothorax, pneumomediastinum) and volutrauma (lung parenchymal injury due to overinflation), although linked to high Ppeak, correlate best with Pplat. A good example of the relationship of Ppeak and Pplat to alveolar distension is demonstrated by the effect of endotracheal tube size on Ppeak and Pplat. As the internal diameter of an endotracheal tube is decreased in a patient receiving volume ventilation, the same tidal volume will result in higher Ppeak, yet Pplat and alveolar distension remain unchanged as the pressure is dissipated across the endotracheal tube. The same tidal volume, regardless of the type of breath, produces the same alveolar distension at end inspiration. To avoid injury in patients receiving mechanical ventilation, inspiratory plateau pressure should be maintained at ≤30 cm H_2O. The relation of peak inspiratory pressure and inspiratory plateau pressure is illustrated in **Figure 5-5.**

Figure 5-5. Relationship of Peak Inspiratory Pressure and Inspiratory Plateau Pressure

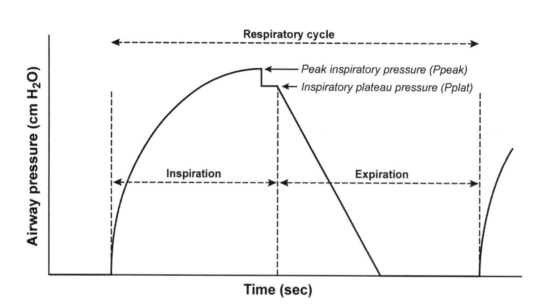

Elevated Pplat may be reduced by the following interventions:

■ Decrease PEEP, which may also decrease oxygenation (if PEEP is used to improve oxygenation).

■ Decrease VT, which may lead to hypercapnia due to a reduction in minute ventilation.

B. Relation of Inspiratory Time to Expiratory Time and Auto-PEEP

The respiratory cycle is the time from the initiation of a breath until the initiation of the next breath (**Figure 5-5**). The respiratory cycle time is calculated by dividing 1 minute (60 seconds) by the respiratory rate. The proportion of time spent in inhalation (inspiratory time) and in exhalation (expiratory time) constitutes the I:E ratio. During spontaneous breathing, the normal I:E ratio is about 1:2; the exhalation time is about twice as long as inhalation time. In chronic lung disease and other conditions associated with expiratory flow limitation, the exhalation time becomes prolonged and the I:E ratio changes (eg, 1:2.5, 1:3). Such changes reflect the pathophysiology of the lung disease and directly influence techniques used during mechanical ventilation.

The inspiratory time during volume breaths (AC or SIMV modes) is usually determined by the V_T, inspiratory flow rate, and inspiratory waveform. A larger V_T takes longer to deliver at the same flow rate, and the same V_T takes longer to deliver at a slower flow rate. In both cases the inspiratory time is longer, but at a constant respiratory rate, the cycle time remains the same. Therefore, the time available for exhalation (the expiratory time) must shorten to fit into the cycle time. Inspiratory time is actively set by adjusting V_T, inspiratory flow rate, and waveform, or by use of inspiratory pauses on the ventilator. The expiratory time, however, is passively determined.

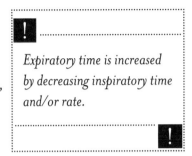

Expiratory time is increased by decreasing inspiratory time and/or rate.

If the expiratory time is too short to allow full exhalation, the previously delivered breath is not completely expired and the next lung inflation is superimposed upon the increased residual gas in the lung. Breath stacking occurs in this situation and results in hyperinflation of the lung and the development of PEEP that is over and above the preset level of PEEP on the ventilator. This increase in end-expiratory pressure is called auto-PEEP, or intrinsic, inadvertent, or occult PEEP. Auto-PEEP can be quantified by using manual methods or through electronic programs within some ventilators. However, it is most easily diagnosed qualitatively by viewing the flow-versus-time graphic waveform tracing available on most mechanical ventilators (**Figure 5-6**). The potentially harmful physiologic effects of auto-PEEP on peak, plateau, and mean airway pressures are the same as those of preset PEEP. In addition, high levels of PEEP may decrease venous return to the heart, resulting in hypotension; increase PCO_2 due to increased dead space; and worsen oxygenation (especially with asymmetric lung disease).

Figure 5-6. Flow-Versus-Time Waveform Tracing

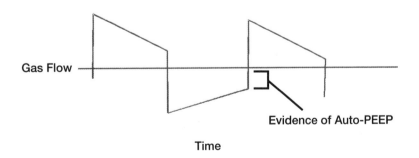

Auto-PEEP is illustrated by the failure of the expiratory flow to return to zero before inspiratory flow is initiated.

Auto-PEEP may be reduced by the following interventions:

■ Decrease respiratory rate by changing the set rate or sedating the patient. These interventions result in fewer inspirations per minute and thus increase the total expiratory time available; this is the most effective way of decreasing auto-PEEP.

■ Decrease V_T, requiring less time to deliver a smaller breath and thus allowing more expiratory time.

■ Increase gas flow rate, delivering the V_T faster and allowing more time in the cycle for exhalation. This intervention has little impact unless the initial flow rate was set at a low level.

The first 2 interventions, as discussed earlier, may lead to hypercapnia due to a reduction in minute ventilation; however, the benefits of a decrease in auto-PEEP despite the lower minute ventilation may lead to little change in $PaCO_2$. When severe air trapping occurs, allowing sufficient expiratory time may improve ventilation and CO_2 removal. The clinician may accept CO_2 retention as a necessary result of lower tidal volumes or minute ventilation. Hypercapnia and a controlled reduction in pH (permissive hypercapnia) may be acceptable in some clinical conditions but requires expert consultation. This approach may not be suitable for patients with intracranial hypertension because hypercapnia causes cerebral vasodilation and further increases in the intracranial pressure.

C. F$_I$O$_2$

High levels of inspired oxygen may be harmful to lung parenchyma after prolonged exposure. Although the precise threshold for concern is not known, it is desirable to reduce the F_IO_2 to ≤0.5 (50% oxygen) as soon as possible (ideally within the first 24 hours). However, hypoxemia is always considered a greater risk to the patient than high F_IO_2 levels.

The primary determinants of oxygenation during mechanical ventilation are the F_IO_2 and mean airway pressure ($\overline{Paw}$). In the patient with acute lung injury (ALI and ARDS), PEEP becomes an additional independent determinant. Tidal volume, I:E ratio, inspiratory flow rate, PEEP, auto-PEEP, use of inspiratory pause, and the inspiratory flow waveform pattern (volume breaths) all interact to affect $\overline{Paw}$. The interrelationships of these various parameters, as already demonstrated, often lead to complex adjustments within the plan for mechanical ventilation.

D. Minute Ventilation and Alveolar Minute Ventilation

Minute ventilation is defined as the amount of gas exchanged by an individual in 1 minute and is calculated as the respiratory rate multiplied by mean tidal volume. The primary determinant of CO_2 exchange during mechanical ventilation is alveolar minute ventilation, calculated as

$$V_A = (V_T - V_D)f$$

where V_D is dead space and f is respiratory rate (**Chapter 4**). The V_T, the respiratory rate, and their interrelationships with other ventilatory parameters have already been discussed. Physiologic V_D represents, in general, lung units that are relatively well ventilated but underperfused. The physiologic effect of high amounts of V_D is hypercapnia. Dead space may result from the pathologic process in the lung or from mechanical ventilation complicated by high airway pressures, low intravascular volume, or low cardiac output. It may be necessary to use a low V_T to avoid high airway pressure and/or a low respiratory rate to avoid auto-PEEP, thus permitting hypoventilation and hypercapnia. This permissive hypercapnia technique should be initiated only with the support of an appropriate consultant.

As previously discussed, adequate ventilation is assessed by consideration of both the $PaCO_2$ and the pH. Hyperventilation resulting in a low $PaCO_2$ level may be an appropriate short-term compensatory goal during metabolic acidosis while the primary etiology is corrected. Similarly, a patient with chronic hypercapnia has an increased baseline $PaCO_2$ and maintains a near-normal pH by renal compensation (increased bicarbonate production). Patients with chronic compensated hypercapnia should receive sufficient minute ventilation during mechanical ventilation to maintain the $PaCO_2$ at their usual level to avoid severe alkalemia and loss of retained bicarbonate.

E. Humidification

Gases delivered by mechanical ventilators are typically dry, and the upper airways are bypassed by artificial airways. These circumstances result in loss of heat and moisture from the respiratory tract. Heating and humidification of gases are routinely provided during mechanical ventilation to prevent mucosal damage and minimize inspissation of secretions. Available systems include passive humidifiers (artificial nose) or active, microprocessor-controlled heat and humidifying systems (heated humidifiers). The passive humidifiers are contraindicated in the presence of copious secretions, minute ventilation >12 L/min, air leaks of greater than 15% of delivered tidal volume, or blood in the airway.

VII. SEDATION, ANALGESIA, AND NEUROMUSCULAR BLOCKADE

Endotracheal intubation and mechanical ventilation can be uncomfortable and anxiety provoking. To improve patient comfort and relieve anxiety, anxiolytics, sedative, and analgesics may be administered. Neuromuscular blocking agents should be used with caution. Guidelines for the use of these agents are outlined in SCCM's *Clinical Practice Guidelines for Sustained Neuromuscular Blockade in Critically Ill Adults* (http://www.sccm.org/professional_resources/guidelines/table_of_contents/Documents/NeuromuscularBlockade.pdf). The amnestic properties of benzodiazepines are particularly beneficial. Caution should be taken with use of sedation in nonintubated patients with acute respiratory insufficiency or impending respiratory failure. Before initiating therapy with neuromuscular blocking agents, expert consultation should be sought.

VIII. VENTILATORY GUIDELINES FOR SPECIFIC CLINICAL SITUATIONS

A. Acute Lung Injury/Acute Respiratory Distress Syndrome

 Case Study

An 18-year-old female patient is brought to the emergency department after being found unresponsive at a party where alcohol was consumed. The paramedics reported vomitus in the oral cavity and a difficult intubation due to copious foreign matter. In spite of bag-mask ventilation with 100% oxygen, her oxyhemoglobin saturation remained 87% to 88% during transport. The initial assessment reveals diffuse crackles, more prominent on the right hemithorax, and a chest radiograph shows diffuse bilateral infiltrates. The ventilator is constantly alarming for high pressure.

– What ventilator settings are recommended for this patient?

– What steps should be taken to avoid triggering the pressure alarm?

– What parameters should be measured and monitored?

Acute lung injury (ALI) and ARDS cause a decrease in lung compliance, making the lungs more stiff and difficult to inflate, and produce hypoxemic respiratory failure (**Chapter 4**). Guidelines for mechanical ventilation in ALI and ARDS are outlined in **Tables 5-8** and **5-9.** High peak and plateau airway pressures complicate mechanical ventilation because of the low lung compliance or high airway resistance. Lower V_T is required and the Pplat should be maintained at the desired level of ≤30 cm H_2O. Permissive hypercapnia may be required to accomplish that goal. The FiO_2 is increased as necessary to prevent hypoxemia but reduced as soon as other ventilatory interventions are effective. Because of increased shunt in ARDS, hypoxemia may be severe. Positive end-expiratory pressure is the most effective way to improve oxygenation and is typically applied in the range of 8 to 15 cm H_2O, based on the severity of hypoxemia. Higher PEEP levels may be indicated in severe lung injury. Although patients with ARDS are somewhat less likely to develop auto-PEEP because expiratory time requirements are reduced due to decreased lung compliance (stiffness), the presence of auto-PEEP should be monitored, especially at higher I:E ratios.

Table 5-8. Mechanical Ventilation in ALI/ARDS

Goals

- PaO$_2$: 55-80 mm Hg (7.3-10.7 kPa)

- Pplat: ≤30 cm H$_2$O

- V$_T$: 6 mL/kg PBW

- pH: >7.15 is acceptable

Start With Assist/Control With VT of 8 mL/kg PBW

- Decrease by 1 mL/kg at a time over the next 4 hours until V$_T$ 6 mL/kg is reached.

- If Pplat >30 cm H$_2$O, decrease V$_T$ by 1 mL/kg at a time until V$_T$ is 4 mL/kg or arterial pH reaches 7.15.

- If using V$_T$ of 4 mL/kg and Pplat is <25 cm H$_2$O, V$_T$ can be increased 1 mL/kg at a time until Pplat is 25 cm H$_2$O or V$_T$ is 6 mL/kg again.

- If a Pplat of ≤30 cm H$_2$O has been achieved with a V$_T$ >6 mL/kg and a lower V$_T$ is clinically problematic (ie, need for increased sedation), it is acceptable to maintain the higher V$_T$.

Initiation of PEEP in ARDS

- Initiate PEEP at 5 cm H$_2$O and titrate up in increments of 2 cm H$_2$O, according to **Table 5-9.**
- Full recruitment effect may not be apparent for several hours.
- Monitor blood pressure, heart rate, and PaO$_2$ or pulse oximetry during PEEP titration and at intervals while the patient is receiving PEEP therapy.
- Optimal PEEP settings are typically 8-15 cm H$_2$O.

NOTE: These guidelines are summarized to facilitate early intervention in critical patients. The treating physician should be familiar with these situations and seek appropriate specialist advice as soon as possible.

Abbreviations: ALI, acute lung injury; ARDS, acute respiratory distress syndrome. PBW, predicted body weight.

Table 5-9. Suggested Combinations of PEEP and FiO$_2$ to Reach Goal PaO$_2$

FiO$_2$	0.3	0.4	0.4	0.5	0.5	0.6	0.7	0.7	0.7	0.8	0.9	0.9	0.9	1.0	1.0	1.0	1.0
PEEP (cm H$_2$O)	5-14	5-14	8-16	8-16	10-20	10-20	10-20	12-20	14-20	14-22	14-22	14-22	16-22	18-22	20-22	22	24

B. Obstructive Airway Disease

 # Case Study

A 70-year-old patient with a long history of smoking has been kept on an observation unit where a trial of noninvasive positive-pressure ventilation has lasted 4 hours. The patient's breathing difficulty has progressively worsened, and he has become uncooperative and agitated. He was recently sedated, intubated, and placed on mechanical ventilation. A low blood pressure alarm is now sounding.

– What ventilator settings are recommended for this patient?

– What are the possible causes of this patient's hypotension?

– What immediate interventions should be performed?

Mechanical ventilation for patients with asthma and chronic obstructive pulmonary disease (COPD) is designed to support oxygenation and assist ventilation until airway obstruction has improved. Mechanical ventilation of patients with obstructive airway disease may produce hyperinflation, auto-PEEP, and resultant hypotension. Therefore, careful attention is needed to balance cycle, inspiratory, and expiratory times.

The initial V_T should be ~8 to 10 mL/kg, and the minute ventilation should be adjusted to a low normal pH. With volume ventilation, the inspiratory flow rate should be set to optimize the I:E ratio and allow complete exhalation. Such management reduces breath stacking and the potential for auto-PEEP. It should be noted that as flow rate increases, there may be an increase in peak inspiratory pressure, which is not mirrored in the plateau pressure. This is a function of airways resistance and not an indication of worsening lung compliance.

While the patient is supported with mechanical ventilation, airway obstruction should be aggressively treated with bronchodilators (**Chapter 4**). As airflow obstruction improves, the patient will tolerate higher V_T levels and longer inspiratory times.

C. Asymmetric Lung Disease

Asymmetric lung disease or injury that occurs after aspiration, contusion, or a localized pneumonia may cause abnormal distribution of ventilation and gas exchange during mechanical ventilation. Because the conditioned gas from the ventilator follows the path of least resistance along the bronchi, the V_T is distributed primarily to the less-affected (more-compliant) lung and may overexpand it. Overdistension of the less-affected lung and poor expansion of the diseased/injured lung worsen ventilation-perfusion relationships in both lungs, and hypoxemia and hypercapnia may occur, persist, or worsen. Standard settings and principles of ventilatory support should be initiated. However, if this attempt is unsuccessful, expert consultation should be obtained to facilitate further efforts at patient management. Putting the less-involved lung in the gravitationally dependent (decubitus) position may be helpful in directing pulmonary blood flow to lung units receiving better ventilation. Other techniques, such as differential lung ventilation, may be required.

D. Heart Disease

The major goal of ventilatory support in patients with myocardial ischemia is to decrease the work of breathing and ensure adequate oxygen delivery to the heart. Decreasing the work of breathing will reduce the consumption of oxygen by respiratory muscles, thus increasing oxygen availability to the heart. Patients with cardiogenic pulmonary edema may also benefit from the mechanical ventilation–induced increase in intrathoracic pressure. Increased intrathoracic pressure decreases left ventricular filling by decreasing right ventricular filling. Afterload also decreases through application of positive juxtacardiac pressure during systole.

E. Neuromuscular Disease

Patients with peripheral neuromuscular disease typically have an intact respiratory drive and normal lungs. These patients may require a higher V_T level to avoid the sensation of dyspnea. Adjustments are made in other ventilatory parameters to ensure a normal arterial pH.

IX. MONITORING MECHANICAL VENTILATORY SUPPORT

Patients who receive mechanical ventilatory support require continuous monitoring to assess the beneficial and adverse effects of treatment (**Table 5-10**). Arterial blood gas measurements provide valuable information about the adequacy of oxygenation, ventilation, and acid-base balance. This information is essential during the initial phases of ventilatory support and during periods of patient instability. If available, a pulse oximeter (**Chapter 6**) and end-tidal capnometer (for measuring end-tidal CO_2) can be used to further monitor the patient's progress.

Ventilators are equipped with sophisticated alarms and monitors to assist with patient management and detection of adverse events. When initiating ventilatory support, the respiratory care practitioner usually establishes alarm parameters for low and high minute ventilation, high inspiratory pressures, and low exhaled volumes and pressures. Many ventilators allow for the measurement of auto-PEEP.

Table 5-10.	Recommendations for Monitoring Mechanical Ventilatory Support

1. Obtain a chest radiograph after intubation and additional chest radiographs as indicated to evaluate any deterioration in status.
2. Obtain arterial blood gas measurements after initiation of mechanical ventilation and intermittently, based on patient status.
3. Frequently measure vital signs and directly observe the patient (including patient-ventilator interaction).
4. Measure inspiratory plateau pressure as clinically appropriate.
5. Use pulse oximetry to monitor oxygenation.
6. Use ventilator alarms to monitor key physiologic and ventilator parameters.

The low-pressure alarm is intended to alert the clinician to a leak in the circuit or to ventilator disconnection. A high-pressure alarm alerts the clinician that the set maximum peak airway pressure has been exceeded. This alarm is usually set 10 cm H_2O above the patient's baseline peak airway pressure. If a patient receiving volume ventilation develops mucus plugging or a marked change in airway or lung compliance, the peak pressure will acutely rise. If the peak pressure alarm sounds with volume ventilation, it implies that the patient is not receiving the set tidal volume, as inspiration ends when the pressure alarm limit is exceeded. Some ventilators have substituted a low minute ventilation alarm in place of the low pressure alarm to alert the clinician to leaks in the circuit or ventilator disconnection.

X. HYPOTENSION ASSOCIATED WITH INITIATION OF MECHANICAL VENTILATION

A. Tension Pneumothorax

When hypotension occurs immediately after initiation of mechanical ventilation, tension pneumothorax should be one of the first considerations. Diagnosis of tension pneumothorax is based on a physical examination that finds decreased or absent breath sounds and tympany to percussion on the side of the pneumothorax. Tracheal deviation away from the side of the pneumothorax may be observed, although it is uncommon after placement of an endotracheal tube. Treatment includes emergent decompression by inserting a large-bore catheter or needle into the second or third intercostal space in the midclavicular line (**Appendix 8**). Treatment should not be delayed to wait for a chest radiograph. The insertion of a catheter or needle is both diagnostic and therapeutic: it improves blood pressure and reverses the findings of physical examination. The insertion of the catheter or needle must be followed by chest tube placement.

B. Conversion From Negative to Positive Intrathoracic Pressure

Normal intrathoracic pressure is slightly negative relative to the atmosphere. When positive pressure ventilation is initiated, intrathoracic pressure becomes positive. As intrathoracic pressure rises, right atrial pressure rises and the intravascular pressure gradient for return of blood from the large extrathoracic veins into the right heart decreases. As a result, blood return to the heart may be reduced. Left ventricular preload, stroke volume, cardiac output, and blood pressure may then decrease in sequence. Underlying intravascular volume depletion exacerbates the deleterious effects of the increased intrathoracic pressure on cardiac output and blood pressure. Treatment of this common complication includes volume resuscitation by means of rapidly infused fluid boluses to raise extrathoracic venous pressure and increase venous return to the right heart until the blood pressure increases. Oxygen saturation should be monitored to avoid overly aggressive fluid resuscitation. Use of ventilation techniques associated with high $\overline{Paw}$ may exacerbate the deleterious hemodynamic consequences of mechanical ventilation.

C. Auto-PEEP

Auto-PEEP occurs when the combination of ventilator settings and patient physiology results in an inadequate expiratory time, as discussed earlier in this chapter. Excessive end-expiratory pressure may increase intrathoracic pressure and cause hypotension due to decreased venous return to the heart. Although auto-PEEP may occur in any patient, patients with obstructive airway disease are particularly predisposed to this condition. Assessment and treatment of auto-PEEP are performed as previously described.

D. Acute Myocardial Ischemia/Infarction

Stress from the cause of acute respiratory failure, as well as the stress of intubation itself, may lead to increased myocardial oxygen demand and to acute myocardial ischemia, infarction, and subsequent hypotension. Patients at high risk should be evaluated with serial ECGs and myocardial markers of injury.

Mechanical Ventilation

■ The primary goals of noninvasive and invasive positive-pressure ventilation are to support ventilation and oxygenation, and to reduce work of breathing while ensuring patient comfort.

■ Noninvasive positive-pressure ventilation is best utilized in the alert, cooperative patient whose respiratory condition is expected to improve in 48 to 72 hours.

■ The advantages and disadvantages of the different modes of invasive mechanical ventilation must be considered when determining the optimal ventilatory support for the patient's clinical condition.

■ Guidelines for initiating mechanical ventilation should be carefully followed, with adjustments made based on patient assessment and monitoring.

■ The complex interactions of inspiratory pressures, I:E ratio, FiO_2, and PEEP must be appreciated to evaluate the potential benefits and harmful effects in each patient.

■ The primary determinants of oxygenation are FiO_2 and mean airway pressure, whereas alveolar ventilation primarily affects CO_2 exchange.

■ During mechanical ventilation, a patient must be closely monitored using the ventilator alarm systems, continuous pulse oximetry, attentive physical assessment, measurement of inspiratory plateau pressure (as clinically appropriate), and intermittent arterial blood gases and chest radiographs as needed.

■ The inspiratory plateau pressure should be maintained ≤30 cm H_2O.

■ Hypotension occurring immediately after initiation of invasive mechanical ventilation should prompt evaluation for tension pneumothorax, decreased venous blood return due to intrathoracic pressure, auto-PEEP, or myocardial ischemia.

 Suggested Readings

1. Acute Respiratory Distress Syndrome Network. Ventilation with lower tidal volumes as compared with traditional tidal volumes for acute lung injury and the acute respiratory distress syndrome. *N Engl J Med.* 2000;342:1301.

2. Caples SM, Gay PC. Noninvasive positive pressure ventilation in the intensive care unit: a concise review. *Crit Care Med.* 2005;33:2651.

3. Fink M, Abraham E, Vincent J, et al, eds. Controlled mechanical ventilation. In: *Textbook of Critical Care.* 5th ed. Philadelphia, PA: WB Saunders Co; 2005:chap 66.

4. Fink M, Abraham E, Vincent J, et al, eds. Patient-ventilator interaction. In: *Textbook of Critical Care.* 5th ed. Philadelphia, PA: WB Saunders Co; 2005:chap 67.

5. Hess DR, Kacmarek RM. *Essentials of Mechanical Ventilation.* 2nd ed. New York, NY: McGraw-Hill Companies; 2002.

6. Kallet RH, Jasmer RM, Pittet J-F, et al. Clinical implementation of the ARDS network protocol is associated with reduced hospital mortality compared with historical controls. *Crit Care Med.* 2005;33:925.

7. Leisching T, Kwok H, Hill NS. Acute applications of noninvasive positive pressure ventilation. *Chest.* 2003;124:699.

8. MacIntyre N. Ventilatory management of ALI/ARDS. *Semin Resp Crit Care Med.* 2006;27:396.

9. MacIntyre N, Branson RD. *Mechanical Ventilation.* Philadelphia, PA: WB Saunders Co; 2000.

10. Marini JJ, Gattinoni L. Ventilatory management of acute respiratory distress syndrome: a consensus of two. *Crit Care Med.* 2004;1:250.

11. Petrucci N, Iacovelli W. Ventilation with smaller tidal volumes: a quantitative systematic review of randomized controlled trials. *Anesth Analg.* 2004;1:193.

12. Tobin MJ. Advances in mechanical ventilation. *N Engl J Med.* 2001;344:1986.

13. Tobin MJ. *Principles and Practice of Mechanical Ventilation.* Rev. ed. New York, NY: McGraw-Hill Companies; 2006.

14. Murray MJ, Cowen J, DeBlock H, et al. Clinical practice guidelines for sustained neuromuscular blockade in critically ill adults. *Crit Care Med.* 2002;30(1):142. Available online at http://www.sccm.org/professional_resources/guidelines/table_of_contents/Documents/NeuromuscularBlockade.pdf.

Chapter 6:

Monitoring Blood Flow, Oxygenation, and Acid-Base Status

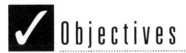 Objectives

■ Outline the determinants of oxygen balance.

■ Recognize disorders of blood flow and oxygenation.

■ Identify the principles and limitations of techniques for monitoring oxygen balance.

■ Explain the use of acid-base status as a monitor in the seriously ill patient.

Case Study

A previously healthy 40-year-old man presents to the emergency department with complaints of general malaise and lethargy after caring for his flu-stricken son. His vital signs at the triage desk are heart rate 145/min, blood pressure 118/82 mm Hg, respiratory rate 22/min, and SpO_2 98% while receiving room air. As the evaluation is initiated, he is noted to be more tachypneic and anxious.

- What monitoring should be immediately implemented?

- What additional parameters should be assessed to determine if blood flow and oxygen utilization are adequate?

I. Introduction

Monitoring is never therapeutic, and information from monitors must be integrated with patient assessment and clinical judgment to determine optimal care. In addition, the clinician must be aware of the risk-benefit ratio of a monitoring system. Monitoring may be as simple as measuring the pulse or temperature or as complex as invasive hemodynamic techniques with direct and calculated measurements. More invasive monitoring strategies that carry a higher risk should be considered if they provide sufficient new information to guide therapy. As an example, neuroendocrine responses to physiologic stress lead to early effects on heart rate, respiratory rate, vascular tone, and blood pressure. These combined signs are neither sensitive nor specific for the adequacy of oxygen balance, but they may provide a signal suggesting the need for more intensive monitoring to appropriately evaluate and treat the patient. This chapter will emphasize basic monitoring techniques that can be accomplished in most care environments.

The goals of monitoring in seriously ill patients are to recognize physiologic abnormalities and to guide interventions to ensure adequate blood flow and oxygen utilization for maintenance of cellular and organ function. Tissue oxygenation cannot be directly measured or monitored, but estimates of the adequacy of oxygenation can be made based on knowledge of oxygen balance, which includes oxygen delivery and oxygen consumption. An understanding of these principles is required to appreciate the usefulness and limitations of various monitoring tools.

II. PRINCIPLES OF OXYGEN DELIVERY

Oxygen delivery is the amount of oxygen presented to the tissues, and it is the component of oxygen balance that can most often be altered by interventions in the seriously ill patient. Normally, the amount of oxygen delivered to the tissues is 3 to 4 times greater than the tissue needs. In critical illness, physiologic derangements that result in an absolute decrease in the oxygen delivered or an increase in tissue oxygen demand may compromise this margin of safety. Oxygen delivery is dependent on cardiac output (blood flow) and the oxygen content of arterial blood. Invasive and/or more complex monitoring is required for exact measurement of cardiac output. However, an understanding of the variables that determine oxygen content of blood and cardiac output along with less invasive monitoring may guide appropriate treatment.

A. Oxygen Content of Arterial Blood

Arterial oxygen content (CaO_2) is defined as the amount of oxygen carried bound to hemoglobin plus the amount of oxygen dissolved in arterial blood. The components of arterial oxygen content are related by the formula

$$CaO_2 = (\text{Hemoglobin Concentration} \times 1.34 \times SaO_2) + (0.0031 \times PaO_2),$$

where SaO_2 is the arterial oxyhemoglobin saturation and PaO_2 is the partial pressure of oxygen in arterial blood. Each gram of hemoglobin that is fully saturated with oxygen transports approximately 1.34 milliliters of oxygen. The amount of oxygen may vary from 1.34 to 1.39 milliliters depending on the affinity of hemoglobin for oxygen. Hemoglobin is the major contributor of oxygen for tissue demands and releases bound oxygen based on cellular uptake of dissolved oxygen as blood flows through the capillaries. The ability of hemoglobin to release more oxygen when oxygen supply is inadequate or cellular demand is increased is one of the main compensatory mechanisms to sustain cellular function. The oxyhemoglobin dissociation curve shows the relationship of hemoglobin saturation and partial pressures of oxygen (PO_2; **Figure 6-1**). When the PO_2 drops to approximately 40 mm Hg (5.3 kPa) in the capillaries, the decrease in oxyhemoglobin saturation to 75% reflects the amount of oxygen released to the tissues. During physiologic stress, oxyhemoglobin saturation at the tissue level may decrease to <20%, reflecting the release of additional oxygen to tissues. Acidosis and fever will shift this curve to the right, resulting in a lower affinity of oxygen for hemoglobin and greater delivery of oxygen to the tissues.

> *The usual arterial oxygen content is 18–20 mL/dL when hemoglobin concentration and saturation are normal.*

> *Calculated CaO_2 reflects oxygen that is available in the arterial circulation and not necessarily the oxygen that is delivered to or consumed by specific tissues.*

Arterial oxygen content can be estimated by direct measurement of the hemoglobin concentration and arterial oxyhemoglobin saturation in intermittent blood samples as dissolved oxygen contributes minimally to oxygen content. Although hemoglobin is not monitored continuously, oxyhemoglobin saturation measured by pulse oximetry (SpO_2) allows continuous assessment of this determinant of arterial oxygen content.

Figure 6-1. Oxyhemoglobin Dissociation Curve

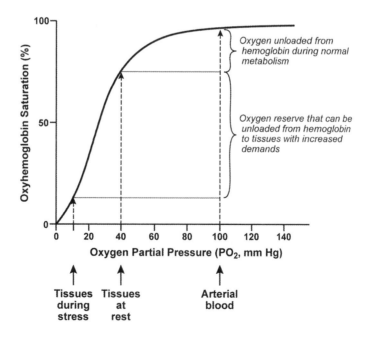

The oxyhemoglobin dissociation curve relates the partial pressure of oxygen (PO_2) to oxyhemoglobin saturation. Near-maximal saturation of hemoglobin occurs at a PO_2 of 60 mm Hg (8.0 kPa). PO_2 values above this point provide only a modest increase in oxyhemoglobin saturation. Note, however, that a rapid decrease in oxyhemoglobin saturation occurs when the PO_2 drops below 60 mm Hg (8.0 kPa). Reproduced with permission from Mayo Clinic.

B. Cardiac Output

If the oxygen content of arterial blood is optimum, then an appropriate cardiac output is needed to ensure delivery of oxygen to the tissues. Cardiac output is the product of heart rate and stroke volume. Variables that affect stroke volume are preload, afterload, and contractile function. The first compensatory mechanism to increase oxygen delivery is an increase in heart rate. Patients who are unable to increase their heart rate (eg, beta blockade) will have a limited

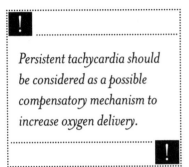

Persistent tachycardia should be considered as a possible compensatory mechanism to increase oxygen delivery.

ability to compensate. Although heart rate is easily measured and evaluated, an evaluation of stroke volume must be performed with echocardiography or invasive methods. The option of measuring cardiac output depends on the expertise and resources available. The clinician caring for the patient must be aware of the limitations of any chosen technique. If cardiac output is not directly measured, an indirect assessment of variables involved in determining cardiac output (see **Table 6-1**) and knowledge of hemodynamic principles may be useful.

Table 6-1. Determinants of Cardiac Output and Assessment

Variable	Method of Assessment
Heart rate and rhythm	Finger on the pulse
	Pulse oximetry
	Electrocardiography
Preload	
Right heart	Neck vein distension, liver enlargement, dependent edema
	Central venous pressure
Left heart	Presence of dyspnea on exertion, orthopnea
	Pulmonary edema, rales on lung examination
	Pulmonary artery occlusion pressure
Afterload (left heart)	Mean arterial blood pressure
	Systemic vascular resistance
Contractility	Ejection fraction
	Echocardiography

1. Contractility

Contractility is the ability of myocardial fibers to shorten during systole. Contractility is highly dependent on preload and afterload and is difficult to measure as an independent variable. Additional factors that can affect contractility in the critically ill patient are endogenous sympathetic activation, acidosis, ischemia, inflammatory mediators, and vasoactive agents. There are no readily available methods for monitoring the contractile state of the myocardium in the acutely ill patient.

2. Preload

Preload is a measure or estimate of the ventricular volume at the end of diastole. The distensibility of the ventricle and the volume load it can accept are the basis for the Frank-Starling curve. In general, a greater end-diastolic volume (EDV) leads to increased stretch on the myocardium, resulting in a larger stroke volume (**Figure 6-2**). Because it is difficult to measure volume, preload is most often estimated from the ventricular end-diastolic pressure (EDP), which is transmitted and reflected in the atrial pressure. The atrial pressure is estimated by measurement of pressure in a central vein or the pulmonary artery. Thus, right ventricular preload is estimated by measurement of the central venous pressure (CVP) and left ventricular preload by measurement of pulmonary artery occlusion pressure (PAOP). These pressures indirectly reflect the end-diastolic volume as well as the compliance of the ventricular wall.

Figure 6-2. Relationship Between Ventricular Preload and Stroke Volume

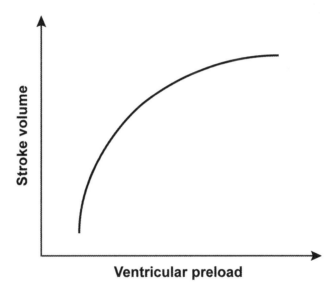

When end-diastolic volume of the ventricle (preload) increases, stroke volume usually increases proportionately. Reproduced with permission from Mayo Clinic.

The implied equivalency between the measured pressure and volume in the ventricular chambers may not be correct and depends upon the compliance or distensibility of the ventricle. During myocardial ischemia, sepsis, valvular dysfunction, and even in simple tachycardia, the ventricles may become less compliant and may not fully relax during diastole. This diastolic dysfunction reduces the ventricular volume at end diastole but may be associated with a higher filling pressure; therefore the clinician may misinterpret pressure measurements to indicate adequate volume loading. Changes in intrathoracic pressures (eg, tension pneumothorax, positive pressure ventilation) may also affect the filling pressures.

3. Afterload

Afterload is the myocardial wall tension required to overcome the resistance, or pressure load, that opposes ejection of blood from the ventricle during systole. The higher the afterload, the more tension the ventricle must develop, the more work is performed, and the less efficient the contraction may become. Afterload is usually estimated by calculations of vascular resistance.

III. ASSESSMENT OF OXYGEN BALANCE

In addition to oxygen delivery, oxygen consumption by the tissues affects oxygen balance. However, less is known about the factors that determine oxygen utilization at the cellular and tissue levels, and no direct routine measures of oxygen consumption are available. Indirect calculated measurement of oxygen consumption requires invasive or complex techniques. Measures of oxygen consumption reflect global oxygen utilization and do not provide information on oxygen utilization by specific tissues or organs.

Measurements of global oxygen balance that may be useful to monitor in the seriously ill patient include central venous oxyhemoglobin saturation ($ScvO_2$) and lactate concentrations. Central venous oxyhemoglobin saturation can be obtained continuously or intermittently from a catheter placed in the internal jugular or subclavian vein and correlates with the mixed venous oxyhemoglobin saturation (SvO_2) obtained from a pulmonary artery catheter. The SvO_2 measures the oxyhemoglobin saturation of blood from the superior vena cava and the inferior vena cava that has been mixed in the right ventricle. These measures of venous oxyhemoglobin saturation represent the amount of oxygen still bound to hemoglobin after traversing the tissue capillaries; the decrease from the SaO_2 estimates the amount of oxygen utilized (**Figure 6-3**). In normal individuals, the SvO_2 is >65% and the $ScvO_2$ is 2% to 3% lower. However, in patients with shock and/or hypoperfusion the $ScvO_2$ may be 5% to 7% higher than the SvO_2 due to greater desaturation of venous blood from the gastrointestinal tract contributing to SvO_2. Low values of $ScvO_2$ suggest an imbalance in the oxygen supply and demand. This imbalance may be due to alterations in cardiac output, hemoglobin concentration, arterial oxyhemoglobin saturation, or tissue oxygen consumption. A normal $ScvO_2$ may still be associated with tissue hypoxia in conditions such as severe sepsis and certain poisonings (eg, cyanide).

Figure 6-3. Determinants of Oxygen Balance

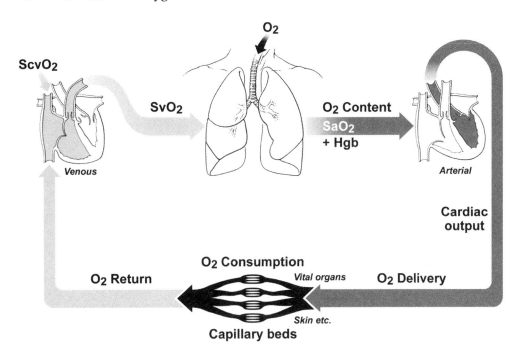

Oxygen balance depends on the oxygen delivered to the tissues and the metabolic needs of the tissues. An estimate of the oxygen utilized by the tissues is provided by the $ScvO_2$ and SvO_2. Abbreviations: Hgb, hemoglobin; SVO_2, arterial oxyhemoglobin saturation. Reproduced with permission from Mayo Clinic.

Lactate is another indicator of overall oxygen balance. Lactate is produced during anaerobic metabolism when cellular hypoxia occurs. The elevation of blood lactate in shock and hypoperfusion may be due to inadequate oxygen supply to tissue but also may be affected by altered hepatic metabolism, use of vasoactive drugs, and other factors. Lactate concentrations do not have high sensitivity or specificity for inadequate tissue oxygenation, but elevated concentrations often are associated with tissue hypoperfusion. A decreasing lactate concentration may be a useful indicator of the success of interventions.

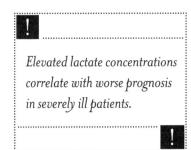

Elevated lactate concentrations correlate with worse prognosis in severely ill patients.

IV. MONITORING DETERMINANTS OF OXYGEN BALANCE

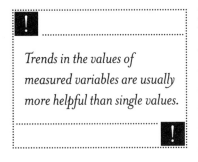

Trends in the values of measured variables are usually more helpful than single values.

Precise monitoring of oxygen balance is not easily accomplished because techniques may not be available to assess some variables (contractility, tissue oxygen consumption) or special expertise and resources are required (pulmonary artery catheter, echocardiography). However, monitoring of variables such as oxyhemoglobin saturation, blood pressure, central venous pressure, $ScvO_2$, and lactate concentration combined with other clinical information may provide guidance in evaluating the adequacy of oxygenation in seriously ill patients.

A. Monitoring of Oxyhemoglobin Saturation

1. Principles

The pulse oximeter is a simple, noninvasive device that *estimates* arterial oxyhemoglobin saturation. The transmission of red and infrared light through the capillary bed creates several signals throughout the pulsatile cardiac cycle. These signals measure the absorption of the transmitted light by the tissue or venous and arterial blood. Calculations made from the processed signals provide estimates of the oxygen saturation of hemoglobin, expressed as a percentage. This is *not* the same as the PaO_2 (partial pressure of oxygen) in the blood, although PaO_2 is a primary determinant of the saturation of hemoglobin. The oxyhemoglobin saturation also does not reflect adequacy of oxygen delivery. The value measured by the device is commonly called the SpO_2 to distinguish it as the oxyhemoglobin saturation measurement by a pulse oximeter rather than the SaO_2, which is determined directly from an arterial blood sample by co-oximetry.

2. Clinical Issues

Studies have shown that to ensure a PaO_2 of 60 mm Hg (8.0 kPa), an SpO_2 of 92% should be maintained in patients with light skin, whereas 94% saturation may be needed in patients with dark skin. Oximetry sensors can be applied to the finger, toe, earlobe, bridge of nose, mouth, or any skin surface from which a reliable signal can be obtained. Factors that can affect signal detection or fidelity are listed in **Table 6-2.** Pulse oximeters display a digital heart rate derived from the pulsatile signal detected by the sensor. This rate should equal the patient's heart rate as measured by another method. Therefore, these 2 pulse rates should be compared as the first step in the analysis of an SpO_2 reading.

Table 6-2. Factors That Affect Accuracy of Pulse Oximetry	
Anatomic or Physiologic Factors	**External Factors**
Dark skin	Lipid suspensions, propofol (falsely elevate the SpO_2)
False nails	Bright room lighting
Nail polish	Electrical interference
Hypothermia	Poorly adherent probe
Vasoconstriction	Excessive motion of the sensor
Hypotension	
Poor regional perfusion	
Hematocrit <15%	
Hyperlipidemia	
Carboxyhemoglobin	

B. Blood Pressure Monitoring

Although blood pressure is not a direct determinant of oxygen balance, an appropriate driving pressure is necessary for oxygen delivery at the tissue level. Blood pressure is determined by the cardiac output and systemic vascular resistance according to the following relationship:

Blood Pressure = Cardiac Output × Systemic Vascular Resistance

Blood pressure may be monitored invasively or noninvasively.

1. Automated Noninvasive Devices

a. Principles

Automated blood pressure devices are frequently used to obtain intermittent blood pressure measurements. These devices use one of several methods to measure systolic and diastolic pressure, but the most common method is oscillometry. Systolic and diastolic pressures and the mean arterial pressure (MAP) are directly measured via appearance, disappearance, and amplitude of oscillating waves. The arm is the preferred measurement site in adults, but alternative sites include the calf, thigh, or forearm. The thigh is the least comfortable site for patients. The cuff should not be placed on an extremity that is being used for intravenous infusion or in an area susceptible to circulatory compromise. The appropriate cuff size is necessary for accurate measurements. A cuff that is too large will underestimate the true blood pressure and a cuff that is too small yields artificially high blood pressure measurements.

b. Clinical Issues

Automated blood pressure devices are less accurate in clinical situations commonly encountered with the critically ill patient, such as shock, vasoconstriction, mechanical ventilation, and arrhythmias. Shivering and movement of the extremity can lead to erroneous measurements. Malfunction of the device can also distract the attention of the caregiver from the patient. It is important to remember that an adequate blood pressure does not ensure adequate tissue perfusion. Blood pressure monitoring via an arterial catheter is preferable to the use of an automated blood pressure device in hemodynamically unstable patients.

2. Arterial Cannulation

a. Principles

An indwelling arterial catheter allows for continuous measurement of blood pressure, pulse volume or pressure, and mean arterial pressure (**Figure 6-3**) by transduction of pressure via a specialized monitoring setup. It may also be used for continuous arterial blood gas measurement. The primary indications for insertion of an arterial cannula are the need for frequent arterial samples and continuous assessment of arterial blood pressure. Use of an arterial catheter should be considered for arterial blood sampling if more than 4 samples are required in 24 hours. The complication rate is lower for inserting a 20-gauge, 2-inch radial artery catheter than for performing four 22-gauge needle sticks in a single artery. Arterial pressure monitoring may also be used with special systems to evaluate cardiac output, stroke volume, and/or systolic pressure variation (as an estimate of volume responsiveness).

Figure 6-4. Appearance of Arterial Pressure Wave With Invasive Monitoring

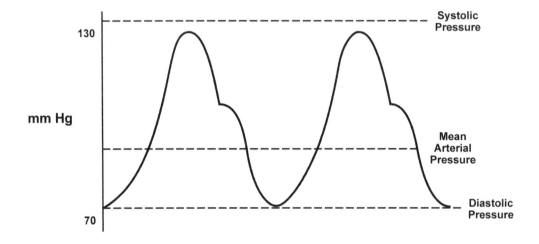

When invasive monitoring is used, the calculation of the mean arterial pressure is based on the area under the curve. Reproduced with permission from Mayo Clinic.

The most common insertion sites for arterial catheters are (in order of preference for adults) the radial, femoral, axillary, and dorsalis pedis arteries. Shorter catheters are used for radial and dorsalis pedis artery insertion and longer catheters for insertion in femoral and axillary sites. Preferred sites have alternative collateral circulations. The choice of site is based on palpable pulses, general hemodynamic state, and other anatomic or physiologic factors unique to each patient. (See **Appendix 9** for insertion techniques.)

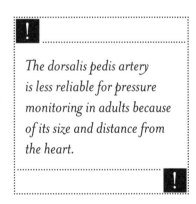

! *The dorsalis pedis artery is less reliable for pressure monitoring in adults because of its size and distance from the heart.* !

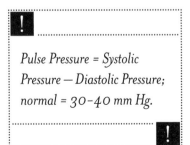

! *Pulse Pressure = Systolic Pressure − Diastolic Pressure; normal = 30–40 mm Hg.* !

b. Clinical Issues

The arterial catheter is never used for infusion of any medications or fluids and must be continuously monitored. When there is concern about the accuracy of the intra-arterial pressure measurements, a return-to-flow assessment with a manual blood pressure cuff should be performed (**Appendix 9**).

Several technical and anatomic factors may affect the accuracy of the pressures obtained from the catheter system. Distortion of the arterial waveform signal may occur due to vascular alterations, the hydraulic coupling system of the transducer, the calibration of the transducer, or the maintenance of the pressurized system tubing. Inspection of the waveform may show an overdamped and domed waveform or the high-spiking, "overshoot or ringing" pattern of the underdamped waveform (**Appendix 9**). Both distortions have the greatest effect on the systolic and diastolic pressures, whereas the MAP is less affected.

As with noninvasive monitoring, intra-arterial blood pressure monitoring may not be a sensitive indicator of hypoperfusion because of compensatory vasoconstriction. Additional clinical information regarding volume status can be obtained by inspection of the blood pressure waveform in mechanically ventilated patients (**Figure 6-5**). Positive pressure during inspiration may decrease the stroke volume in patients with inadequate intravascular volume due to decreased venous return. The decrease in stroke volume leads to a decreased pressure that is visually represented as a systolic variation of blood pressure.

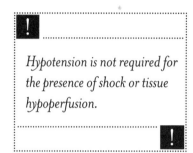

Hypotension is not required for the presence of shock or tissue hypoperfusion.

Figure 6-5. Variation of Blood Pressure in a Mechanically Ventilated Patient with Hypovolemia

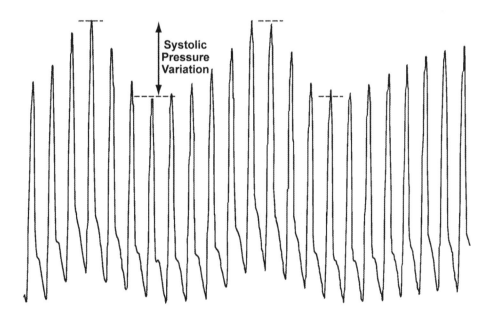

With positive pressure applied during inspiration, the decrease in systolic pressure is greater than the decrease in diastolic pressure. Reproduced with permission from Mayo Clinic.

Possible complications associated with arterial catheter insertion are listed in **Table 6-3.** These can be minimized by careful insertion technique, appropriate catheter size for the artery selected, proper site care, and a continuous flush system. The arterial waveform must be continuously monitored and displayed, with alarm settings to prevent inadvertent blood loss through a catheter that is accidentally opened to the atmosphere. The extremity with the arterial catheter should be inspected frequently for evidence of ischemia or infection. Any sign of ischemia distal to the catheter or infection at the site of insertion requires immediate removal of the catheter.

Table 6-3.	Possible Complications of Arterial Catheters
	Hematoma formation
	Blood loss
	Arterial thrombosis
	Proximal or distal embolization
	Arterial pseudoaneurysm
	Infection
	Accidental administration of fluids or medications

C. Monitoring Right Ventricular Filling Pressures and Central Venous Oxyhemoglobin Saturation

A central venous catheter in the internal jugular or subclavian vein allows measurement of CVP and $ScvO_2$. Placement of a central venous catheter may be indicated for other reasons as well (**Table 6-4**). **Appendix 10** reviews both the techniques for catheter insertion in common locations and potential complications. Confirmation of catheter placement in the internal jugular or subclavian vein by chest radiography is recommended to ensure accurate measurements of CVP and $ScvO_2$ and to detect complications of the procedure.

Table 6-4.	Common Indications for Central Venous Cannulation
	Measurement of mean central venous pressure
	Measurement of $ScvO_2$
	Large-bore venous access
	Difficult or long-term venous access
	Administration of irritating drugs and/or parenteral nutrition
	Hemodialysis
	Placement of a temporary pacing wire
	Placement of a pulmonary artery catheter

Central venous pressure, obtained from an appropriately positioned catheter, estimates the right ventricular filling pressure as a reflection of preload (end-diastolic volume). Normal values for CVP are 2 to 8 mm Hg, and measurements should be made at the end of expiration. Significant variation of the CVP waveform may occur during spontaneous breathing and mechanical ventilation, requiring visual assessment of the waveform to identify the end of expiration (**Figure 6-6**). In general, a low CVP indicates a low intravascular volume associated with a low preload. Normal or high CVP measurements must be evaluated cautiously, as they may not predict adequate or increased preload volume due to changes in intrathoracic pressures or ventricular compliance. Additional clinical assessment is required to estimate preload with normal or elevated CVP measurements.

Figure 6-6. Typical Cyclic Pattern for CVP Waveform

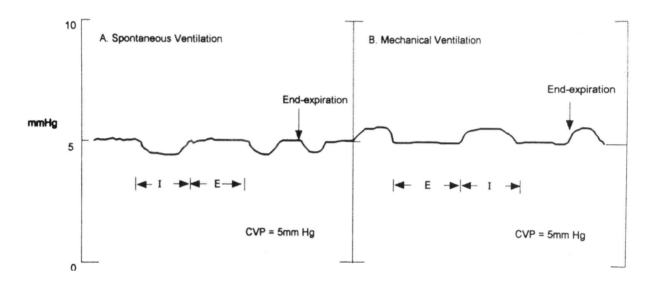

Typical cyclic pattern for CVP waveform that shows inspiration (I) and expiration (E). A, Respiratory variation during spontaneous ventilation: CVP decreases during spontaneous inspiration as intrapleural pressure decreases. B, Respiratory variation during positive pressure mechanical ventilation: CVP increases during delivery of the mechanical breath as positive pressure is transmitted from the airway to the intrapleural space and great vessels. The vertical arrows denote the point of end-expiration during spontaneous and mechanical ventilation.

Central venous oxyhemoglobin saturation ($ScvO_2$) can be monitored intermittently by withdrawal of blood for laboratory analysis or continuously with a catheter containing an oximeter to evaluate oxygen balance. Clinical protocols have used $ScvO_2$ measurements along with other parameters to determine adequacy of resuscitation. Normal values for $ScvO_2$ are usually >65%.

D. Measuring Left Ventricular Filling Pressures

Left ventricular filling pressures are estimated from measurement of the pulmonary artery occlusion pressure (PAOP). A pulmonary artery catheter (PAC) is necessary to obtain this information but requires expertise in insertion, data collection, and data interpretation. The clinician should consult with a critical care practitioner if invasive monitoring with a PAC is needed to obtain additional hemodynamic information.

E. Measuring Cardiac Output

Cardiac output plays a key role in determining oxygen delivery to the tissues. Methods to measure cardiac output, such as thermodilution with a PAC, esophageal Doppler ultrasonography, and arterial waveform pulse contour analysis, require varying degrees of invasiveness as well as special expertise. In the absence of direct measurement of cardiac output, less specific indicators of tissue oxygenation, such as lactate concentration and $ScvO_2$, may guide specific interventions until critical care expertise is available.

V. ACID-BASE DISORDERS

Acid-base disorders are common in the critically ill patient, and assessment of acid-base status may indicate specific diagnoses and/or therapeutic interventions. The presence of an acidosis should suggest hypoperfusion and prompt further assessment of the adequacy of oxygen balance. Appropriate evaluation of acid-base status requires accurate interpretation of simultaneous measurements of electrolytes, albumin, and arterial blood gases, as well as knowledge of compensatory physiologic responses.

A. Evaluation of Acid-Base Disorders

Analysis of acid-base disorders in seriously ill patients requires a systematic approach. Although several methods of evaluating acid-base disorders can be utilized (base excess, strong ion difference), the approach below relies on traditional analysis using formulas based on hydrogen ion (H) and bicarbonate (HCO_3).

1. Determine the overall acid-base condition by measuring pH. Is acidemia or alkalemia present?

2. If an abnormality is present, determine if the primary process is metabolic (change in [HCO_3]) or respiratory (change in $PaCO_2$).

3. If a respiratory disturbance is present, determine if it is an acute or a chronic process.

4. If a metabolic disturbance is present, determine if respiratory compensation is adequate.

5. Calculate the anion gap (AG).

6. If an AG metabolic acidosis is present, calculate the delta gap (Δgap) to determine if other metabolic disturbances are present.

B. Metabolic Acidosis

Metabolic acidosis results from an increase in endogenous acid production that overwhelms renal excretion (eg, ketoacidosis, lactic acidosis), exogenous acid input (eg, toxin ingestion), excessive loss of bicarbonate (eg, diarrhea), or decreased renal excretion of endogenous acids (eg, renal failure). Compensation is achieved primarily by increasing minute ventilation to eliminate CO_2. The adequacy of respiratory compensation can be estimated by the following formulas:

appropriate $PaCO_2 = 1.5 \times [HCO_3] + 8 \pm 2$; or $\Delta PaCO_2 = 1.2 \times \Delta[HCO_3]$

The lower limit of respiratory compensation is $PaCO_2$ of approximately 10 mm Hg.

Metabolic acidosis is further characterized by the anion gap. Normally, unmeasured anions exceed unmeasured cations, and the difference results in the AG. The anion gap is estimated by the following formula:

$AG = [Na] - ([Cl] + [HCO_3]) = 10 \pm 4$

An increased AG indicates an increase in unmeasured anions and/or a decrease in unmeasured cations. The AG has limitations as the sole indicator of a metabolic acidosis. In patients with severe hypoalbuminemia, an AG acidosis can exist even when a normal AG is measured. In such patients, the expected AG may be as low as 4 to 5 mmol/L. For every decrease of 1 g/dL in albumin, a decrease of 2.5 to 3 mmol in AG will occur. Another exception can occur when an elevated AG does not reflect an underlying acidosis. In patients with significant alkalemia (usually pH >7.5), albumin is more negatively charged, which increases unmeasured anions.

In an uncomplicated AG metabolic acidosis, every increase of 1 mmol/L in the AG should result in a concomitant decrease of 1 mmol/L in [HCO_3]. Deviation from this relationship suggests a mixed acid-base disorder. The difference between these 2 values has been termed the delta gap (Δgap), and can be expressed as follows: Δgap = (deviation of AG from normal) – (deviation of [HCO_3] from normal). The normal value for Δgap should be 0. However, variance in measurements can result in a Δgap of 0 ± 6. If the Δgap is positive, then a simultaneous metabolic alkalosis exists. If the decrease in [HCO_3] is greater than the increase in AG, which results in a negative Δgap, then a concomitant normal AG acidosis (hyperchloremic) may exist. Small deviations of the Δgap may not indicate mixed acid-base disorders, and clinical information must always be considered in the evaluation.

The most common causes of metabolic acidosis with an increased AG in seriously ill patients are lactic acidosis, renal failure, and diabetic ketoacidosis. Metabolic acidosis with a normal AG, often called hyperchloremic acidosis, may result from gastrointestinal or renal loss of HCO_3 and volume resuscitation with normal saline.

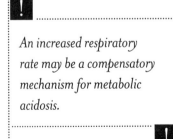

An increased respiratory rate may be a compensatory mechanism for metabolic acidosis.

C. Metabolic Alkalosis

Metabolic alkaloses are usually characterized as chloride-depleted (hypovolemic) and chloride-expanded (hypervolemic). Hypokalemia is common to both types of metabolic alkalosis. Measurement of urine chloride is helpful in distinguishing the 2 categories, with urine chloride <20 mmol/L in chloride-depleted metabolic alkaloses and urine chloride >20 mmol/L in chloride-expanded metabolic alkaloses. Normal compensation for metabolic alkalosis is hypoventilation, which is limited by hypoxemia as $PaCO_2$ increases. $PaCO_2$ may rise 6 to 7 mm Hg for every increase of 10 mmol/L in $[HCO_3]$. Treatment includes volume replacement for chloride-depleted states and assessment of the renal-adrenal axis for chloride-expanded conditions. Potassium deficiencies should be corrected. Severe alkalemia is associated with high mortality and requires aggressive treatment.

D. Respiratory Acidosis

Respiratory acidosis is most commonly due to ineffective alveolar ventilation. If the respiratory acidosis is acute, the pH decreases by 0.08 units for each increase of 10 mm Hg in $PaCO_2$. A very small increase in plasma $[HCO_3]$ can be seen acutely because of titration of intracellular nonbicarbonate buffers. For each acute increase of 10 mm Hg in $PaCO_2$, the $[HCO_3]$ increases by 1 mmol/L to a maximum of 30 to 32 mmol/L. In chronic respiratory acidosis, the pH decreases 0.03 units and the $[HCO_3]$ increases 3.5 mmol/L for each increase of 10 mm Hg in $PaCO_2$. The limit of normal renal compensation in chronic respiratory acidosis is a $[HCO_3]$ of approximately 45 mmol/L. Higher values suggest an associated metabolic alkalosis.

Treatment of respiratory acidosis involves the rapid identification of the etiology and implementation of corrective action. In some circumstances, intubation and mechanical ventilation may be necessary to support alveolar ventilation.

E. Respiratory Alkalosis

Respiratory alkalosis results from primary hyperventilation due to a variety of etiologies. Acute pulmonary processes or an acidosis should be considered in the seriously ill patient. Similar to changes noted in respiratory acidosis, pH increases 0.08 for every decrease of 10 mm Hg in $PaCO_2$ in acute respiratory alkalosis, and pH increases 0.03 for each decrease of 10 mm Hg in $PaCO_2$ in chronic respiratory alkalosis. The $[HCO_3]$ decreases 2 mmol/L in acute respiratory alkalosis and 5 mmol/L in chronic respiratory alkalosis for each decrease of 10 mm Hg in $PaCO_2$. Chronic respiratory alkalosis is unique among acid-base disorders in that pH may return to normal if the condition is prolonged. Therapy is directed to the underlying cause.

F. Complex Acid-Base Disorders

Simple acid-base disorders result from a single process such as metabolic alkalosis. In many critically ill patients, multiple acid-base disturbances exist concurrently and result in complex acid-base disorders. For example, septic shock often presents with respiratory alkalosis and metabolic acidosis. A systematic approach to acid-base analysis is needed to identify the ongoing disturbances and determine appropriate diagnoses and interventions. Formulas that are helpful in evaluating acid-base status are listed in **Table 6-5.**

Table 6-5. Acid-Base Formulas

Acid-Base Disorder	Equation
Respiratory Acidosis	
Acute	Decrease in pH $= 0.08 \times \dfrac{(PaCO_2 - 40)}{10}$
	Increase in $[HCO_3] = \dfrac{\Delta PaCO_2 \pm 3}{10}$
Chronic	Decrease in pH $= 0.03 \times \dfrac{(PaCO_2 - 40)}{10}$
	Increase in $[HCO_3] = 3.5 \times \dfrac{\Delta PaCO_2}{10}$
Respiratory ~~Acidosis~~ *Alkalosis*	
Acute	Increase in pH $= 0.08 \times \dfrac{(40 - PaCO_2)}{10}$
	Decrease in $[HCO_3] = 2 \times \dfrac{\Delta PaCO_2}{10}$
Chronic	Increase in pH $= 0.03 \times \dfrac{(40 - PaCO_2)}{10}$
	Decrease in $[HCO_3] = \left(5\text{~~#~~}\right) \times \dfrac{\Delta PaCO_2}{10}$
Metabolic Acidosis	Anion Gap $= [Na] - ([Cl] + [HCO_3])$
	Expected $PaCO_2 = 1.5 \times [HCO_3] + 8 \pm 2$ or expected $\Delta PCO_2 = 1.2 \times \Delta[HCO_3]$
	Δgap $= $ (Measured Anion Gap $-$ Normal Anion Gap) $- (24 - [HCO_3])$
Metabolic Alkalosis	Increase in $PaCO_2 = 0.6 - 0.7 \times \Delta[HCO_3]$

(handwritten: 12)

(handwritten: ⊕ = met Alk
⊖ = NonAG metA *)*

(handwritten calculations:
6.0
1.2
─── 120
60
─── 720

40
−7.2
─── 7.33 *)*

Key Points

Monitoring Blood Flow, Oxygenation, and Acid-base Status

■ Oxygen delivery is dependent on cardiac output (blood flow) and the oxygen content of arterial blood.

■ Hemoglobin is the major contributor of oxygen for tissue demands.

■ Normal ventricular filling pressure measurements may not indicate adequate preload volume.

■ Measurements of global oxygen balance that may be useful to monitor in the seriously ill patient include central venous oxyhemoglobin saturation ($ScvO_2$) and lactate concentrations.

■ Low values of $ScvO_2$ suggest an oxygen imbalance that may be due to alterations in cardiac output, hemoglobin concentrations, arterial oxyhemoglobin saturation, or tissue oxygen consumption.

■ The pulse oximeter estimates arterial oxyhemoglobin saturation but does not reflect adequacy of oxygen delivery.

■ Blood pressure monitoring via an arterial catheter is preferable to the use of an automated blood pressure device in unstable patients.

■ Assessment of acid-base status may suggest specific diagnoses and/or therapeutic interventions.

Suggested Readings

1. Huang Y-C T. Monitoring oxygen delivery in the critically ill. *Chest.* 2005;128:554S.

2. Magder S. Central venous pressure monitoring. *Curr Opin Crit Care.* 2006;12:219.

3. Marx G, Reinhart K. Venous oximetry. *Curr Opin Crit Care.* 2006;12:263.

4. McMorrow RCN, Mythen MG. Pulse oximetry. *Curr Opin Crit Care.* 2006;12:269.

5. Nguyen HB, Rivers EP, Knoblich BP, et al. Early lactate clearance is associated with improved outcome in severe sepsis and septic shock. *Crit Care Med.* 2004;32:1637.

Chapter 7:

Diagnosis and Management of Shock

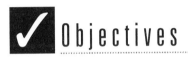

Objectives

■ Identify the 4 main categories of shock.

■ Discuss goals of resuscitation in shock.

■ Summarize the general principles of shock management.

■ Describe the physiologic effects of vasopressor and inotropic agents.

■ Discuss the differential diagnosis of oliguria.

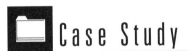

Case Study

A 25-year-old woman with no prior history presents to the emergency department complaining of a cough productive of tenacious greenish yellow mucous. Vital signs are temperature 101.8°F (38.8°C), heart rate 129/min, respiratory rate 27/min, and blood pressure 112/68 mm Hg.

    – What information is needed to determine if this patient has shock?

    – What initial interventions are needed to stabilize the patient?

I. INTRODUCTION

Shock is a syndrome of impaired tissue oxygenation and perfusion due to a variety of etiologies. Prompt recognition of shock and early, effective intervention is needed to prevent irreversible injury, organ dysfunction, and death. Inadequate tissue oxygenation and perfusion may result from 1 or more of the following mechanisms:

■ An absolute or relative decrease in systemic oxygen delivery (inadequate cardiac output, low blood oxygen content)

■ Ineffective tissue perfusion (maldistribution of blood flow to tissues)

■ Impaired utilization of delivered oxygen (cellular or mitochondrial dysfunction)

Basically, shock results when oxygen balance is disturbed and demand exceeds supply. Shock is not defined by hypotension, although hypotension is frequently associated with shock. Initially, blood pressure may be normal in some patients with shock even though it has significantly dropped from baseline, or blood pressure may be preserved due to compensatory sympathetic responses. Management of shock should be directed toward correcting oxygen balance and hypoperfusion as the primary end points.

II. CLINICAL ALTERATIONS IN SHOCK

The presentation of patients with shock may be subtle (mild confusion, tachycardia) or easily identifiable (profound hypotension, anuria). Shock may be the initial manifestation of an underlying condition or it may develop as the condition progresses. A strong index of suspicion and vigilant clinical assessment are needed to identify the early signs of shock and initiate appropriate treatment. The clinical manifestations of shock result from inadequate tissue oxygenation and perfusion, compensatory responses, and the specific etiology of shock. Hypoperfusion of end organs may result in hypotension, altered mental status, oliguria/anuria, and other organ dysfunction. In addition, hypoperfusion is associated with some degree of inflammatory response that may contribute to organ injury. Direct and indirect effects of hypoperfusion may be reflected in laboratory findings of abnormal oxygenation, blood urea nitrogen (BUN), creatinine, bilirubin, hepatic transaminases, and coagulation parameters. An anion gap metabolic acidosis is one of the most common findings of hypoperfusion. The acidosis is often associated with an elevated lactate concentration. Although neither sensitive nor specific for the diagnosis of shock, the lactate concentration is an indicator of hypoperfusion and a relevant monitoring tool for assessment of therapeutic interventions.

Compensatory mechanisms in shock involve complex neuroendocrine responses that attempt to increase tissue perfusion and oxygenation. In many forms of shock, sympathetically mediated vasoconstriction redirects blood flow from low-oxygen-requiring organs such as the skin toward oxygen-dependent organs such as the brain and heart. Compensatory vasoconstriction can maintain blood pressure early in shock and lead to an increase in the diastolic pressure and a

> **!**
>
> *The increased systemic vascular resistance present in cardiogenic, hemorrhagic, and obstructive shock is the body's attempt to maintain blood pressure (perfusion pressure).*
>
> **!**

narrowing of the pulse pressure. Intense vasoconstriction correlates with cold, clammy extremities and contributes to organ hypoperfusion. Hypothermia may also be a manifestation of severe vasoconstriction. Patients with distributive shock (see below) often have vasodilation and warm extremities, but other signs of hypoperfusion are usually present. Tachycardia, mediated by the sympathetic response, reflects an attempt to increase cardiac output in shock. Tachypnea may be a compensatory response to metabolic acidosis, a response to lung injury, or due to direct stimulation of the respiratory center.

Additional alterations in shock occur to increase oxygenation at the tissue level. As discussed in **Chapter 6,** hemoglobin will release more oxygen as it traverses the capillaries in order to meet tissue demands. A rightward shift of the oxyhemoglobin saturation curve due to acidosis or increased temperature facilitates release of hemoglobin-bound oxygen. The greater extraction of oxygen is reflected in lower SvO_2 or $ScvO_2$ measurements in many forms of shock. However, a normal value of venous oxyhemoglobin saturation does not imply that tissue oxygenation is adequate because some forms of shock (eg, septic shock) may lead to impaired tissue or cellular utilization of oxygen or result in maldistribution of blood flow.

III. CLASSIFICATION OF SHOCK

There are 4 main categories of shock based on cardiovascular characteristics: hypovolemic, distributive, cardiogenic, and obstructive, as outlined in **Table 7-1.** A careful history and a physical examination often provide information that is helpful in determining the likely cause of shock. However, many patients will have components of more than one type of shock (mixed shock). Septic shock is a form of distributive shock, but it may have a hypovolemic component prior to fluid resuscitation. Likewise, myocardial dysfunction may be present in septic shock and hypovolemic shock.

Table 7-1.	Classifications of Shock
Hypovolemic	**Cardiogenic**
Hemorrhagic	Myopathic (ie, ischemic)
Nonhemorrhagic	Mechanical (ie, valvular)
	Arrhythmic
Distributive	**Obstructive**
Septic	Massive pulmonary embolism
Adrenal crisis	Tension pneumothorax
Neurogenic (spinal shock)	Cardiac tamponade
Anaphylactic	Constrictive pericarditis

Knowledge of the expected hemodynamic profiles associated with different types of shock is helpful in determining appropriate therapy, even when specific measurements are not available. **Table 7-2** presents the usual hemodynamic profiles for more common forms of shock, but variations occur depending on the specific etiology, cardiac function, and resuscitation status of the patient.

Table 7-2.	Hemodynamic Profiles of Shock					
Type of Shock	**Heart Rate**	**Cardiac Output**	**Ventricular Filling Pressures**	**Systemic Vascular Resistance**	**Pulse Pressure**	**SvO$_2$/ScvO$_2$**
Cardiogenic	↑	↓	↑	↑	↓	↓
Hypovolemic	↑	↓	↓	↑	↓	↓
Distributive	↑	↑ or N[a]	↓ or N[b]	↓	↑	↑ or N[a]
Obstructive	↑	↓	↑	↑	↓	↓

Abbreviations: SvO$_2$, mixed venous oxyhemoglobin saturation; N, normal; ScvO$_2$, central venous oxyhemoglobin saturation.

[a]May be decreased prior to or early in resuscitation
[b]Left ventricular filling pressures may be normal or low in massive pulmonary embolism.

A. Hypovolemic Shock

Hypovolemic shock occurs when intravascular volume is depleted relative to the vascular capacity as a result of hemorrhage, gastrointestinal or urinary fluid losses, dehydration, or third-space fluid losses. Third-space fluid losses resulting from interstitial fluid redistribution may be prominent in burn injury, trauma, pancreatitis, and any severe form of shock. The hemodynamic findings in hypovolemic shock are decreased cardiac output, decreased right and left ventricular filling pressures (preload), and an increased afterload (systemic vascular resistance [SVR]) due to compensatory vasoconstriction. The SvO$_2$ or ScvO$_2$ is decreased as a result of decreased cardiac output with unchanged or increased tissue oxygen demands and potentially decreased hemoglobin concentration (hemorrhage). In addition to the usual clinical findings, patients with hypovolemic shock have flat, nondistended jugular veins.

B. Distributive Shock

Distributive shock is characterized by loss of peripheral vascular tone (vasodilation). However, patients with distributive shock often have components of hypovolemic shock and cardiogenic shock. The most common form of distributive shock is septic shock, with neurogenic shock and anaphylactic shock being much less common. The hemodynamic profile usually includes a normal or increased cardiac output with a low SVR and low to normal ventricular filling pressures. A decreased cardiac output may result if intravascular volume is not optimized. ScvO$_2$ or SvO$_2$ may be normal or increased due to shunting of blood in the microvasculature or the inability of tissue to utilize oxygen. In contrast to other forms of shock, the vasodilation of fluid-resuscitated distributive shock results in warm extremities, decreased diastolic pressure, and increased pulse pressure. Neurogenic shock may be associated with bradycardia rather than tachycardia. Fever may be present in septic shock and adrenal crisis.

C. Cardiogenic Shock

In cardiogenic shock, forward blood flow is inadequate because of cardiac pump failure due to loss of functional myocardium (ischemia, cardiomyopathy), a mechanical or structural defect (valvular failure, septal defect), or arrhythmias. Most commonly, cardiogenic shock results from acute myocardial infarction (MI) or a subsequent complication. Cardiogenic shock is the most severe form of heart failure and is distinguished from less severe chronic heart failure by the presence of hypoperfusion, hypotension, and the need for different therapeutic interventions (**Chapter 10**). The typical hemodynamic characteristics are decreased cardiac output, elevated ventricular filling pressures, and increased afterload (SVR). When cardiac output is low, the SvO_2 or $ScvO_2$ declines due to increased extraction of oxygen from hemoglobin at the tissue level. Clinical manifestations associated with cardiogenic shock may include distended jugular veins, pulmonary edema, and S_3 gallop.

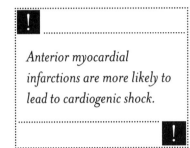

Anterior myocardial infarctions are more likely to lead to cardiogenic shock.

D. Obstructive Shock

The common features in obstructive shock are obstruction to flow due to impaired cardiac filling and excessive afterload. Cardiac tamponade and constrictive pericarditis impair diastolic filling of the right ventricle, while tension pneumothorax limits right ventricular filling by obstruction of venous return. Massive pulmonary emboli increase right ventricular afterload. The hemodynamic profile is characterized by decreased cardiac output, increased afterload, and variable left ventricular filling pressures, depending on the etiology. In cardiac tamponade, the pressures of the right heart chambers, the pulmonary artery, and the left heart chambers equilibrate in diastole. A drop of >10 mm Hg in systolic blood pressure during inspiration (pulsus paradoxus) is an important clinical finding in patients with suspected cardiac tamponade. Distended jugular veins may be present in obstructive shock, depending on the time course of development and intravascular volume status.

IV. GENERAL PRINCIPLES OF SHOCK MANAGEMENT

The overall goal of shock management is to improve oxygen delivery or utilization in order to prevent cellular and organ injury. Effective therapy requires treatment of the underlying etiology, restoration of adequate perfusion, monitoring, and comprehensive supportive care. Interventions to restore perfusion center on achieving an adequate blood pressure, increasing cardiac output, and/or optimizing the oxygen content of blood. Oxygen demand should also be decreased when possible. These goals are usually accomplished with a combination of interventions, as summarized in **Table 7-3.**

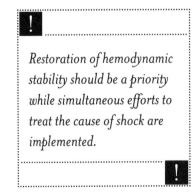

Restoration of hemodynamic stability should be a priority while simultaneous efforts to treat the cause of shock are implemented.

Table 7-3.	Interventions for Managing Shock

Component	Intervention
Blood pressure	Fluids, vasopressor or vasodilator agents[a]
Cardiac Output	
Preload	Fluids, vasodilator agents[a]
Contractility	Inotropic agents
Afterload	Vasopressor or vasodilator agents[a]
Oxygen Content	
Hemoglobin	Blood transfusion
Hemoglobin saturation	Supplemental oxygen, mechanical ventilation
Oxygen demand	Mechanical ventilation, sedation, analgesia, antipyretics

[a] Vasodilator agents are used only when blood pressure is adequate (see text).

The first goal in treating hypotensive shock is to achieve a minimum blood pressure (driving pressure). A minimum blood pressure is needed to maintain blood flow to the heart and other organs while optimizing other components of oxygen delivery. A mean arterial pressure (MAP) ≥65 mm Hg is usually recommended as an initial goal. A higher MAP may be needed in patients with myocardial ischemia or chronic hypertension, but an increase in blood pressure is beneficial only if it translates into improved perfusion. Otherwise, higher blood pressures may increase myocardial oxygen demands. Following initial resuscitation, the MAP goal should be individualized based on further assessment of the adequacy of systemic and organ perfusion. A blood pressure goal is usually achieved with fluids and/or vasoactive agents (see "Fluid Therapy" and "Vasoactive Agents," below).

The next goal in the management of shock is to optimize oxygen delivery. As outlined in **Chapter 6,** oxygen delivery can be enhanced by increasing cardiac output, hemoglobin concentration, or oxyhemoglobin saturation. In the absence of specific measurement of cardiac output, an assessment of adequacy depends on the etiology of shock and the presence of hypoperfusion abnormalities (see "Monitoring," below). Fluids and/or vasoactive agents are often needed to optimize cardiac output. The determinants of the oxygen content of blood (hemoglobin and oxyhemoglobin saturation) can be easily measured and optimized when indicated. Increasing hemoglobin concentration by transfusion may be one of the most efficient ways of improving oxygen delivery in some patients with shock. For example, increasing the hemoglobin concentration from 7 g/dL to 9 g/dL increases oxygen delivery by almost 30%, even if cardiac output remains constant. The oxyhemoglobin saturation can be increased by increasing the PaO_2 with oxygen supplementation and mechanical ventilation. However, once the PaO_2 has been increased to a range of 60 to 70 mm Hg (8-9.3 kPa), little additional benefit is gained by increasing the PaO_2 further. An oxyhemoglobin saturation ≥95% is recommended in patients with shock.

!
Almost all patients with shock require intubation.
!

A. Monitoring

Patients with shock require monitoring to determine the appropriate interventions and to assess their response to interventions (**Chapter 6**). Continuous electrocardiographic monitoring is needed to assess changes in heart rate and rhythm. Blood pressure is best monitored with an arterial catheter due to the inaccuracy of noninvasive devices in patients with shock. Pulse oximetry should be routinely monitored to ensure adequate oxyhemoglobin saturation. Monitoring of central venous pressure may be helpful in selected patients as an indicator of right ventricular preload. Measurement of $ScvO_2$ via a central venous catheter may be useful as an indicator of oxygen balance. However, a normal $ScvO_2$ value does not rule out hypoperfusion. A urinary catheter should be inserted to monitor urine output as an indicator of renal perfusion, with a suggested goal of 0.5 to 1 mL/kg/h. Lactate concentrations should be measured initially and monitored at appropriate intervals. A normal or decreasing lactate concentration suggests improved oxygen balance. Other laboratory data should be monitored with the goal of assessing progression or improvement of organ dysfunction.

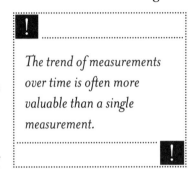

The trend of measurements over time is often more valuable than a single measurement.

B. Fluid Therapy

The initial therapy for most forms of shock is replacement of intravascular volume. Physical examination may provide valuable information about the intravascular volume status. Diffuse or dependent crackles, as well as distended neck veins, suggest high ventricular filling pressures, unless acute respiratory distress syndrome or diffuse pneumonia is present. Clear lung fields and flat neck veins suggest inadequate preload in the hypotensive patient. Although orthostatic changes in blood pressure and heart rate may be helpful in assessing the degree of volume depletion, patients with hypotension or severe tachycardia should not be subjected to such positional changes. The nature and degree of fluid deficit should be determined to identify the necessary type of fluid replacement.

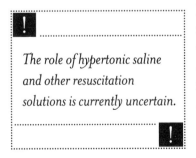

The role of hypertonic saline and other resuscitation solutions is currently uncertain.

Intravascular volume deficiency in the patient who is not anemic may be replenished with either crystalloid or colloid solutions. Crystalloids are less expensive than colloids and typically accomplish the same goals. Crystalloid solutions for volume resuscitation include lactated Ringer's and normal saline. Dextrose 5% in water does not offer any expansion of intravascular volume since it is quickly distributed throughout body fluid compartments and should not be used to treat hypovolemic shock. For the same reasons, 0.45% saline is not appropriate for volume expansion. Colloid solutions include hetastarch, albumin, and gelatins. Crystalloids and colloids appear to be equally effective when infused to physiologic end points. Crystalloid in titrated boluses of 500 to 1000 milliliters or colloid in titrated boluses of 300 to 500 milliliters may be given initially to most adult patients and repeated as necessary while appropriate parameters are closely monitored. Smaller bolus amounts are indicated for patients with suspected or known cardiogenic shock.

In addition to crystalloid or colloid solutions, packed red blood cells are indicated to increase oxygen-carrying capacity in the patient with significant bleeding or anemia. In many critically ill patients, a hemoglobin concentration of 7 to 9 g/dL may be adequate after stabilization, but a higher hemoglobin may be needed during acute resuscitation. Fresh frozen plasma should be used only for correction of a coagulopathy and not for volume replacement. Priorities in the administration of fluids are resuscitation and then replacement of ongoing losses. As the patient's clinical course continues, the solution that most closely approximates the patient's losses should be used with serum electrolytes guiding therapy.

The first target in fluid resuscitation is correction of hypotension. Once hypotension is corrected, further fluid resuscitation will decrease elevated heart rate and correct hypoperfusion abnormalities, thus achieving the true end point of effective shock treatment. The potential deleterious effect of overly aggressive fluid resuscitation is deterioration of oxygenation due to an increase in pulmonary capillary pressure, which can result in pulmonary edema. Therefore, frequent auscultation of the chest for the presence of crackles and monitoring of PaO_2 or oxyhemoglobin saturation by pulse oximetry should be performed during fluid resuscitation. In the absence of invasive hemodynamic monitoring, volume therapy can be administered vigilantly in patients with persistent hypotension and/or hypoperfusion until a significant drop in arterial oxygenation is noted or until the abnormalities are corrected. This approach to volume therapy presents minimal risk in patients with adequate oxygenation.

C. Vasoactive Agents

Vasoactive agents for the acute management of the patient with shock include medications with vasopressor, inotropic, and vasodilator effects. Many agents have more than one hemodynamic effect, and effects may vary with dose. Based on knowledge of the pharmacology of the individual agents, the clinician should choose the vasoactive agent that is most likely to achieve the hemodynamic effect desired for an individual patient. The goals of resuscitation are usually more important than the specific agent chosen.

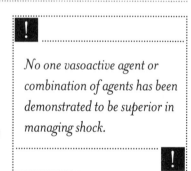

No one vasoactive agent or combination of agents has been demonstrated to be superior in managing shock.

1. Dopamine

Dopamine is a frequently used vasoactive agent with inotropic and vasopressor effects. Although dose response varies greatly among patients, some generalization can be helpful about dose and anticipated effect. At low rates of infusion (2-3 µg/kg/min), dopamine has modest inotropic and chronotropic effects. At this dose range, dopamine acts on the dopaminergic receptors in the kidney and may increase urine output. However, the use of low doses of dopamine for renal effects is not recommended, because it does not prevent renal dysfunction or improve outcomes. At intermediate rates of infusion (4-10 µg/kg/min), dopamine has primarily inotropic effects and loses its effect on the kidney. At higher infusion rates (≥10 µg/kg/min), dopamine has significant α-agonist effects that produce dose related vasoconstriction. At infusion rates ≥25 µg/kg/min, dopamine usually offers no advantage over norepinephrine, which may have greater vasopressor effect. Potential adverse effects include arrhythmias and tachycardia.

2. Norepinephrine

Norepinephrine is a potent α-adrenergic vasopressor. Norepinephrine also has β-adrenergic, inotropic, and chronotropic effects. In adults, the infusion rate of norepinephrine starts at 0.05 µg/kg/min and is titrated to desired effects. As with other vasopressors, cardiac output may decrease as afterload and blood pressure are increased. Norepinephrine usually increases renal blood flow in patients with adequate volume resuscitation. An increase in heart rate is uncommon with use of norepinephrine.

3. Epinephrine

Epinephrine has both α-adrenergic and β-adrenergic effects. It has potent inotropic and chronotropic effects, and, at higher doses, it has vasopressor effects. Doses start at 0.1 µg/kg/min and can be titrated to desired effects. The epinephrine-induced increase in myocardial oxygen consumption may limit the use of this agent in adults, especially in the presence of coronary artery disease. Mesenteric ischemia is also more common with epinephrine than with other vasopressors.

4. Vasopressin

Vasopressin is a potent vasopressor that acts through V1 receptors to produce vasoconstriction. As blood pressure is increased, cardiac output may decrease, similar to the effect of norepinephrine. The recommended dose in adults is 0.01 to 0.04 units/min. Higher doses may lead to ischemic events. Vasopressin may be considered for use in hypotensive shock refractory to other agents and fluid resuscitation. Further study is needed to define the role of vasopressin in the management of shock.

5. Dobutamine

Dobutamine is a β-adrenergic agonist with inotropic effects. Dobutamine is used in doses of 5 to 20 µg/kg/min and is usually associated with an increase in cardiac output. Arterial blood pressure may remain unchanged, decrease, or increase slightly. Dobutamine must be introduced with care in the hypotensive patient. In the face of inadequate intravascular volume replacement, blood pressure can drop precipitously, and tachycardia may be problematic. This agent has variable chronotropic effects.

V. MANAGEMENT OF SPECIFIC TYPES OF SHOCK

A. Hypovolemic Shock

The treatment goals for hypovolemic shock are restoration of intravascular volume and prevention of further volume loss. Therapy of hypovolemic shock should be targeted to reestablish normal blood pressure, pulse, and organ perfusion. For initial resuscitation, either colloid or crystalloid fluids are effective if given in sufficient volume. Subsequently, the fluid that is used should replace the fluid that has been lost. For example, blood products may be needed to replace blood loss (**Chapter 9**), and crystalloid should be used for vomiting and dehydration. For hypotension, the crystalloid choice is normal saline or lactated Ringer's solution because of the osmolality needed to restore intravascular volume. In large volume resuscitation, however, normal saline infusion may produce hyperchloremic metabolic acidosis. Vasopressors should be considered only as a temporizing measure while fluid resuscitation is ongoing or when hypotension persists despite adequate volume resuscitation. Central venous pressure monitoring may be helpful to guide fluid resuscitation in patients without significant heart or lung disease.

B. Distributive Shock

The initial approach to the patient with septic shock is restoration and maintenance of adequate intravascular volume. Prompt institution of appropriate antibiotics is essential, as are other interventions to control the infection (removal of catheter, surgery, drainage, debridement). Early goal-directed therapy using central venous pressure (CVP) monitoring and measurement of $ScvO_2$ has been shown to reduce mortality in severe sepsis and septic shock. (See the protocol in **Figure 7-1.**) Volume expansion can be initiated with isotonic crystalloid or colloid solutions. Vasodilation and diffuse capillary leak are common in septic shock, and fluid requirements may be large. The evaluation of fluid input and output measurements is therefore not helpful in determining aggressiveness of volume resuscitation because the measured volumes do not reflect fluid movement into the extravascular space. If the patient with septic shock remains hypotensive despite adequate fluid resuscitation, dopamine or norepinephrine are recommended as initial vasopressors. Low-dose vasopressin or epinephrine can be considered for patients who fail to respond adequately to first-line vasopressors. Dobutamine should be considered in patients with adequate blood pressure who have hypoperfusion and low cardiac output with adequate ventricular preload. Reversible myocardial dysfunction with ventricular dilation and decrease in ejection fraction frequently occurs in septic shock. An initial MAP <65 mm Hg may require initiation of vasopressor therapy until fluid resuscitation is optimized. Corticosteroids (hydrocortisone 200-300 mg in 24 hours administered as boluses or continuous infusion) should be considered in patients with septic shock when the blood pressure is poorly responsive to fluids and vasopressors. Results of an adrenocorticotropic hormone (ACTH) stimulation test are not required to initiate corticosteroid therapy. Anaphylactic shock is treated with volume resuscitation and subcutaneous epinephrine. In circumstances of very low blood pressure and poor peripheral perfusion, titrated intravenous epinephrine is indicated. Acute adrenal insufficiency is treated with volume therapy, intravenous corticosteroids, and vasopressors, if needed (**Chapter 12**). See **Chapter 9** for information about the management of neurogenic shock.

Figure 7-1. Protocol for Early Goal-Directed Resuscitation in Severe Sepsis and Septic Shock[a]

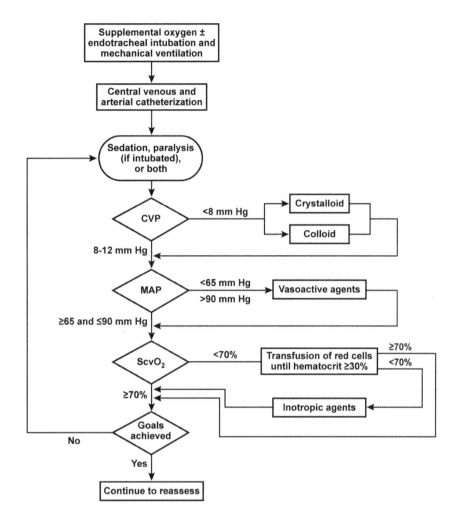

[a] Modified from Rivers E, Nguyen B, Havstad S, et al. Early goal-directed therapy in the treatment of severe sepsis and septic shock. *N Engl J Med.* 2001;345:1371. Abbreviations: CVP, central venous pressure; MAP, mean arterial pressure.

C. Cardiogenic Shock

The primary goal in treating cardiogenic shock is to improve myocardial function. Arrhythmias should be treated promptly. Reperfusion by percutaneous intervention is the treatment of choice in cardiogenic shock due to myocardial ischemia (**Chapter 10**). Diastolic dysfunction during myocardial ischemia may decrease ventricular compliance and elevate the left ventricular filling pressures, falsely indicating adequate preload. Therefore, a cautious trial of fluid administration may be warranted (250 mL bolus amounts). When blood pressure is decreased in cardiogenic shock, initial therapy with a single agent that has inotropic and vasopressor effects (eg, norepinephrine or dopamine) is indicated. Severely hypotensive patients (systolic arterial pressure <70 mm Hg) should be treated with norepinephrine to rapidly raise the systolic arterial pressure. If the systolic arterial pressure is 70 to 90 mm Hg, dopamine may be considered initially. The addition of an intravenous inotrope, such as dobutamine (or dopexamine, which is available in some countries), may be considered to augment myocardial contractility after blood pressure stabilizes, with the goal of decreasing vasopressor therapy. If moderate hypotension is not responsive to initial therapy, consultation should be obtained for consideration of intra-aortic balloon counterpulsation, left/right ventricular assist devices, etc.

The elevated afterload (SVR) may also impair cardiac output if it is a primary hemodynamic alteration, as occurs in chronic congestive heart failure. Often in acute cardiogenic shock, the SVR is secondarily elevated to maintain vascular perfusion pressure. Treatment aimed primarily at reducing afterload with a vasodilator, such as nitroprusside, should be initiated very cautiously and only in patients with hypoperfusion accompanied by adequate blood pressure.

When cardiac failure is characterized by low cardiac output, normal or elevated blood pressure, and hypoxemia due to high pulmonary capillary pressure, reduction of preload and afterload is helpful in improving hypoxemia. High pulmonary capillary pressure is diagnosed clinically.

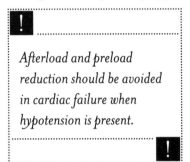

Afterload and preload reduction should be avoided in cardiac failure when hypotension is present.

Preload reduction is accomplished with loop diuretics (furosemide or bumetanide) and venodilators (nitroglycerin and morphine). Afterload reduction is accomplished with arterial vasodilators (angiotensin-converting enzyme inhibitors or, occasionally, nitroprusside). If the blood pressure can be increased to normal levels with inotropes, then the cautious addition of afterload and preload reduction is feasible in the presence of low cardiac output or high pulmonary capillary pressure.

D. Obstructive Shock

In the patient with obstructive shock, relief of the obstruction is the treatment of choice. If cardiac tamponade is present, pericardiocentesis may be lifesaving. Tension pneumothorax must be treated promptly. Maintenance of intravascular volume is vitally important in patients with all forms of obstructive shock. Fluid resuscitation may improve the patient's cardiac output and hypotension temporarily. Inotropes or vasopressors have a minimal role in the management of obstructive shock, and these agents provide only temporary improvement, if any.

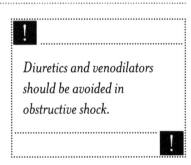

Diuretics and venodilators should be avoided in obstructive shock.

VI. OLIGURIA

Oliguria, defined as urine output <0.5 mL/kg/h for >2 hours, is an important manifestation of hypoperfusion. Oliguria may also be due to inherent renal injury or postrenal obstruction, in which case urine output cannot be used as a goal of adequate resuscitation of shock. Causes of oliguria are categorized as prerenal, renal, and postrenal, as outlined in **Table 7-4**.

Table 7-4. Differential Diagnosis of Oliguria

Prerenal

- Decreased cardiac output (eg, volume depletion, cardiac failure, tamponade)
- Redistribution of blood flow (distributive shock) with peripheral vasodilation and/or shunting

Renal

- Glomerular disease (glomerulonephritis)
- Vascular disease (eg, vasculitis)
- Interstitial disease (eg, antibiotics)
- Renal tubular disease
- Ischemia
- Nephrotoxic drugs

Postrenal (Obstructive)

- Bilateral ureteral obstruction
- Urethral stricture
- Bladder outlet obstruction
- Urinary catheter obstruction

Assessment of volume status by physical examination is often difficult in the critically ill patient, and invasive hemodynamic monitoring may be of benefit. Additional laboratory tests can help differentiate prerenal causes of oliguria from acute tubular necrosis (ATN). Some laboratory tests of renal function are shown in **Table 7-5.** Results of these tests should be obtained before the administration of diuretics.

Table 7-5. Laboratory Tests to Distinguish Prerenal Conditions From Acute Tubular Necrosis

Laboratory Test	Prerenal	ATN
Blood urea nitrogen/creatinine ratio	>20	10–20
Urine specific gravity	>1.020	>1.010
Urine osmolality (mOsm/L)	>500	<350
Urinary sodium (mmol/L)	<20	>40
Fractional excretion of sodium (%)[a]	<1	>2

[a] Fractional excretion of sodium (FENa) = ([urine sodium ÷ serum sodium] ÷ [urine creatinine ÷ serum creatinine]) × 100.

VII. MANAGEMENT OF ACUTE RENAL INSUFFICIENCY

Shock-induced hypoperfusion may lead to renal insufficiency or failure, as may other direct renal insults associated with critical illness. Reversible causes of acute renal insufficiency should always be excluded. A urinary catheter and renal ultrasound will exclude urinary obstruction in most patients. The urinary catheter is also a useful device to monitor urine output. Intravascular volume should be optimized with crystalloid and/or colloid solutions. If the patient remains oliguric after an adequate fluid challenge, a high dose of a loop diuretic (eg, furosemide 200 mg slow IV push) will often induce a nonoliguric state. Although the conversion to a nonoliguric state may not change outcome, fluid management is usually easier and dialysis may be avoided. There is no evidence to support the use of low-dose dopamine in oliguric patients. Once oliguric acute renal failure is confirmed, fluids should be restricted to the replacement of ongoing losses (including insensible losses). In disease states associated with ongoing loss of intravascular volume, fluid administration is necessary to maintain adequate left ventricular preload. These losses may be substantial, as in pancreatitis, severe sepsis, and large open wounds.

Because there is no specific treatment for most cases of acute renal failure, expectant and supportive care is maintained. Drug dosages need adjustment not only for glomerular filtration rate but also for the type of renal replacement therapy that is utilized. Nephrotoxic drugs should be avoided if possible. Problems with extracellular fluid overload, hyperkalemia, and hypermagnesemia should be anticipated and avoided if possible. Hyperkalemia usually can be managed medically until dialysis is available (**Chapter 12**). Bleeding may require the use of red cell transfusion or desmopressin (DDAVP). Nutritional supplements must also be adjusted for renal function.

Renal replacement therapy (RRT) is necessary when uremic symptoms develop or whenever extracellular volume excess, hyperkalemia, or metabolic acidosis is refractory to medical therapy. Various intermittent or continuous therapies are available to accomplish fluid removal (ultrafiltration) or solute removal (dialysis, hemofiltration, hemodiafiltration). Selection of a particular RRT depends on the circumstances of the individual patient and the resources available. Consultation with a nephrology expert is advised to assist with determining the most appropriate RRT.

Diagnosis and Management of Shock

■ Shock is characterized by impaired tissue oxygenation and hypoperfusion.

■ The 4 major categories of shock with characteristic hemodynamic patterns are hypovolemic, distributive, cardiogenic, and obstructive.

■ The clinical manifestations of shock result from inadequate tissue oxygenation and perfusion, compensatory responses, and the specific etiology of shock.

■ Interventions to restore perfusion center on achieving an adequate blood pressure, increasing cardiac output, optimizing the oxygen content of blood, and/or decreasing oxygen demand.

■ The initial therapy for most forms of shock is replacement of intravascular volume with crystalloid or colloid solutions.

■ The selection of a vasoactive agent to treat shock should be based on the hemodynamic effect desired for an individual patient and knowledge of the pharmacology of available agents

■ Reversible causes of acute oliguria should always be excluded and intravascular volume should be optimized with crystalloid and/or colloid solutions.

 Suggested Readings

1. The Albumin Reviewers (Alderson P, Bunn F, Li Wan Po A, Li L, Roberts I, Schierhout G). Human albumin solution for resuscitation and volume expansion in critically ill patients. *Cochrane Database Syst Rev.* 2004;(4):CD001208. doi:10.1002/14651858. CD001208.pub2.

2. American Thoracic Society. Evidence-based colloid use in the critically ill: American Thoracic Society consensus statement. *Am J Respir Crit Care Med.* 2004;170:1247.

3. Annane D, Sebille V, Charpentier C, et al. Effect of treatment with low doses of hydrocortisone and fludrocortisone on mortality in patients with septic shock. *JAMA.* 2002;288:862.

4. Dabrowski GP, Steinberg SM, Ferrara JJ, Flint LM. A critical assessment of endpoints of shock resuscitation. *Surg Clin North Am.* 2000;80:825.

5. Dellinger RP, Carlet JM, Masur H, et al. Surviving Sepsis Campaign guidelines for management of severe sepsis and septic shock. *Crit Care Med.* 2004;32:858.

6. Finfer S, Bellomo R, Boyce N, et al. A comparison of albumin and saline for fluid resuscitation in the intensive care unit. *N Engl J Med.* 2004;350:2247.

7. Gutierrez G, Reines HD, Wulf-Gutierrez ME. Clinical review: hemorrhagic shock. *Crit Care.* 2004;8:373.

8. Hébert PC, Wells G, Blajchman MA, et al. A multicenter, randomized, controlled clinical trial of transfusion requirements in critical care. *N Engl J Med.* 1999;340:409.

9. Lameire N, Van Biesen W, Vanholder R. Acute renal failure. *Lancet.* 2005;365:417.

10. Müller M, Urbanek B, Havel C, et al. Vasopressors for shock [review]. *Cochrane Database Syst Rev.* 2004;(3):CD003709. doi:10.1002/14651858.CD003709.pub2.

11. Rivers E, Nguyen B, Havstad S, et al. Early goal-directed therapy in the treatment of severe sepsis and septic shock. *N Engl J Med.* 2001;345:1368.

12. Singri N, Ahya SN, Levin ML. Acute renal failure. *JAMA.* 2003;289:747.

Web Site

Surviving Sepsis Campaign. www.survivingsepsis.org. This Web site contains guidelines for the management of severe sepsis and septic shock, information on the Surviving Sepsis Campaign, and sepsis-related information and resources for healthcare professionals, patients, and the general public.

Chapter 8

NEUROLOGIC SUPPORT

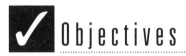 Objectives

■ Review the principles of primary and secondary brain insult and the common mechanisms of neuronal injury.

■ Apply the concepts of intracranial hypertension and brain oxygen delivery and consumption to the management of the brain-injured patient.

■ Review the clinical and diagnostic assessment of a brain-injured patient.

■ List general treatments that are common in brain injury.

■ Review specific management principles and options for selected pathophysiologic conditions.

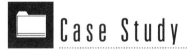 Case Study

A 16-year-old male, riding his bicycle without a helmet, struck the post of a traffic sign and was thrown to the ground. According to bystanders, he was unconscious for approximately 30 to 45 seconds, then got up and began to walk around the scene. When paramedics arrived, his vital signs were heart rate 110/min, respiratory rate 20/min, and blood pressure 124/62 mm Hg. He was oriented to name, place, and time but was slow to respond; his pupils were equal and reactive, and he showed no focal neurologic deficits. He was transported to the emergency department and after a brief, unchanged neurological examination, an emergent CT of his head without contrast was completed. Approximately 30 minutes later, the patient became less responsive, did not follow commands, and was moving his left arm significantly less than his right arm.

    – What type of primary brain injury is likely to be present?

    – What are the immediate concerns?

    – What interventions and monitoring should be instituted for the patient in addition to the CT scan?

I. INTRODUCTION

Primary injuries to the brain include ischemic events, trauma, hemorrhage, and anoxia, which may occur either in isolation or in combination. Mechanisms for these and other primary injuries are shown in **Table 8-1**.

Table 8-1.	Common Mechanisms of Primary Brain Injuries

- Trauma: concussion, contusion, shear and penetrating injury
- Ischemia: global (eg, cardiac arrest with anoxia) or regional (eg, vasospasm, compression of blood vessels, stroke)
- Inflammation: meningitis, encephalitis
- Compression: tumor, cerebral edema, hematoma (eg, epidural, subdural, or intraparenchymal)
- Metabolism: encephalopathies (eg, hepatic, Reye's syndrome, electrolytes, drugs, toxins)

Often, little can be done to reverse the immediate and frequently devastating effects of the primary cerebral insult that produces neuronal injury or death. In some circumstances, the immediate effects of an injury may be reversed by prompt surgical intervention. Analogous to the injury seen in myocardial infarction, many types of brain insults produce a region of maximum injury associated with a surrounding area of tissue, or penumbra, that may survive and potentially recover if further damage can be prevented. Common mechanisms of secondary injury are shown in **Table 8-2**. Note that some also occur as primary injuries, as indicated in **Table 8-1**. The mechanisms of secondary brain injury may evolve over time from other primary insults. For example, edema after head trauma commonly develops and produces secondary brain compression, vasospasm after subarachnoid hemorrhage (SAH) may cause regional ischemia and stroke, or secondary hemorrhagic conversion after an ischemic stroke may induce compression and further ischemia.

Table 8-2.	Common Mechanisms of Secondary Brain Injuries

- Hypoperfusion: global (ie, secondary to high intracranial pressure [ICP], systemic arterial hypotension, or severe anemia) or regional (eg, secondary to high ICP, local edema, or vasospasm)
- Hypoxia: systemic hypoxemia, regional hypoperfusion, or high tissue consumption (ie, seizures, hyperthermia)
- Electrolyte or acid base changes from systemic or regional ischemia
- Reperfusion injury with free radical formation

II. PRINCIPLES OF MANAGING BRAIN INJURY

The focus of treatment for a neurologically compromised patient is the same as that for patients with other illnesses and injuries, that is, to ensure a balance between oxygen delivery and demand to meet the needs of both the damaged and the undamaged brain tissue. Put simply, *the primary goal is the prevention of secondary injury.* The initial care team must take early and aggressive action to ensure that secondary brain injury is prevented, minimized, or reversed with careful monitoring and treatment, particularly prevention and early treatment of hypoxia and hypotension. Optimizing oxygen delivery to the brain requires attention to oxygenation, hemoglobin concentration, cardiac output, and blood pressure. Prevention and early treatment of fever, seizures, pain, agitation, and anxiety can minimize oxygen demands.

A. Intracranial Hypertension

Intracranial pressure is a reflection of the overall balance of volume-control mechanisms within the fixed and noncompliant cerebral compartment. Because the brain is enclosed within a rigid structure (skull and dura), with tissue and water that are incompressible (Monroe-Kellie hypothesis), control of extravascular intracranial volume is essential in maintaining brain homeostasis, controlling intracranial pressure, and maintaining cerebral perfusion. The critical compartment relationship depends on the space occupied by each component. The increased occupation of space by one component (brain volume) must be accompanied by a decrease in another component (blood flow, lymphatic flow, or cerebrospinal fluid [CSF]). When the compensatory mechanisms are overwhelmed, intracranial pressure (ICP) increases and injury ensues (usually with ICP >20 mm Hg).

An intensivist or a neurosurgeon should be consulted if intracranial hypertension is suspected. The patient may need a catheter inserted into a lateral ventricle for monitoring and drainage of CSF or into the brain parenchyma for monitoring only (**Table 8-3**). Intracranial pressure, temperature, and/or brain oxygen can then be closely monitored. Intracranial pressure is clinically relevant because pathologic increases, especially when acute, can cause significant brain ischemia and mechanical compression, which can lead to increased loss of brain function, herniation syndromes, and, ultimately, death.

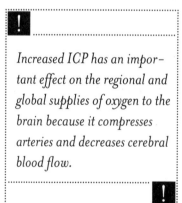

Increased ICP has an important effect on the regional and global supplies of oxygen to the brain because it compresses arteries and decreases cerebral blood flow.

Table 8-3.	Conditions Associated With Potential Need for Invasive ICP Monitoring

- Severe traumatic brain injury (Glasgow Coma Scale <8) plus abnormal CT scan
- Acute subarachnoid hemorrhage with coma or clinical deterioration
- Intracranial hemorrhage with intraventricular blood
- Ischemic stroke (middle cerebral artery)
- Fulminant hepatic failure
- Global brain ischemia/anoxia with increasing edema

Measurements of cerebral oxygen consumption and delivery usually require special equipment and expertise that are not available in most facilities. When direct measures are not available, the initial care team must proceed with treatment on the basis of commonly accepted principles of oxygen supply and demand.

B. Hypoperfusion: Cerebral Blood Flow

Cerebral autoregulation is the normal prearteriolar dilation or constriction that controls regional cerebral blood flow (CBF) and links oxygen delivery to the demands of oxygen consumption; thus, global cerebral blood flow normally remains constant over a wide range of mean arterial pressures. Loss of autoregulation may occur in a variety of pathologic conditions and may lead to regional vasodilatation and local edema formation, which can further increase ICP. Increases in blood flow will also profoundly affect the pressure inside the noncompliant cranial vault.

Cerebral blood flow is usually evaluated by the cerebral perfusion pressure (CPP), which is the mean arterial pressure (MAP, the driving pressure) minus the ICP (the pressure impeding blood flow):

$$CPP = MAP - ICP$$

Normal CPP is between 60 and 100 mm Hg. If ICP increases without a change in MAP, CPP decreases and CBF will also decrease if autoregulation has failed. The decrease in CBF increases the risk of brain ischemia. Clinicians should pay particular attention to changes in mental status, as these may indicate hypoperfusion and changes in CBF.

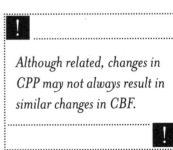

Although related, changes in CPP may not always result in similar changes in CBF.

C. Recommendations for Therapy

To minimize damage to the brain, therapies are primarily designed to minimize oxygen demand and increase CBF and oxygen delivery. The concepts of promoting and/or restoring sufficient flow may be simple, but in practice they may be very difficult to achieve.

Table 8-4 summarizes commonly accepted principles and therapeutic guidelines for treating a variety of primary brain insults and avoiding secondary brain injury. Note the focus on factors that minimize oxygen consumption and maximize oxygen delivery.

Table 8-4 General Principles of Managing Brain Injury

Prevent Abnormal Oxygen Demands

1. Avoid fever. The goal is normothermia. Fever increases metabolic demand, resulting in elevation of ICP.

2. Avoid seizures. Prophylactic anticonvulsant administration is indicated after head trauma to prevent seizures in the first week, but the available evidence does not support longer use in head trauma or use for other neurologic injuries.

3. Avoid anxiety, agitation, or pain. Neuronal oxygen consumption may be decreased by anxiolysis, sedation, and analgesia.

4. Avoid shivering.

5. Minimize stimulation, particularly for the first 72 hours.

Promote Oxygen Delivery

1. Ensure systemic oxygen transport with adequate oxygenation, hemoglobin concentration, and cardiac output. Catecholamine release during brain injury may cause ECG changes, myocardial ischemia, and arrhythmias.

2. Ensure optimal blood pressure. Many primary insults are associated with hypertension that may be a physiologic compensation or may be injurious. Higher blood pressures may be undesirable in patients with unsecured aneurysms and recent intracranial hemorrhage (ICH). *However, excessive lowering of blood pressure may result in secondary ischemia.*

3. Avoid prophylactic or routine hyperventilation because an increase in extracellular brain pH constricts responsive vessels and may reduce CBF to ischemic zones. Brief hyperventilation while instituting other methods to lower elevated ICP may be lifesaving in the patient with evidence of herniation.

4. Ensure euvolemia because hypovolemia may result in systemic hypotension and hypoperfusion of brain tissue.

5. Rapid-sequence intubation can be used for patients with increased ICP. Consider administration of intravenous lidocaine (1.5 mg/kg) or intravenous thiopental (5 mg/kg) to blunt the rise in ICP associated with intubation.

6. Nimodipine should be instituted immediately in patients with SAH.

III. ASSESSMENT

After appropriate management of airway, breathing, and hemodynamic concerns, the priority in neurologic assessment is to distinguish among ischemic, structural, and metabolic/infectious injuries. Suspected ischemic stroke requires an immediate decision regarding thrombolytic therapy, and emergent neurologic consultation should be obtained. The presence of an expanding mass lesion accompanied by significant brain shift may indicate the need for immediate surgical evaluation and possible intervention. The most common causes of such an event include epidural, subdural, and intracerebral hematomas. Intracranial hematomas should be suspected in the settings of head trauma, recent neurosurgery, anticoagulant therapy, alcohol abuse, coagulopathies, and chronic or acute hypertension. The diagnostic procedure of choice, CT scan of the brain, characterizes the extent of structural injury. Medical treatment may be a temporizing option until more definitive therapy is available and implemented.

> **!**
>
> *Early identification of patients with ischemic stroke or potential surgical lesions provides the best opportunity to minimize secondary brain injury.*
>
> **!**

Serial examinations are necessary to detect the possible sequelae of many brain insults. Subtle changes in neurologic function are rarely diagnostic of the specific cause, but any change in the examination is a sensitive indicator of deterioration and should prompt an immediate and thorough reevaluation. For example, a decreased level of consciousness without other lateralizing findings may be due to elevated ICP, hydrocephalus, fever, toxic ingestants, or worsening of a primary encephalopathy, among other possible explanations.

> **!**
>
> *When physical examination or CT scan suggests significant brain compression, medical therapy to reduce ICP should be instituted immediately while awaiting definitive treatment.*
>
> **!**

The GCS score is widely used in the initial and serial assessment of patients with head trauma and is often considered useful in evaluating other brain insults. **Table 8-5** lists its components.

| Table 8-5. | Components of Glasgow Coma Scale Score | |

Clinical Parameter	Adults	Points
Eye opening	Spontaneous	4
	Response to speech	3
	Response to pain	2
	No response	1
Verbal response	Oriented and appropriate	5
	Disoriented and confused	4
	Inappropriate words	3
	Incomprehensible sounds	2
	No response	1
Best motor response	Obeys commands	6
	Localizes pain	5
	Withdraws from pain	4
	Flexor response	3
	Extensor response	2
	No response	1

Total Glasgow Coma Scale Score = eye and verbal and motor scores; best possible score = 15 and worst possible score = 3.

Serial examinations, including evaluation of brainstem and cranial nerve function, should be performed. Pupillary asymmetry is an important sign of serious horizontal shift of the brain, which commonly precedes downward herniation in patients with supratentorial masses. Disconjugate eye movements, a change in respiratory pattern, or deterioration in motor response may suggest an increase in intracranial mass effect and should be investigated immediately.

> **!**
> *Cushing's reflex with increased pulse pressure, bradycardia, and systolic hypertension may be an indication of brain herniation.*
> **!**

When clinical findings suggest herniation, emergent administration of mannitol or hypertonic saline should be initiated to lower ICP, and emergent neurosurgical assistance should be obtained. A brief period of hyperventilation may be considered. Whether repetition of an imaging study or immediate surgical therapy is required depends upon the nature, location, and progression of the pathologic process.

Neurosurgical consultation is advised for any patient who (1) is at risk for developing an expanding intracranial mass lesion; (2) has an open or depressed skull fracture or acute ventricular obstruction; (3) demonstrates blood in the fourth ventricle, cerebellar bleeding, or subarachnoid hemorrhage; or (4) has cerebrospinal fluid leakage. Nontraumatic disease processes, such as spontaneous intracerebral hematoma, large brain tumors, or brain abscesses, require urgent neurosurgical consultation if clinical findings or an imaging study indicate significant mass effect (midline deviation, ventricular obliteration, brainstem or basal cistern compression).

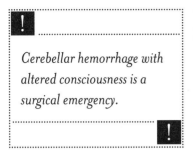

Cerebellar hemorrhage with altered consciousness is a surgical emergency.

Urgent neurosurgical consultation should be obtained for cerebellar hemorrhages and infarcts regardless of the patient's level of consciousness. Although such patients may have few findings on initial clinical examination, progressive swelling around the lesion may necessitate emergent surgical decompression. Typically, any cerebellar mass >3 cm in diameter with hydrocephalus or brainstem compression will require evacuation.

IV. SPECIFIC DIAGNOSES AND CONSIDERATIONS

A. Head Trauma

Approximately 25% of patients who experience blunt head trauma require urgent evacuation of a subdural hematoma (shown in **Figure 8-1A**) or an epidural hematoma (**Figure 8-1B**) to relieve compression of the brain. Consider neurosurgical consultation early.

Figure 8-1A. Subdural Hematoma

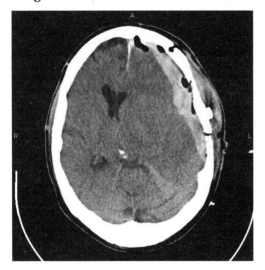

Figure 8-1B. Epidural Hematoma

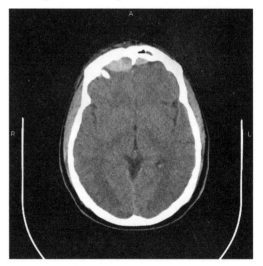

Used with permission from Scot Nolan and Scripps Mercy Hospital, San Diego Campus.

Penetrating and nonpenetrating head injuries are often associated with the formation of cerebral edema, brain contusions, or hemorrhage within the parenchyma. Because the skull cannot expand to accommodate increased intracranial volume and the compensatory space in the subarachnoid space of the spinal canal is very limited, the ICP commonly becomes elevated. Monitoring and treatment of increased ICP is considered an important process in such patients.

Guidelines for the management of severe traumatic brain injury have been developed by the Brain Trauma Foundation on the basis of established evidence. These principles are included in the recommendations in **Table 8-6**.

Table 8-6. General Principles for Treatment of Head Trauma

- Ensure the ABCs of resuscitation.

- Avoid hypotension and maintain systolic blood pressure (SBP) >90 mm Hg. Although it may be valuable to maintain MAP higher than the pressure represented by the SBP, the actual value to target is not clear from current evidence.

- Hypoxemia (PaO_2 <60 mm Hg [8.0 kPa] or SpO_2 <90%) should be avoided while adequate oxygenation is maintained.

- Maintain alignment between head and trunk to avoid jugular compression.

- Keep the head of the bed at 30° to 45° elevation unless the patient is hypotensive. Elevation of the head promotes venous drainage and CSF displacement to the spinal compartment. Avoid or adjust any devices that may constrict the neck.

- Maintain the $PaCO_2$ at 35 to 40 mm Hg (4.7-5.3 kPa). Prophylactic hyperventilation is not recommended. Hyperventilation is recommended as a temporizing measure for reduction of elevated ICP. CBF is often reduced in the first 24 hours after head trauma, and hyperventilation should be avoided in this period to prevent further reductions in CBF.

- Use normal saline as the primary maintenance fluid. Dextrose administration is avoided unless the patient is hypoglycemic. Hypotonic solutions should be avoided.

- Actively treat fever to maintain body temperature at normal levels.

- Sedation may be necessary to control harmful agitation. Use medications with a relatively short half-life to facilitate reliable and ongoing neurologic assessments.

- Maintain usual electrolyte homeostasis and treat hyperglycemia/hypoglycemia.

- Assess and treat coagulation defects.

- Provide nutrition to attain full caloric replacement by day 7 after injury.

- Prophylactic use of anticonvulsants (phenytoin, valproate) for preventing late posttraumatic seizures is not indicated. Although prophylactic anticonvulsants prevent early seizures, they do not improve mortality. If seizures occur, they should be aggressively treated.

- Mannitol (0.25-1 g/kg intravenous push) should be given for signs of herniation or if neurologic deterioration occurs that is not attributable to other factors. There are no specific recommendations for use of hypertonic saline, and expert consultation should be obtained if this type of hyperosmolar therapy is considered.

- Steroids are contraindicated in patients with head trauma.

- ICP monitoring is appropriate
    - For a salvageable patient with a GCS score of 3 to 8 after resuscitation and an abnormal CT scan (hematoma, contusion, edema, herniation, or compressed basal cisterns)
    - For a patient who has normal CT scan results but has at least 2 of the following factors:
        1. Age >40 years
        2. Systolic blood pressure <90 mm Hg
        3. Unilateral or bilateral motor posturing (decerebrate/decorticate)

- Pentobarbital coma should be induced only in the presence of intracranial hypertension that cannot be controlled by other means and requires consultation with experts in neurosurgery and critical care medicine.

- The target CPP is in the range of 50 to 70 mm Hg, although patients with intact autoregulation may tolerate higher CPP values. The ideal CPP is the pressure that provides adequate cerebral perfusion and oxygenation while ICP is maintained <20 mm Hg. This approach emphasizes maintaining the lowest perfusion pressure compatible with adequate CBF.

B. Intracerebral Hemorrhage

Patients with intracerebral hemorrhage (hemorrhagic stroke) frequently have a history of hypertension and may be of advanced age. Blood pressure control is controversial in these cases.

Elevated blood pressure levels may contribute to rebleeding and edema formation but may also preserve regional CPP. If the elevated blood pressure is causing considerable systemic effects, such as cardiac stress, *modest* reductions may be safe. The target blood pressure should take into account the patient's age, baseline blood pressure, presumed cause of hemorrhage, and intracranial pressure (if known). If elevated intracranial pressure is suspected, expert consultation is advised for assistance with blood pressure management. Preferred agents include α-blockers and β-blockers, such as labetalol, and calcium channel blockers such as nicardipine. Venodilators and ganglionic blockers should be avoided. Primary arterial vasodilators remain controversial, but drugs that cause substantial intracranial vasodilation (eg, nitroprusside, nitroglycerin) and the potential for increased bleeding should be avoided.

Expansion of the hematoma may occur in one third of patients, especially patients who are taking anticoagulants, have liver disease or low platelet counts, and those whose original hemorrhage is large or irregular. Some neurosurgeons may consider removal of the hematoma, especially in a young, clinically deteriorating patient with a large lobar hemorrhage or when the hemorrhage is associated with a surgically accessible lesion, such as an aneurysm, arteriovenous malformation, or cavernous angioma.

C. Subarachnoid Hemorrhage

Characteristic historical ("worst headache of their life") and CT findings usually confirm the diagnosis of subarachnoid hemorrhage. Classification systems (eg, the Hunt and Hess scale) have been used to categorize findings and suggest prognosis in relation to surgical therapy but do not alter the care provided by the primary team, as outlined in **Table 8-7.**

Table 8-7. **Treatment of Subarachnoid Hemorrhage**

- Ensure the ABCs of resuscitation.
- Control blood pressure early, prior to definitive surgical therapy. Rebleeding is the major early complication until the aneurysm is clipped or coiled. A variety of intravenous antihypertensive agents have been useful. Labetalol and nicardipine have been selectively advocated. Nitroprusside should be avoided because of its tendency to induce cerebral vasodilation. Consider the effects of nimodipine on blood pressure when using other antihypertensive agents.
- Initiate oral nimodipine 60 mg every 4 hours. (An intravenous preparation is available in some countries.) Hypotension should be avoided.
- Maintain euvolemia. Some advocate gentle intravascular volume expansion. Significant cardiac injury can occur as a result of high circulating catecholamine levels; thus, careful attention to arrhythmias and cardiac function is necessary.
- Avoid hyponatremia, which is commonly encountered. Normal saline should be used as the primary intravenous fluid. Hyponatremia in SAH patients usually reflects cerebral salt wasting rather than the syndrome of inappropriate antidiuretic hormone (SIADH) release. Cerebral salt wasting should not be treated with the volume restriction utilized for SIADH. Both groups of patients will have inappropriately high urine osmolalities, so this marker cannot be used to indicate SIADH. If salt administration is indicated for cerebral salt wasting, small amounts of hypertonic saline may be necessary. Hyponatremia should be corrected slowly, as central pontine myelinolysis can occur from rapid and aggressive sodium correction.
- Rapid evaluation of the aneurysm location for surgical clipping or coiling requires urgent neurosurgical and/or neurointerventional radiology consultation.
- Patients with SAH are best managed in centers with the capacity for clipping, coiling, and vasospasm management.

D. Ischemic Stroke

Ischemic stroke usually occurs due to the thromboembolic obstruction of arteries. Evidence supports the use of intravenous recombinant tissue plasminogen activator (rtPA) during the first 3 hours of the onset of ischemic stroke in an attempt to dissolve the obstruction and restore blood flow, as advocated by the American Academy of Neurology and the American Heart Association (AHA).

Onset of symptoms or the last time the patient was reported to be seen without symptoms (or at baseline) is the time used to determine whether a patient is a candidate for thrombolytic therapy. After the initial CT scan rules out the presence of hemorrhage, intravenous rtPA should be administered in a dosage of 0.9 mg/kg (10% as a bolus over 1 minute and 90% in a 1-hour infusion). Personnel who are not familiar with the use of rtPA for the acute treatment of nonhemorrhagic stroke should seek immediate neurologic consultation prior to administering therapy.

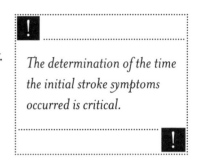

The determination of the time the initial stroke symptoms occurred is critical.

Supportive care includes management of hypertension. Although elevated blood pressure is often present early, a decrease in pressure usually occurs in the first hours after stroke without specific medical treatment. There is no evidence to define a level of blood pressure that requires emergent intervention. Consensus recommendations from the AHA and the American Stroke Association are presented in **Table 8-8** for patients that are candidates for thrombolytic therapy. Emergency administration of antihypertensive agents is not indicated in other patients unless the diastolic blood pressure (DBP) is >120 mm Hg, systolic blood pressure (SBP) is >220 mm Hg or there is evidence of end-organ injury (pulmonary edema, myocardial ischemia, etc). If treatment is indicated, the blood pressure should be lowered cautiously with a reasonable goal of lowering the pressure approximately 15% in the first 24 hours after stroke onset.

Urgent anticoagulation with unfractionated or low-molecular-weight heparin is not indicated in acute stroke. Prophylactic heparin should be administered to immobilized patients to prevent venous thromboembolism but the ideal time to start this therapy is not known. Aspirin administration within 24 to 48 hours of stroke onset is recommended for most patients after hemorrhage is excluded, but clopidogrel administration is not recommended. Significant edema formation, typically within the first 72 hours, or extensive hemorrhage within the ischemic zone may require ICP monitoring or emergent craniectomy.

Table 8-8.	Blood Pressure Management in Patients Eligible for rtPA Treatment
Blood Pressure	**Treatment**
Pretreatment	
SBP >185 or DBP >110 mm Hg	Labetalol 10-20 mg IV bolus as 1-2 doses
	Nitroglycerin paste 1-2 in
	Nicardipine infusion 5 mg/h titrated to goal BP
	(maximum 15 mg/h); reduce infusion to 3 mg/h when goal BP attained
Posttreatment	
SBP >230 mm Hg or DBP 121-140 mm Hg	Labetalol 10-20 mg IV bolus; may repeat every 10-20 min to maximum 300 mg
	Labetalol 10 mg IV bolus followed by infusion at 2-8 mg/min
	Nicardipine 5 mg/h IV infusion and titrate (maximum 15 mg/h)
SBP 180-230 mm Hg or DBP 105-120 mm Hg	Labetalol 10 mg IV bolus; may repeat every 10-20 min to maximum 300 mg
	Labetalol 10 mg IV bolus followed by infusion at 2-8 mg/min

Abbreviations: SBP, systolic blood pressure; DBP, diastolic blood pressure.
Adapted from Adams HP, del Zoppo G, Alberts MJ, et al. Guidelines for the early management of adults with ischemic stroke. *Stroke*. 2007;38:1655.

E. Anoxic Injury

Relative anoxia may be a part of other injuries and may be due to airway loss, systemic hypoxemia, hypoperfusion, and other causes. Anoxia may also be the primary brain insult, as occurs during cardiac arrest. Neuronal injury or death may occur as a direct result of the primary insult of hypoxemia or hypoperfusion or may occur secondarily due to glial swelling, cytotoxic edema, or other causes of the no-reflow phenomenon. Similarly, reperfusion-induced cytotoxic mediators may secondarily injure the brain.

The primary care team should maintain the usual standards of optimal oxygen delivery. Despite extensive studies of many agents and therapy options, none has proven selectively beneficial, nor has the poor prognosis from anoxic brain injury improved over time. Monitoring of ICP is rarely pursued. Systemic cooling to approximately 33°C for 12 to 24 hours improves neurologic outcome in coma after out-of-hospital ventricular fibrillation cardiac arrest.

F. Metabolic Abnormalities, Infectious Emergencies, and Seizures

In adult patients with depressed consciousness after initial resuscitation, the use of 50% dextrose (50 mL intravenously) and thiamine (100 mg intravenously) should be considered for the treatment of potential hypoglycemia and the prevention of Wernicke's encephalopathy if an immediate determination of the blood glucose concentration is not available. Intravenous naloxone should be administered if narcotic intoxication is a possibility. Other metabolic abnormalities, such as electrolyte disorders (ie, acute hyponatremia, hypercalcemia), liver failure,

> **!**
>
> *In the absence of papilledema or focal neurologic signs, a lumbar puncture may be performed without a prior CT scan for evaluation of meningitis.*
>
> **!**

or uremia may also cause coma. Because headache or altered state of consciousness accompanied by fever, nuchal rigidity, and leukocytosis suggests meningitis or encephalitis, the cerebrospinal fluid should be submitted for physical, chemical, and bacteriologic (culture and Gram's stain) studies. If clinical examination suggests a mass lesion or elevated ICP, a CT scan should be performed before lumbar puncture. If the CT scan reveals evidence of mass effect or generalized cerebral edema, a lumbar puncture may precipitate a herniation syndrome and should be postponed. When infection is part of the differential diagnosis, appropriate antibacterial and antiviral treatment should be initiated before performing the imaging study because early therapy for bacterial meningitis or encephalitis may be lifesaving. Antibiotics should also be given if lumbar puncture is delayed for any other reason. Treatment recommendations for adults are outlined in **Chapter 11** and those for children are in **Chapter 16**.

Seizure activity after an acute brain injury increases cerebral oxygen requirements and may elevate the ICP if intracranial compliance is reduced. Appropriate therapy should be administered to terminate seizure activity as soon as possible. The intravenous administration of anticonvulsants, many of which have a potent sedative effect, may depress respiratory function and requires appropriate supportive therapy. In addition, hypotension may occur, requiring additional intravenous fluids and/or vasopressors to preserve MAP and CPP. If neuromuscular-blocking agents must be administered, continuous electroencephalographic (EEG) monitoring is necessary to determine if seizures are continuing to occur despite pharmacologic muscle paralysis.

> **!**
>
> *Avoid the use of neuromuscular–blocking agents in patients at risk for seizure because these agents obscure detection of seizure activity.*
>
> **!**

Intravenous benzodiazepines are administered at the onset of seizure activity and lorazepam at an initial dose of 2 mg in adults may terminate the seizure. Persistent seizure activity indicates status epilepticus and requires emergent neurologic consultation. Lorazepam in a dosage of 0.1 mg/kg should be administered for status epilepticus in adults. Subsequently, a full intravenous loading dose of phenytoin (18-20 mg/kg in glucose-free solution, infused no faster than 50 mg/min) or an equivalent dose of fosphenytoin should be administered. Alternative anticonvulsants used in status epilepticus include propofol (3 mg/kg loading dose, then infusion of 1-5 mg/kg/h) or midazolam (0.1 mg/kg loading dose, then infusion of 1-20 µg/kg/min) with EEG and other ICU monitoring.

G. Brain Death Criteria and Organ Donation

Despite the best efforts of the medical and surgical teams, massive injury, cerebral infarction, or hemorrhage may result in a loss of all cerebral and brainstem functions. Evaluation of brain death and the guidelines for organ donation are variable, depending on the country, state, and facility.

Measures of brain death may include a combination of cortical and brainstem function testing, apnea evaluation, and confirmatory tests such as transcranial Doppler ultrasonography or EEG. Wide variations in evaluation techniques and criteria for diagnosis of brain death may exist from state to state and from country to country. For more information about brain death and organ donation, see **Appendix 11**.

Neurologic Support

Key Points

- Brain injury occurs as a consequence of a primary insult and secondary injury. The prevention of secondary brain injury is a critical goal for the primary care team.

- The most significant mechanisms for secondary injury in brain injured patients are hypotension and hypoxia.

- Optimizing oxygen delivery while controlling oxygen consumption is a general treatment principle for all types of brain injury.

- Important principles/guidelines for initial treatment apply to all types of primary brain injury to prevent harmful secondary sequelae.

- Blood pressure management is dependent on the initial brain injury. However, excessive lowering of blood pressure in any acute brain injury may induce secondary ischemia.

- Avoid prophylactic or routine hyperventilation in patients with brain injuries. Mannitol should be given and hyperventilation initiated for signs of herniation or if neurologic deterioration occurs that is not attributable to other factors.

- Ensure euvolemia using normal saline as the primary maintenance fluid. Use only glucose-free intravenous fluids.

- Seizure activity after acute brain injury should be terminated with an intravenous dose of a benzodiazepine followed by an intravenous loading dose of phenytoin or fosphenytoin.

Suggested Readings

1. Adams HP, del Zoppo G, Alberts MJ, et al. Guidelines for the early management of adults with ischemic stroke. *Stroke.* 2007;38:1655. Available online at www.stroke-site.org.

2. Adelson PD, Bratton SL, Carney NA, et al. Guidelines for the acute medical management of severe traumatic brain injury in infants, children, and adolescents. *Pediatr Crit Care Med.* 2003;4(3)(suppl):S1. Available online at www.braintrauma.org.

3. Brain Trauma Foundation, American Association of Neurological Surgeons, Congress of Neurological Surgeons, AANS/CNS Joint Section on Neurotrauma and Critical Care. Guidelines for the management of severe traumatic brain injury. 3rd ed. *J Neurotrauma.* 2007;24(suppl 1). Available online at www.braintrauma.org.

4. Brisman JL, Song JK, Newell DW. Cerebral aneurysms. *N Engl J Med.* 2006;255:928.

5. Broderick J, Connolly S, Feldman E, et al. Guidelines for the management of spontaneous intracerebral hemorrhage in adults. 2007 update. *Stroke.* 2007;38:2001. Available online at www.stroke-site.org.

6. Marik PE, Varon J. The management of status epilepticus. *Chest.* 2004;126:582.

7. Qureshi AI, Tuhrim S, Broderick JP, et al. Spontaneous intracerebral hemorrhage. *N Engl J Med.* 2001;344:1450.

8. Prasad K, Al-Roomi K, Krishnan PR, Sequiera R. Anticonvulsant therapy for status epilepticus (review). Cochrane Database Syst Rev. 2007;(2):CD003723.

9. Royal College of Physicians. National Clinical Guidelines for Stroke, 2nd ed. Prepared by the Intercollegiate Stroke Working Party. London, RCP, 2004. Available online at www.rcplondon.ac.uk.

10. Suarez JI, Tarr RW, Selman WR. Aneurysmal subarachnoid hemorrhage. *N Engl J Med.* 2006;354:387.

▣ Web Sites

1. Brain Trauma Foundation. http://www.braintrauma.org. In addition to guidelines for management of traumatic brain injury, this site offers Internet-based continuing education programs, including recorded presentations, live Web-based lectures, and interactive learning modules based on the latest scientific-evidence, and professional and academic resources for people interested in learning more about traumatic brain injury and quality improvement in healthcare.

2. Brain Attack Coalition. http://www.stroke-site.org. This Web site contains such practical information for professionals as guidelines for the diagnosis of strokes, order sets and checklists from a variety of institutions, and pathways—step-by-step approaches to the management of stroke. It also provides information and resources for stroke patients, families, and caregivers.

Chapter 9:

BASIC TRAUMA AND BURN SUPPORT

✓ Objectives

- Prioritize and initiate a timely assessment of the traumatized patient.

- Initiate treatment of life-threatening traumatic injury.

- Utilize radiography in identifying significant traumatic injury.

- Identify and respond to significant changes in the status of a patient after traumatic injury.

- Initiate early burn management.

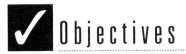 Case Study

A middle-aged man has been brought to the emergency department after his car collided with a semitrailer. He was not wearing a seatbelt and was ejected. He is making incoherent sounds and has oral secretions that he is unable to clear. He has an open femur fracture with hemorrhage as well as blood coming from a scalp laceration. Contusions are present over the left chest wall and upper quadrant of the abdomen. Vital signs include a blood pressure of 90/60 mm Hg, pulse rate of 125/min, and respiratory rate of 35/min. The patient is lethargic but moves all extremities voluntarily. His skin is cool and clammy.

- What does the primary survey indicate?

- What are the most urgent initial interventions?

I. INTRODUCTION

It is not the intention of the FCCS program to replace the Advanced Trauma Life Support (ATLS) course provided by the American College of Surgeons. The material presented here is intended to highlight similar issues. Care providers who regularly encounter patients with traumatic injuries are encouraged to enroll in an ATLS course.

A. Death Following Injury

Death due to injury occurs in 1 of 3 time periods. The first time period is within seconds to minutes of injury. During this early period, deaths generally result from severe brain or high spinal-cord injury or rupture of the heart, aorta, or other large blood vessel. Due to the severity of injury, few of these patients can be salvaged, and prevention is the only way to reduce such trauma-related deaths. The second peak occurs within minutes to hours following injury. Deaths occurring during this period are usually due to subdural and epidural hematomas, hemopneumothorax, solid organ rupture (spleen or liver), pelvic fractures, or other injuries associated with blood loss. The "golden hour" after injury is characterized by the need for rapid assessment and resolution of these problems. The third peak occurs days to weeks after the initial injury and is most often due to sepsis with associated multiple organ failure.

Three premises guide the approach to injury. The most important is that the greatest threat to life must be treated first. For example, the inability to breathe kills more quickly than the loss of circulating blood volume. The second premise is that lack of a definitive diagnosis should never impede application of indicated treatment. And the third is that a detailed history is not essential to begin evaluation in the setting of acute injury.

II. TRAUMA MANAGEMENT

Early management of the seriously injured patient requires simultaneous evaluation and treatment. The first goal is to ensure adequate oxygen delivery to vital organs by following an established sequence of priorities that allows identification and treatment of immediately life threatening injuries (primary assessment). The patient's vital functions must be assessed quickly and efficiently. Patient management should consist of a rapid primary evaluation, resuscitation of vital functions, more detailed secondary assessment (from head to toe), and finally, the initiation of definitive care. This process begins with the ABCDE of trauma care, which guides the identification of life-threatening conditions through the initial assessment sequence of airway, breathing, circulation, disability, and exposure (**Table 9-1**).

Table 9-1.	Initial Assessment of Trauma

Airway maintenance with cervical spine precautions

Breathing: ventilation and oxygenation

Circulation with hemorrhage control

Disability: brief neurologic examination

Exposure/environment: undress patient, but avoid hypothermia

A surgeon skilled in trauma management should be consulted early in the course of all serious trauma cases. When a surgeon is not immediately available or when the patient is awaiting transfer, ongoing evaluation (tertiary assessment) and intervention should continue.

A. Primary Assessment: Initial Evaluation and Resuscitation

1. Airway and Breathing

If the patient is able to communicate verbally, the airway is unlikely to be in immediate jeopardy; however, repeated assessment of airway patency is essential. Patients with severe head injury (GCS score of 8 or less) usually require placement of a definitive, protective airway. Nonpurposeful motor responses support the need for immediate airway management.

> !
>
> *Airway patency should be frequently reassessed, particularly in patients with head injury, shock, and facial fractures.*
>
> !

The airway should first be assessed to ascertain patency. Assessment for signs of airway obstruction includes inspection for foreign bodies and facial, mandibular, or tracheal/laryngeal fractures that may result in airway obstruction. It is not uncommon for patients to develop signs of airway obstruction after benign initial presentation in the emergency department.

After blunt trauma, airway control should proceed on the assumption that an unstable fracture of the cervical spine (C-spine) exists. The patency of the airway must be established, supplemental oxygen provided, and adequacy of ventilation ensured, as discussed in **Chapter 2**. If active airway intervention is needed before radiologic evaluation for possible C-spine fracture, the technique chosen for airway control (intubation, adjunctive device, or surgical airway) should take into account the expertise of available personnel, type of equipment available, and patient factors and injuries. If the patient is apneic or deteriorating rapidly, standard orotracheal intubation should be attempted with the use of in-line manual stabilization of the head and neck. Proper in-line stabilization may be accomplished from the front or the side of the patient. One care provider supports the occiput and mandible with both hands to maintain neck alignment without applying traction

> !
>
> *If the patient is combative and needs an airway, a rapid-sequence intubation should be performed.*
>
> !

or distraction. With secure stabilization, the anterior portion of the cervical collar may be removed to allow airway interventions and application of cricoid pressure. In-line stabilization is continued until the cervical collar is replaced and the endotracheal tube or other airway device is secured. If an airway cannot otherwise be secured, a laryngeal mask airway, esophageal-tracheal double-lumen airway device, or surgical cricothyrotomy are indicated.

a. Key Issues in Airway Control

Facial fractures are not an immediate treatment priority unless heavy bleeding or uncontrollable secretions are present. Similarly, facial fractures usually do not require that the patient be intubated. Mandibular fractures, however, are more likely to be associated with soft-tissue injury that may compromise the airway.

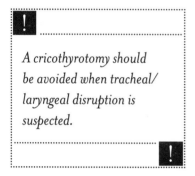

A cricothyrotomy should be avoided when tracheal/laryngeal disruption is suspected.

Tracheal/laryngeal disruption or fracture most commonly occurs at the junction of the larynx and trachea. Signs and symptoms may include hoarseness, subcutaneous air, edema, or ecchymosis of the neck, but the patient may have minimal evidence of injury. Allow the patient to assume a position of comfort, including sitting if spinal injury is unlikely. Airway management by an experienced physician may include an awake tracheostomy. Neurologic examination alone does not exclude a C-spine injury. The following considerations apply to patients at risk for C-spine injury:

■ Presence of paraplegia or quadriplegia is presumptive evidence of spinal instability.

■ Early computed tomographic (CT) scans may facilitate evaluation of the C-spine in any head-injured or intubated patient. Adding CT evaluation of the C-spine to the initial CT scan of the head is an appropriate strategy after injury.

■ Patients with neurologic deficits potentially due to a C-spine injury require neurosurgical consultation.

■ Patients who are alert, awake, and without changes in mental status, neck pain, distracting injuries, or neurologic deficits may be considered to have a stable C-spine and need no radiologic studies.

■ All other patients should have at least a lateral view of the C-spine that includes the base of the occiput to the upper border of the first thoracic vertebra.

■ Exclusion of bony injury does not eliminate the possibility of ligamentous disruption. Magnetic resonance imaging (MRI) is a useful tool to facilitate clearance of ligamentous injury if the examination is not reliable for injury.

Additional details regarding imaging to evaluate for cervical spine injury are given below, under "Radiologic Evaluation."

b. Key Injuries

Rib fractures are often missed on a chest radiograph; however, a fracture may be suspected and documented by tenderness over the fracture during physical examination. Pain control may be required to ensure adequate spontaneous ventilation. High-risk patients, such as the elderly or those with chronic obstructive pulmonary disease, may require epidural analgesia to prevent the deleterious effects of systemic narcotics. Flail chest resulting from rib fractures is manifested by paradoxical movement of the involved portion of the chest wall (ie, inward movement of the segment during inhalation). Frequently, flail chest is associated with contusion of the underlying lung, pain, and hypoxemia.

Pneumothorax is frequently associated with rib fractures and usually requires tube thoracostomy (**Appendix 8**). Suction is routinely applied via the drainage apparatus at approximately 20 cm H_2O. Any patient who has a pneumothorax on plain chest films and is receiving general anesthesia should have a chest tube in place. Tension pneumothorax is evaluated and treated as discussed in **Chapter 5**. Open pneumothorax is generally associated with soft-tissue loss requiring dressing closure and chest-tube placement. Massive hemothorax is suggested by physical examination and chest radiograph. Rapid loss of 1,000 to 2,000 mL of blood or ongoing blood loss of >200 mL/h is an indication for thoracotomy.

2. Circulation

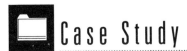

Case Study

A young man arrives in the emergency department with an epigastric stab wound, but the character of the weapon is unknown. Presenting systolic blood pressure is 90 mm Hg and the patient is tachycardiac. His systolic blood pressure improves to >100 mm Hg systolic with administration of intravenous fluids but deteriorates when bolus fluids are stopped. Extremities are cool and the patient is anxious.

    – Is this patient in shock?

    – What is the primary concern?

    – What therapy is recommended?

Hemorrhage is the most likely cause of postinjury shock. Initial empiric treatment in adults consists of crystalloid infusion (2 liters of warmed lactated Ringer's solution) via 2 large-bore intravenous cannulas and control of external hemorrhage by means of manual compression. Targets for empiric volume therapy are normalization of blood pressure, reversal of tachycardia, and maintenance of adequate organ perfusion (see **Chapter 7**). When hypoperfusion and vascular compensation limit peripheral access, cannulation of a central vein (ideally with a 7F, 8.5F, or 9F introducer) is an alternative, as is saphenous vein cutdown. Concomitant diagnostic studies for the source of bleeding if an external source is not apparent can include chest radiograph, pelvic radiograph, focused assessment sonography in trauma (FAST), diagnostic peritoneal lavage (DPL), or CT scan of the abdomen (if the patient stabilizes quickly).

Immediate control of external hemorrhage should proceed simultaneously with aggressive resuscitation. In trauma to an extremity, direct pressure is recommended, whereas blind clamping at bleeding vessels is discouraged to avoid potential injury to adjacent structures (eg, nerves). A urinary catheter should be inserted as soon as practical to monitor urine output as a gauge of renal perfusion, although it is contraindicated in male patients when urethral injury is suspected (e.g. blood at the meatus, scrotal hematoma, or high-riding prostate).

As **Table 9-2** shows, a patient's systolic blood pressure, heart rate, respiratory rate, and mental status can be used to assess blood loss. The American College of Surgeons also validates a decrease in pulse pressure as a sign of occult hypoperfusion. Circulating blood volume corresponds to 7% of normal body weight (70 mL/kg) in an adult and 8% to 9% (80-90 mL/kg) of normal body weight in children. It should be noted that a blood loss up to 1,200 mL may occur in an adult (70 kg) with no hypotension and minimal tachycardia. Class II hemorrhage is uncomplicated shock, but crystalloid resuscitation is required. Class III hemorrhage requires crystalloid resuscitation and often blood replacement. Class IV hemorrhage can be considered preterminal and requires aggressive measures to restore volume and red blood cell mass and to control bleeding. Treatment should be directed by the initial response to therapy rather than by a classification scheme.

> **!**
>
> *If the initial fluid bolus produces only transient improvement or no response, immediate surgical consultation is required.*
>
> **!**

Table 9-2. Hemorrhage Classification[a]

Variable	CLASS			
	I	II	III	IV
Systolic blood pressure (mm Hg)	Normal	Normal	Decreased	Decreased
Pulse (beats/min)	<100	>100	>120	>140
Respiratory rate (breaths/min)	14-20	20-30	30-40	>35
Mental status	Anxious	Agitated	Confused	Lethargic
Blood loss (mL)	<750	750-1500	1500-2000	>2000
Blood loss (%)	<15	15-30	30-40	>40

[a] Adapted from American College of Surgeons Committee on Trauma. Advanced Trauma Life Support for Doctors (ATLS). 7th ed. Chicago, IL: American College of Surgeons; 2004:74.

Crystalloid resuscitation, usually with 2 to 3 liters of lactated Ringer's solution (>50 mL/kg), should be followed by the administration of packed red blood cells (PRBCs). Fully crossmatched blood is rarely available for emergency trauma resuscitation. Uncrossmatched type-specific blood can be safely administered and is available in most hospitals within 15 to 20 minutes after a request is received. If type-specific blood is not available and the patient is unstable, O-negative PRBCs should be used. When O-negative PRBCs are not available, O-positive PRBCs may be used. The patient may become sensitized to the Rh factor, but this is significant only in female patients of childbearing age (who must be treated with Rh_o(D) immune globulin injection to prevent antibody formation).

Transfusion of other blood products, such as fresh frozen plasma, platelets, or cryoprecipitate, is usually not part of the initial resuscitation but may be urgently required if bleeding persists and/ or a coagulopathy develops. In patients with ongoing significant bleeding, serial coagulation profiles (which include prothrombin time, partial thromboplastin time, hemoglobin, hematocrit, and platelet count) should be obtained. Platelet counts <50,000/mm^3 are usually treated with platelet transfusion in the setting of ongoing hemorrhage. Likewise, abnormalities of prothrombin time and partial thromboplastin time in the bleeding patient should be treated with fresh frozen plasma (10-20 mL/kg initially). Surgical bleeding should be addressed directly, usually in the operating room. Massive volume resuscitation, a common cause of reduced coagulation factors and dilutional thrombocytopenia, requires platelet transfusion and factor replacement. Clinical manifestations of clotting dysfunction should be treated empirically with platelets and fresh frozen plasma when laboratory evaluation of these parameters is not available. The use of recombinant factor VIIa for the management of trauma-related coagulopathy is still under investigation.

> **!**
>
> *Citrate in PRBCs may chelate calcium, promoting a coagulation defect in patients receiving massive transfusion. Ionized calcium levels should be monitored and calcium administered as needed.*
>
> **!**

3. Disability/Exposure

Rapid neurologic evaluation is performed in the emergency department and includes determination of level of consciousness, pupillary size and reaction, lateralizing signs, and level of spinal cord injury. The Glasgow Coma Scale score is a quick, simple method for determining the level of consciousness and is predictive of outcome (particularly the best motor response). A decrease in the level of consciousness may reflect decreased cerebral oxygenation or perfusion or may be due to direct brain injury. An altered level of consciousness indicates the need for immediate reevaluation of oxygenation, ventilation, and tissue perfusion. Hypoglycemia, ethanol, narcotics, and other drugs may also affect the level of consciousness. Changes in the level of consciousness should be considered as due to intracerebral conditions until proven otherwise.

Throughout the initial resuscitation period, efforts should be made to control and prevent hypothermia. Patients are often hypothermic after environmental exposure, and the body temperature may fall even more after administration of room temperature resuscitation fluids and cold blood, removal of clothing for examination purposes, loss of normal temperature-regulating reflexes in shock, or some medications. Hypothermia contributes to coagulation abnormalities, cardiovascular collapse, and poor outcome, and should be avoided and treated. Warm intravenous fluids, heated respiratory gases if the patient is mechanically ventilated, warm rooms, insulating covers, and heating lamps can be used.

4. Monitoring

Improvements in parameters such as heart rate, blood pressure, pulse pressure, ventilatory rate, acid-base status, body temperature, and urinary output are the best guides to adequacy of resuscitation. Early evaluation begins during the initial survey and reevaluation should be done periodically. Pulse oximetry is another valuable adjunct for monitoring oxygenation in injured patients, but it is not useful for evaluating the adequacy of ventilation. Finally, blood pressure may be a poor measure of actual tissue perfusion. In addition to the assessment of metabolic acidosis and lactate concentrations, perfusion of extremities must be evaluated. Circulation to extremities may be problematic in elderly patients, and early invasive monitoring of tissue perfusion and/or cardiac function may be needed.

5. Hemorrhagic Shock

As resuscitation proceeds, it is crucial to identify potential causes of hypotension. Following traumatic injury a search for occult blood loss should be undertaken after any external hemorrhage is controlled. The most frequent sites for such blood loss are the chest, abdomen, and pelvis.

a. Hemothorax

A chest radiograph (ideally with the patient in upright or reverse Trendelenburg position if hemodynamically stable) is a reliable screen for intrathoracic bleeding. Ultrasonography of the chest may also reliably detect hemothorax or pericardial fluid. Hemothorax should be drained promptly by tube thoracostomy. A radiograph should be obtained subsequently to verify location of the chest tube, blood evacuation, and lung expansion. As noted earlier, rapid loss ≥1,000 mL of blood via the chest tube and continued losses >200 mL/h for 4 hours may require thoracotomy. If available, autotransfusion devices should be used in patients with rapid hemorrhage.

b. Intra-abdominal Hemorrhage

Abdominal examination is often misleading in the detection of acute hemoperitoneum, especially in patients with lower chest trauma, rib fractures, spinal cord injury, intoxication, or altered level of consciousness. Any patient who has sustained significant blunt torso injury from a direct blow or deceleration or from a penetrating torso injury must be considered to have an abdominal visceral or vascular injury. Focused assessment sonography in trauma and diagnostic peritoneal lavage are the most expedient and reliable methods of identifying significant intraperitoneal hemorrhage, although the FAST exam has largely replaced the use of DPL in most institutions. When readily available and used by trained individuals, FAST has the sensitivity, specificity, and accuracy of DPL in detecting hemoperitoneum. When present, hemoperitoneum requires an immediate surgical evaluation to determine the need for an operative intervention. In many cases, abdominal CT scan may be appropriate in stable patients to identify the source of bleeding. Abdominal hemorrhage frequently comes from liver or splenic laceration, visceral injury, or retroperitoneal hematoma. Patients with unstable or abnormal vital signs are usually not candidates for CT scanning and often require surgery to control damage.

c. Pelvic Hemorrhage

Assessment of bony stability by means of physical examination and plain radiographs of the pelvis is crucial for early identification of major pelvic fractures. Patients with pelvic fractures are at high risk for major bleeding, which is usually venous. Initial management includes vigorous blood volume replacement and, possibly, mechanical tamponade with a sheet wrapped tightly around the pelvis or other strategies to produce circumferential compression. External skeletal fixation may be helpful if the fracture anatomy is appropriate, and an orthopedic surgeon should be consulted early in the course of treatment. In patients with arterial bleeding associated with pelvic injury, CT scanning will reveal a blush of contrast loss. Pelvic angiography for embolization should be considered in the persistently hypotensive patient due to an increased likelihood for arterial bleeding. Angiography may be required in approximately 10% of patients with pelvic fractures.

6. Nonhemorrhagic Shock

The differential diagnosis of nonhemorrhagic shock in the trauma patient includes obstructive shock (tension pneumothorax, cardiac tamponade), blunt cardiac injury, air embolism, and neurogenic shock with acute spinal cord injury. Head injury is a rare cause of hypotension, but when it occurs, it is usually a preterminal event.

a. Tension Pneumothorax

Tension pneumothorax causes hemodynamic compromise and pulmonary dysfunction due to acute compression of the lung parenchyma, space occupation, and a shift of the mediastinum away from the hemithorax with the increased pressure. Do not wait for a chest radiograph to make this diagnosis. Breath sounds will be diminished, lung expansion will be asynchronous, and patients may develop respiratory distress, acute desaturation, bradycardia, and occasionally, distended neck veins. It is important to note, however, that classic venous distension may be absent in the setting of pneumothorax complicated by hypovolemia and that all but gross changes in breath sounds may be difficult to

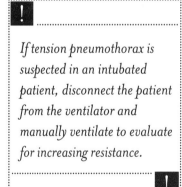

If tension pneumothorax is suspected in an intubated patient, disconnect the patient from the ventilator and manually ventilate to evaluate for increasing resistance.

detect in the resuscitation room. Tracheal shift is a late sign and may not be a presenting finding. In adults, needle thoracostomy is performed via the midclavicular line in the second intercostal space. This is a lifesaving intervention that is followed by placement of a chest tube.

b. Neurogenic Shock

Neurogenic shock occurs when cervical or high thoracic spinal cord injury (above T6 level) causes sympathectomy. It is characterized by hypotension, frequently associated with relative or absolute bradycardia. Flaccid paralysis, loss of extremity reflexes, and priapism may be associated neurologic findings. Treatment for hypotension includes volume resuscitation and vasopressors (phenylephrine, norepinephrine, or dopamine) if volume loading does not reverse hypotension. Atropine is indicated in the presence of bradycardia associated with hemodynamic instability.

c. Cardiac Tamponade

The classic signs of cardiac tamponade—hypotension, distant heart sounds, jugular venous distension, and pulsus paradoxus—may be obscured due to noise in the trauma area and hypovolemia (decreasing jugular distention). Ultrasound (FAST) is a sensitive examination for fluid in the pericardial sac. Pericardiocentesis via a surgical pericardial window should be considered for the patient with refractory shock, persistent central venous hypertension, and a high-risk penetrating wound (between the nipples, above the costal margin, below the clavicles). When surgical expertise is not available, a needle/catheter pericardiocentesis may be performed as a temporizing measure. Occasionally, major blunt chest trauma ruptures the cardiac surface. Most cases involve atrial tears and can be repaired if diagnosed early.

d. Blunt Cardiac Injury

> !
>
> *The right ventricle is most frequently involved in blunt cardiac injury, and volume challenge is the initial therapy for hypotension in the absence of pulmonary edema.*
>
> !

The diagnosis of blunt cardiac injury should be suspected in a patient involved in a high-speed, frontal impact accident who has unexplained hypotension, an unexplained arrhythmia, or, less commonly, cardiogenic shock. Changes in the electrocardiograms (ECGs) are usually nonspecific and can include premature ventricular contractions, bundle branch block, atrial fibrillation, unexplained sinus tachycardia, and ST-segment changes. If blunt cardiac injury is a possibility, a screening ECG should be obtained in the emergency department. Abnormalities other than tachycardia warrant 24 hours of monitoring for possible sudden arrhythmias. Hemodynamically stable individuals without ECG abnormalities need no further cardiac workup or observation. Echocardiography is not indicated in stable patients but may show abnormal wall motion in patients with cardiac injury. Use of cardiac troponins in diagnosing blunt cardiac injury is inconclusive and offers no additional information beyond the ECG. Treatment includes correction of acidosis, hypoxia, and electrolyte abnormalities; judicious administration of fluid; and pharmacologic treatment of life-threatening arrhythmias.

Inotropes may be indicated in some circumstances. It is important to ensure that refractory hypotension is not due to ongoing blood loss. Critical care consultation is important, and a pulmonary artery catheter may provide important information for diagnosis and treatment in this circumstance, particularly in elderly patients or in the setting of preexisting cardiac disease.

B. Secondary Assessment: Diagnosis and Treatment of Other Injuries

Most patients with acute injuries can be resuscitated to a hemodynamically stable state. A good primary survey should immediately identify life-threatening injuries. The next goal is to complete a secondary assessment to identify and treat potentially life-threatening injuries. This assessment is crucial to allow proper triage to the operating room, radiology suite, or ICU.

1. History

Essential components of a patient's history include details of the mechanism of injury, previous medical illness, current medications, allergies, and tetanus immunization.

2. Physical Examination

The patient is examined from head to toe. The skull is carefully inspected to identify occult injuries. The presence or absence of hematotympanum, rhinorrhea, or otorrhea; Battle's sign (ecchymosis of the skin over the mastoid); and raccoon eyes are assessed to evaluate for a basilar skull fracture. Facial bones, mandible, and neck are palpated for tenderness and crepitus. The GCS score and limited neurologic examination from the initial assessment are used to evaluate for head trauma (**Chapter 8**). Extraocular eye movements are checked to exclude muscle or nerve entrapment. The chest is auscultated and palpated for tenderness and crepitus. The patient is log-rolled so that the thoracic and lumbar spine can be palpated for tenderness and other injury can be detected. In penetrating trauma, exclude occult entrance or exit wounds in the axillary, cervical, or inguinal regions. The abdomen is likewise inspected, auscultated, and palpated. The pelvic bones are assessed for stability. The rectum is evaluated for rectal tone and presence or absence of blood and to ensure that the prostate gland is not displaced or nonpalpable. The presence of perineal/scrotal hematoma and blood at the urethral meatus implies urogenital injury, which is a risk for urinary catheter insertion. The extremities are inspected, palpated, and evaluated for range of motion. Additionally, the neurovascular integrity of all extremities is confirmed. Neck pain or tenderness over the cervical spine warrants additional radiographs (see "Radiologic Evaluation," below), spiral CT, or MRI.

3. Laboratory Studies

Minimal testing includes complete blood count, electrolytes, blood glucose, blood alcohol level, and toxicology screening. In any patient with evidence of hypovolemia, blood-group typing and coagulation profile should be performed. In selected patients, blood may be drawn and held until tests are deemed necessary. Arterial blood gas measurements should be analyzed in selected patients to confirm adequate ventilation and metabolic balance (presence of acidosis). An elevated serum amylase level may be an indicator of pancreatic or bowel injury in the patient with blunt abdominal trauma. Be aware that the hematocrit may not reflect the acute status of the patient. Equilibration by transcapillary fluid shifts takes hours to be reflected as a decrease in hematocrit. In general, a fall of 3% in the hematocrit is equivalent to 1 unit of blood loss.

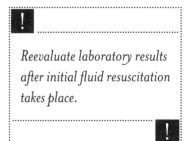

Reevaluate laboratory results after initial fluid resuscitation takes place.

4. Radiologic Evaluation

a. General

In the evaluation of blunt multiple-system trauma, a lateral cervical spine radiograph to the level of T1, a supine chest radiograph, and supine view of the pelvis are obtained as the primary survey is performed; this allows for interpretation of completed radiographs as the secondary survey begins. Plain films of the pelvis are crucial for early identification of major pelvic fractures.

b. Head

Computed tomographic scanning is essential for initial evaluation of a head-injured patient or any patient with a decreased or altered level of consciousness.

c. Spine

The initial lateral C-spine radiograph is valuable in identifying major fractures that would affect decision making and support of catastrophic cervical spinal cord injury. A good-quality lateral C-spine radiograph delineates many unstable C-spine fractures. The most common problems with lateral C spine images are inadequate visualization of C7 to T1 and poor definition of the occiput. Most centers will now obtain at least an anteroposterior, a lateral, and an open-mouth view emphasizing C1 and C2, with CT evaluation of any areas that cannot be cleared or that show possibility of injury. In the patient with increased risk of C-spine injury, cervical immobilization is crucial until these studies are reviewed and correlated with reliable physical examination for evidence of tenderness. If further concern exists, CT scanning of the C-spine should be performed. Magnetic resonance imaging is helpful for disc, spinal cord, and ligament injuries. If a cervical spine fracture is found, a radiographic screening of the spine is indicated since ~10% of these patients will have a second, noncontiguous vertebral column fracture. Anteroposterior and lateral thoracic and lumbar radiographs should be obtained if these areas are tender to palpation, if ecchymosis or palpable irregularities are present, if the physical examination is not reliable, or if the mechanism of injury is suggestive. Computed tomographic scans of chest and abdomen can often be reformatted to provide information on spine injury without the need for additional plain radiographs.

d. Chest

Once the spine is cleared for fractures, an upright (or reverse Trendelenburg) chest radiograph is indicated to better define or identify pneumothorax, hemothorax, mediastinal widening or indistinctness (concern for aortic transection), or fractures and to confirm the position of various tubes. Chest radiographs are inadequate to rule out aortic injury when a significant impact or deceleration injury exists. Suspect this lethal injury where the mediastinum is widened on chest

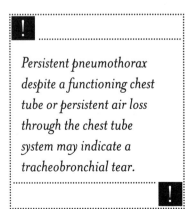

Persistent pneumothorax despite a functioning chest tube or persistent air loss through the chest tube system may indicate a tracheobronchial tear.

radiographs and a decelerating mechanism is present. Aortic angiography remains the standard method for diagnosis of a transected thoracic aorta, although other methods, such as a helical CT scan or a transesophageal echocardiogram, are increasingly used.

e. Abdomen

Plain abdominal radiographs are not usually helpful. In the hemodynamically stable patient, a CT scan of the abdomen with double contrast (oral and IV, if there are no contraindications) is an alternative to DPL for evaluation of blunt trauma. Depending on availability, FAST may be the preferred method in screening for free abdominal fluid (ie, blood) due to its speed and convenience. An equivocal FAST may be followed by abdominal CT or DPL.

f. Genitourinary Tract

Hematuria may be evaluated with a CT scan or other contrast studies. Computed tomography provides anatomic detail about abdominal and retroperitoneal structures and direct injury to the kidney(s). If physical examination suggests that a urethral injury is present, a urethrogram should be obtained before urinary catheterization. A cystogram may be indicated if bladder injury is suspected. Intravenous pyelograms are not commonly performed.

g. Skeletal Fractures

Films of extremities should be obtained on the basis of physical examination or patient complaint. Films should include the joint above and below the site of injury.

5. Other Issues

A nasogastric tube serves to decompress the stomach and may reduce the risk of pulmonary aspiration. However, the tube should be placed orally in patients with midfacial fractures or possible basilar skull fractures. Such placement may decrease the incidence of sinusitis and ventilator-associated pneumonia. Blood in the gastric aspirate may be the only sign of an otherwise occult injury of the stomach or duodenum, and further investigation may be indicated. Tetanus prophylaxis is routine (**Appendix 12**).

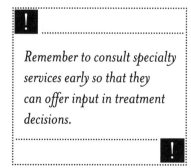

Remember to consult specialty services early so that they can offer input in treatment decisions.

Systemic antibiotics should usually be withheld until a specific indication exists. However, antibiotics are employed in 3 situations involving acute injury: (1) patients with intracranial pressure monitoring or tube thoracostomy frequently receive Gram-positive coverage at the time of device insertion; (2) patients with penetrating abdominal trauma may be given coverage for Gram-negative aerobic and anaerobic organisms for the first 24 hours after injury; and (3) patients with open fractures are given Gram-positive coverage for 24 hours as orthopedic evaluation is arranged.

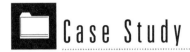

C. TERTIARY ASSESSMENT: ONGOING EVALUATION

Case Study

A middle-aged male sustained multiple liver lacerations in a motor vehicle crash. He also had mesenteric lacerations and bowel resection was performed. The ends of the bowel were stapled, and the abdomen was filled with packs to control venous bleeding from the liver. He continues to require aggressive resuscitation and administration of blood product due to coagulopathy. Several hours after admission to the ICU, increased airway pressures and falling urine output are noted.

– What are possible causes of increased airway pressures?

– Why has urine output fallen?

After life- and limb-threatening injuries have been addressed and metabolic derangements have been corrected, periodic systematic reexaminations are done to identify occult injuries not evident at presentation.

1. Head Injury

Evaluation of the head-injured patient is an ongoing process requiring early neurosurgical consultation. Serial assessment of the GCS scores, pupil size and response, and presence or absence of lateralizing neurologic signs is crucial. Any changes in examination results are noted and acted upon as they are discovered.

Serial CT scans of the head may offer clinically useful information, but the key to patient management is detection of changes in physical examination. Continued resuscitation is imperative to avoid secondary brain injury. Secondary brain injury typically occurs when a patient becomes hypoxic or hypotensive during acute care. These secondary insults increase the likelihood of poor outcome after injury. (**Chapter 8.**)

The administration of atropine or dopamine, as well as mydriatic agents, may dilate the pupils and lead to a false diagnosis of a more severe head injury.

2. Pulmonary Injury

Trauma patients often have a full stomach at the time of injury and therefore may experience aspiration. The acidic gastric contents may cause a chemical pneumonitis initially and predispose patients to an infective pneumonitis or ARDS later. Antibiotics are not indicated in initial management. Steroids and bronchoscopic lavage are not beneficial. Bronchoscopy may be indicated for removal of large particulate matter.

Delayed onset of pneumothorax or hemothorax may follow chest trauma. Additionally, pulmonary contusions and resulting ARDS may not become obvious until later (12-48 hours) in the patient's course. Continued assessment includes physical examination, oximetry and/or arterial blood gas measurements, chest radiographs, and ventilatory mechanics.

3. Cardiac Injury

Continuous ECG monitoring and frequent intermittent measurements of blood pressure, manually or with an automated blood pressure device, are mandatory in the emergency department and intensive care unit. Continuous arterial blood pressure monitoring may be indicated, as discussed in **Chapter 6**. Electrolyte disturbances may lead to cardiac contractile dysfunction or arrhythmias in the aggressively resuscitated trauma patient. Common electrolyte disturbances include hyperchloremia, hypokalemia and hyperkalemia, hypomagnesemia, and hypocalcemia.

4. Abdominal Injury

Substance abuse or neurologic injury may not allow reliable initial abdominal examinations. Perforation of a hollow viscus in blunt trauma is sometimes difficult to diagnose. Free air under the diaphragm on an upright chest radiograph, over the liver on a left lateral decubitus radiograph, or on an abdominal CT prior to FAST or DPL indicates the need for operative exploration. Injury to the pancreas may be subtle. Amylase levels in the serum or DPL fluid may be elevated. Additional evaluation may be accomplished with the administration of radiopaque material through the upper gastrointestinal tract followed by plain radiographs or a CT scan. Computed tomographic scanning also provides information about the retroperitoneum. In the head-injured patient who is undergoing a head CT scan and has a nonoperative neurologic injury, abdominal CT scanning should be considered, as physical examination may be unreliable.

A frequently missed condition is abdominal compartment syndrome. This condition occurs when there is an increase in intra-abdominal pressure due to intraperitoneal or retroperitoneal hemorrhage, ascitic fluid accumulation, edema secondary to massive fluid resuscitation, or intraoperative surgical closure of the abdomen under tension. Increased intra-abdominal pressure decreases cardiac output and compresses the aorta. Both hemidiaphragms are displaced upward by increased intra-abdominal pressure, which results in decreased thoracic volume and compliance. Decreased volume within the pleural cavity predisposes to atelectasis, and ventilated patients with intra-abdominal hypertension require increased airway pressure to deliver a fixed tidal volume. Vascular compression can decrease blood flow to the liver and kidneys with resultant dysfunction. Finally, intra-abdominal hypertension significantly increases intracranial pressure.

Intra-abdominal pressure (IAP) should be expressed in mm Hg and measured at the end of expiration in the supine position with a transducer placed at the level of the midaxillary line after ensuring that abdominal muscle contractions are absent. The current reference standard for IAP measurement is pressure measured via a urinary catheter within the bladder. The aspiration port may be connected to a pressure transducer and intra-abdominal pressure may be read from the bedside monitor. An alternative technique is to read the height of the urine column in urinary catheter drainage tubing. The tubing is clamped just above the urine collection bag and then held 30 to 40 cm above the midaxillary line prior to releasing the clamp; this measurement is read in cm H_2O and must be converted to mm Hg. For either pressure measurement, a maximal volume of 25 mL of sterile, room temperature saline is instilled in the bladder and a stabilization period of 30 to 60 seconds is allowed.

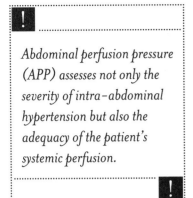

Abdominal perfusion pressure (APP) assesses not only the severity of intra-abdominal hypertension but also the adequacy of the patient's systemic perfusion.

Intra-abdominal hypertension (IAH) is the pathologic elevation of IAP. The IAP can also be used to determine the abdominal perfusion pressure (APP) with the following formula: Abdominal Perfusion Pressure = Mean Arterial Pressure (MAP) – IAP. Intra-abdominal hypertension is defined by sustained or repeated IAP >12 mm Hg or an APP ≤60 mm Hg. Acute intra-abdominal hypertension can develop within hours as a result of trauma or intra-abdominal hemorrhage, or over days as a result of sepsis, capillary leak, or other critical illness.

Abdominal compartment syndrome is present when organ dysfunction occurs as a result of intra-abdominal hypertension. Abdominal compartment syndrome is defined by sustained intra-abdominal pressure >20 mm Hg (with or without an abdominal perfusion pressure <60 mm Hg) in association with new-onset organ dysfunction or failure.

Operative decompression is the method of choice for reducing intra-abdominal pressure in the patient with abdominal compartment syndrome. A surgeon must be consulted when intra-abdominal hypertension is suspected and abdominal compartment syndrome is possible. After decompression, improvements in hemodynamics, pulmonary function, tissue perfusion, and renal function have been demonstrated. To prevent hemodynamic decompensation during a decompression procedure (laparotomy incision), intravascular volume should be maintained and oxygen delivery maximized with correction of hypothermia and coagulation defects.

5. Musculoskeletal Injury

The neurologic and vascular evaluation of the extremities is an ongoing process. A swollen and tense extremity should be watched closely for the development of a compartment syndrome, particularly in patients with decreased responsiveness. In alert patients, serial physical examination is the best monitor. Classical signs include pain, pallor, pulselessness, paresthesia, and/or paralysis. Loss of pulse is a very late finding. The most helpful early signs are complaints of pain out of proportion to physical findings and severe pain on passive stretch of the involved muscle groups. In the unconscious patient or when examination is unreliable, compartment pressure may be monitored using a needle with standard gauge. Pressures >30 mm Hg warrant consideration of fasciotomy.

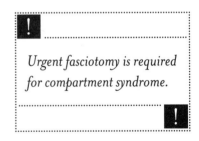

Urgent fasciotomy is required for compartment syndrome.

Musculoskeletal examination should be repeated, either as patients recover from other injuries or as their mental status clears, to identify new pain or tenderness. Plain radiographs should then be obtained to identify occult fractures. Commonly missed orthopedic injuries include fractures of the scapula, thoracic and lumbar spine, pelvis, ankle, and wrist.

6. Other Considerations

Resuscitation is an ongoing process. Traditional end points such as normalization of blood pressure, heart rate, and urine output may not always reflect complete correction of the shock state. The attainment of normal vital signs can occur even in the setting of tissue hypoperfusion resulting in a compensated state of shock. Lactate concentration and resolution of metabolic acidosis may provide more definitive end points for adequacy of resuscitation. Since the time to normalization of these parameters is predictive of survival, additional resuscitation in the form of volume replacement, red cell transfusion, or support with vasoactive agents may be indicated within the first 24 hours postinjury despite normal or near-normal vital signs. Persistence of a metabolic acidosis or elevated lactate concentration may be an early indicator of complications, including ongoing hemorrhage or abdominal compartment syndrome.

Damage control surgery (initial operation limited to control of bleeding and decontamination of hollow organ ruptures with spillage) may need to be done during the first 24 to 48 hours, before definitive surgery is performed. Many trauma patients benefit from delayed definitive surgery, particularly the repair of fractures, during this period of ongoing stabilization. Decisions to proceed with surgery should be made after appropriate consultation with the primary surgical service, a critical care physician, and other consultants as indicated.

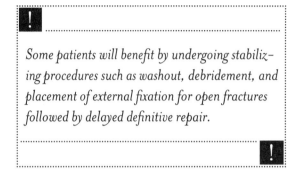

Some patients will benefit by undergoing stabilizing procedures such as washout, debridement, and placement of external fixation for open fractures followed by delayed definitive repair.

In the immediate resuscitation period, it is also vital to ensure that periodic reassessments take place. Once a patient is stabilized, all intravenous access sites should be reassessed. Since full sterile precautions to prevent line-related infections may not be feasible during emergency vascular access, many lines will need to be replaced. If central venous access is no longer indicated, it may be discontinued at this time.

7. Pitfalls to Avoid

The care of patients with multiple injuries requires early surgical consultation. A surgeon should be summoned as soon as it is known that a seriously injured patient is arriving. Early neurosurgical consultation is advised for patients with head injury. Transfer to another institution should not be delayed for additional radiologic studies unless those studies are requested by the accepting physician. The trauma center should be contacted for advice and to discuss potential problems or concerns with transport personnel.

Common pitfalls in the transfer of seriously ill patients include failure to intubate before transfer, failure to recognize the need for transfer to a higher level of care, and, in general, failure to stabilize the patient adequately before transport. Unrecognized ongoing hemorrhage, delayed onset of tension pneumothorax, and reversible/preventable causes of secondary brain injury are also problematic.

III. BURN INJURY: INITIAL EVALUATION AND STABILIZATION

 Case Study

A young male is brought in after a gasoline can exploded as he was burning brush. The patient sustained a full-thickness burn injury to both forearms and showed signs of flash-burn injury to his face. He is in no respiratory distress and has received no fluids since his injury. Although he has no abdominal burns, he complains of abdominal pain. Family members recall that the patient was thrown into a tree stump by the explosion. You are asked to follow up with the patient during his initial wound care in the burn unit.

– What are the initial evaluation priorities?

– What is the greatest risk to this patient?

A. General

Deaths from burn injury occur with greatest frequency as a result of residential fires, particularly in multifamily dwellings and low income areas. Like other forms of injury, burns tend to be most common in the young and the elderly. Scalds are the most common form of childhood injury, whereas electrical and chemical injuries affect adults in the workplace. Factors that affect burn mortality include size of cutaneous injury, patient age, and presence or absence of inhalation injury. Burn injuries should not distract from other potential traumatic injuries. An initial assessment of the patient should be performed as with any trauma patient.

B. Airway/Breathing

Upper airway injury is frequently due to direct heat exposure, whereas laryngeal reflexes usually protect the lung from thermal injury except in high pressure steam exposure. Lower airway injury (below the larynx) is predominantly due to chemical products of combustion carried on particles of soot to the lung.

Aldehydes, oxides of sulfur, and hydrochloric acid may combine with water in the lung to yield corrosive acids and oxygen free radicals. Inhalation injury is also associated with carbon monoxide exposure, although blood carboxyhemoglobin levels may not reflect the true degree of exposure.

Inhalation injury is generally diagnosed by means of bronchoscopy with findings of airway edema, erythema, soot accumulation, and sometimes mucosal loss. More injuries are identified with bronchoscopy than with clinical criteria such as history of closed space burn injury, facial burns with nasal singeing, wheezing, and soot in the sputum. Results of chest radiography are frequently normal at the time of admission, and hypoxemia often is not appreciated.

Three stages of inhalation injury have been identified:

1. Acute hypoxia with asphyxia typically occurs at the scene of the fire.
2. Upper airway and pulmonary edema may evolve during the first hours to days after injury.
3. Infectious complications such as pneumonia that stem from exposure to heat and chemical irritants may appear later.

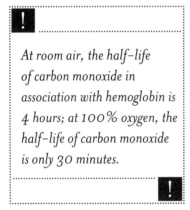

At room air, the half-life of carbon monoxide in association with hemoglobin is 4 hours; at 100% oxygen, the half-life of carbon monoxide is only 30 minutes.

Treatment of inhalation injury is largely supportive. If exposure to carbon monoxide is possible, 100% oxygen should be provided. Early intubation is advocated, especially if the patient will be transferred, because pulmonary and laryngeal injury may quickly evolve even though the initial airway assessment is satisfactory. Caution should be exercised in the use of succinylcholine due to the possibility of clinically significant hyperkalemia. Intravascular resuscitation should not be delayed or withheld because inhalation injury increases resuscitation fluid requirements. Humidification of inhaled gases helps in secretion control and reduces desiccation injury to the airway.

C. Circulation

Large-bore peripheral intravenous catheters should be placed (through the burn, if necessary) and a crystalloid bolus should be initiated immediately. The preferred resuscitation fluid is lactated Ringer's solution. If there is circumferential burn injury to an extremity or the thorax, it may be necessary to divide the burn wound at the lateral aspects of the extremities or the torso to facilitate perfusion or chest wall movement. Division of wound eschar for this purpose is termed escharotomy. Usually the need for escharotomy is clear within 48 hours of injury. Progressive tissue edema during resuscitation may create the need for escharotomy, even if initial perfusion of distal extremities or chest wall movement appears to be adequate. Abdominal wall escharotomy or laparotomy for abdominal compartment syndrome with respiratory compromise is sometimes required. Abdominal compartment syndrome related to edema formation and capillary leak may occur even if the abdomen was not injured or burned.

D. Assessment of Injury

Remove all of the patient's clothing. Depending upon the history of injury leading to burn trauma, the patient may have other injuries and should be assessed for trauma in accordance with the guidelines above.

1. Depth of Burns

There are 3 burn depths:

1. First-degree superficial: erythematous, painful
2. Second-degree (partial thickness): red, swollen, blistered, weeping, very painful
3. Third-degree (full thickness): white, leathery, painless

Third-degree, or full-thickness, injuries involve all layers of the epidermis and dermis and require surgical reconstruction. Burns that involve structures deep to the skin, such as tendon, muscle, and bone, have been called fourth-degree burns.

2. Burn Area (Rule of Nines)

The rule of nines is commonly used to estimate the extent of total body surface area (TBSA) that has been burned (**Figure 9-1**). The head and upper extremities each represent 9% of the TBSA. The anterior and posterior trunk and the lower extremities each represent 18%, and the perineum represents 1% of the TBSA. Alternatively, the patient's hand, which equals roughly 1% of TBSA, may be used to estimate the size of a small or irregular burn. A common mistake is to use the palm of the hand minus the fingers in the calculation, but doing so may lead to overestimation of burn size.

E. Resuscitation

Burn shock presents with profound hypovolemia, which has both interstitial and intracellular components. Increased capillary permeability is one of the key components of the burn shock response. In small burns, maximal edema is seen in as little as 8 to 12 hours after injury; larger burns manifest additional edema at 12 to 24 hours. Plasma volume loss, manifested as hypovolemia, coincides with edema formation and increased extracellular fluid.

Edema formation is affected by fluid administration during resuscitation. Replace fluid and electrolytes as dictated by organ perfusion indicators and electrolyte imbalance. Because fluid and electrolyte losses in burns are primarily insensible, one cannot accurately determine amounts of loss. The American Burn Association recommends the consensus formula of 2 to 4 mL/kg/% burn. Beginning with 2 mL/kg/% burn may reduce edema and extravascular complications such as abdominal compartment syndrome.

Figure 9-1. Rule of Nines

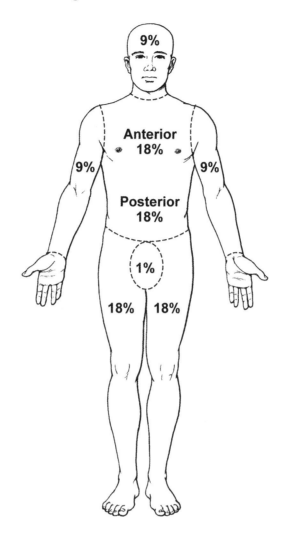

Reproduced with permission from Mayo Clinic.

Any ongoing losses, such as active bleeding, should be added to this starting point. Half of the crystalloid resuscitation should be administered in the first 8 hours and the remaining half over the next 16 hours. Ensure adequate venous access and place a urinary catheter. Urine output (0.5-1 mL/kg/h) is the primary guide to fluid replacement. Vital sign goals may lead to volume overload because heart rate may remain elevated despite adequate resuscitation.

F. Carbon Monoxide Exposure

Consider evaluating a carboxyhemoglobin level for the possibility of significant carbon monoxide exposure, and administer 100% oxygen to facilitate rapid reversal/clearance of carboxyhemoglobin. Early use of hyperbaric oxygen for patients with high carboxyhemoglobin levels (>40%) or evidence of significant neurologic or cardiovascular toxicity has been recommended, but data supporting this recommendation are limited.

G. Burn Wound

Local care of the burn wound begins with serial debridement of nonviable tissue and blisters by appropriate surgical consultants. Little care is required for the burn wound prior to transfer to the burn center or surgical consultation. If gross contamination is present, a gentle washing and coverage with clean linen may be appropriate. If the patient cannot be rapidly transferred to a burn center, it may be necessary to apply silver sulfadiazine (or appropriate antibiotic ointment) and occlusive dressings to help prevent evaporative heat loss.

H. Other Considerations

Place a nasogastric tube if the patient vomits, requires intubation, or has a burn >20% of TBSA. Use doses of intravenous morphine for pain. Remove rings and bracelets.

I. Special Considerations

1. Chemical Burns

Chemical burns may be caused by acid (cleaning products, industrial applications), alkali (hydrides of sodium, potassium, and sodas of ammonia), or organic compounds (petroleum products). Severity of injury relates to the agent involved, the concentration of the agent, and the duration of contact. Initial care requires immediate removal of the patient from the source of chemical injury. In general, removal of clothing is essential. Brush off dry substances and then irrigate copiously with water. Do not use neutralizing agents as they may increase the severity of burn.

Contact with petroleum products is associated with rapid skin penetration and late multiple-organ failure. Patients may be exposed to petroleum from spilled gasoline at the scene of a motor vehicle crash. Rapid removal of the patient from the petroleum source and vigorous irrigation of exposed surfaces are warranted. Advice regarding chemical burns is available from regional burn centers.

2. Electrical Injury

Electrical injury is a syndrome with a variety of presentations. Exposure of the patient to an electrical source <1,000 volts produces a low voltage injury similar to other cutaneous burns. When exposure exceeds 1,000 volts, a greater potential for deep as well as cutaneous injury exists.

Three types of injury to the skin can occur with electrocution:

1. Entrance and exit wounds, typically circumscribed, deep lesions, occur at points of contact with the electrical source or ground (usually on hands and feet).
2. Cutaneous burns, similar to those seen with flame, may be caused by arc injury from the primary site to adjacent body parts.
3. The standard pattern of injury seen with flame exposure may be created by ignition of clothing.

Beware of pneumothorax, airway compromise, cardiac arrest, and blunt injury secondary to falls and violent muscle contraction. Muscle compartment pressures may increase, necessitating fasciotomy, not just escharotomy. If myoglobin is present in the urine or creatine kinase concentrations are elevated, provide adequate intravascular volume to increase the urine output to 70 to 100 mL/h until resolution of the rhabdomyolysis. Patients may have ileus after electrocution. Check the ECG in electrical injury.

The initial priority in the management of electrocution is removal of necrotic tissue and decompression of compromised deep tissue compartments, particularly muscle. Resuscitation is begun at 4 mL/kg/% TBSA cutaneous injury and titrated to maintain urine output of 0.5 to 1 mL/kg/h unless rhabdomyolysis is present and higher urine output is desirable. Aggressive fluid resuscitation potentiates filtering of pigment and dilution of iron (nephrotoxic). Alkalinization of the urine may be considered to decrease the nephrotoxic potential despite lack of supportive evidence. If large areas of soft-tissue injury are present, surgical consultation should be requested. As with other burns, infection is the chief risk in electrical injury. Other potential problems that follow electrocution are myocardial and vascular injury, encephalopathy, cataracts, and gut perforation.

Lightning injury may be thought of as massive exposure to direct current. Most injury is topical because exposure times are extremely brief. Mortality associated with lightning relates to early cardiac and respiratory arrest. Aggressive basic and advanced life support may be lifesaving for these patients.

Basic Trauma and Burn Support

■ The first goal in trauma management is to identify and treat immediately life-threatening injuries by following the ABCDE sequence of priorities.

■ After blunt trauma, airway control should proceed on the assumption that an unstable C-spine fracture exists.

■ A diagnosis of tension pneumothorax should be based on clinical criteria and not on a chest radiograph.

■ Hemorrhage is the most likely cause of shock after injury, and initial empiric treatment consists of crystalloid infusion to normalize blood pressure, reverse tachycardia, and maintain adequate organ perfusion.

■ In general, blood should be added to resuscitation fluids when crystalloid infusion is >50 mL/kg. Uncrossmatched, type-specific blood can be safely administered.

■ A secondary assessment includes a head-to-toe examination to identify and treat potentially life-threatening injuries.

■ Computed tomographic scanning is essential for the initial evaluation of head-injured patients with depressed level of consciousness.

■ Abdominal compartment syndrome may occur due to intraperitoneal or retroperitoneal hemorrhage, ascitic fluid accumulation, edema secondary to fluid resuscitation, or surgical closure of the abdomen under tension.

■ Transfer to a specialized care setting should not be delayed for additional radiologic studies unless the accepting physician requests the studies.

■ Burn resuscitation is proportional to the area sustaining second- and third-degree burns and is titrated to signs of perfusion, including urine output.

■ Closed-space smoke-inhalation injury places the patient at high risk for upper airway and lung injury that may not be obvious at the time of initial patient presentation.

Suggested Readings

1. American College of Surgeons Committee on Trauma. *Advanced Trauma Life Support for Doctors* (ATLS). 7th ed. Chicago, IL: American College of Surgeons; 2004

2. Bagley LJ. Imaging of spinal trauma. *Radiol Clin N Am*. 2006;44:1.

3. Brain Trauma Foundation. Management and prognosis of severe traumatic brain injury. *J Neurotrauma*. 2000;17:449.

4. Chan O, Wilson A, Walsh M. Major trauma. *BMJ*. 2005;330:1136.

5. Cheatham ML, Malbrain MLNG, Kirkpatrick A, et al. Results from the International Conference of Experts on Intra-abdominal Hypertension and Abdominal Compartment Syndrome, II: recommendations. *Intensive Care Med*. 2007;33:951.

6. Elliott DC. An evaluation of the end points of resuscitation. *J Am Coll Surg*. 1998;187:536.

7. Herndon DN, ed. *Total Burn Care. 2nd ed*. London, UK: WB Saunders; 2002.

8. Johnson JW, Gracias VH, Schwab CW, et al. Evolution in damage control for exsanguinating penetrating abdominal injury. *J Trauma*. 2001;51:261.

9. Malbrain MLNG. Different techniques to measure intra-abdominal pressure (IAP): time for a critical re-appraisal. *Intensive Care Med*. 2004;30:357.

10. Malbrain MLNG, Cheatham ML , Kirkpatrick A, et al. Results from the International Conference of Experts on Intra-abdominal Hypertension and Abdominal Compartment Syndrome, I: definitions. *Intensive Care Med*. 2006;3:1722.

11. Moore EE, Feliciano DV, Mattox KL, eds. *Trauma*. 5th ed. New York, NY: McGraw-Hill; 2004.

12. Pryor JP, Braslow B, Reilly PM, et al. The evolving role of interventional radiology in trauma care. *J Trauma*. 2005;59:102.

13. Rhee P, Nunley MK, Demetriades D, et al. Tetanus and trauma: a review and recommendations. *J Trauma*. 2005;58:1082.

14. Sarrafzadeh AS, Peltonen EE, Kaisers U, et al. Secondary insults in severe head injury: Do multiply-injured patients do worse? *Crit Care Med*. 2001;29:1116.

15. Sheridan RL. Burns. *Crit Care Med*. 2002;30(suppl):S500.

16. Stengel D, Bauwens K, Sehouli J, et al. Emergency ultrasound-based algorithms for diagnosing blunt abdominal trauma. *Cochrane Database of Syst Rev*. 2005;(2): CD004446. doi: 10.1002/14651858.CD004446.pub2.

Web Sites

1. Eastern Association for the Surgery of Trauma. http://www.east.org/tpg.html. Best site for evidence-based trauma care guidelines.

2. Trauma.org. http://www.trauma.org. Image bank and links.

3. World Society of the Abdominal Compartment Syndrome. http://www.wsacs.org. Consensus information on abdominal compartment syndrome.

Chapter 10:

ACUTE CORONARY SYNDROMES

✓ Objectives

■ Identify patients with acute coronary syndromes (ACS) with different electrocardiographic and clinical presentations.

■ Outline diagnostic procedures and the acute management of unstable angina (UA), non–ST-elevation myocardial infarction (NSTEMI), and ST-elevation myocardial infarction (STEMI).

■ Identify appropriate reperfusion interventions for patients with ST-elevation myocardial infarction and high-risk patients with UA and NSTEMI.

■ Recognize the complications of myocardial infarction and outline appropriate management.

Case Study

A 64-year-old man with type II diabetes and hypertension awoke with chest pressure. One hour later, when the pain failed to resolve, his wife drove him to the local emergency department. His vital signs on arrival are blood pressure 158/94 mm Hg, heart rate 98/min, respiratory rate 28/min, and SpO$_2$ 97% on room air. His physical examination is remarkable only for a fourth heart sound (S$_4$) and mild diaphoresis.

– What information is needed to determine the type of ACS this patient may have?

– What immediate interventions should be performed?

I. INTRODUCTION

Acute coronary syndromes (ACSs) encompass overlapping clinical conditions of myocardial ischemia that include unstable angina (UA) and acute myocardial infarction, both non–ST-elevation myocardial infarction (NSTEMI) and ST-elevation myocardial infarction (STEMI; **Figure 10-1**). An important distinction is made clinically between patients with ACS that have ST-segment elevation on electrocardiogram (ECG) and those who do not have ST-segment elevation. In most patients, ST elevation evolves into Q-wave (transmural) myocardial infarction (MI), and these patients should be considered for immediate reperfusion.

Figure 10-1. Overlapping Spectrum of Acute Coronary Syndromes

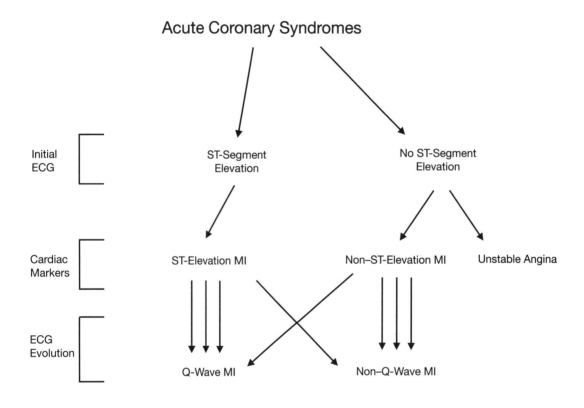

Acute coronary syndromes are distinguished by initial ECG findings, cardiac markers, and evolution of the ECG.

Unstable angina and NSTEMI are grouped together as unstable coronary syndromes that differ in the severity of ischemia and myocardial damage. Myocardial damage resulting in elevation of biochemical markers of myocardial injury establishes the diagnosis of NSTEMI. Although UA and NSTEMI are managed initially with pharmacologic interventions, high-risk patients may also require urgent reperfusion. Unstable angina and NSTEMI are characterized pathologically by various degrees of coronary artery occlusion that result in decreased myocardial oxygen supply relative to myocardial oxygen demand. Rupture or erosion of atherosclerotic plaques leads to a complex process of inflammation, platelet activation and aggregation, thrombus formation, and microembolization to distal vasculature. The specific syndrome manifested by the patient depends on the severity and duration of occlusion. Myocardial ischemia less commonly results from severe anemia or hypoxemia that limits myocardial oxygen delivery.

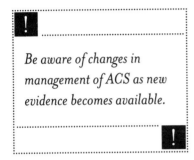

Be aware of changes in management of ACS as new evidence becomes available.

Hospitals should establish multiprofessional teams (including primary care physicians, emergency medicine physicians, cardiologists, and nurses) to develop evidence-based protocols for triaging and managing patients with symptoms suggestive of ACS. The care of patients with ACS continually evolves as information becomes available from clinical trials. Those caring for such patients must periodically update protocols based on the best current evidence.

Identification of patients at risk for ACS includes an assessment of risk factors for coronary artery disease, as summarized in **Table 10-1,** and identification of previous myocardial ischemia. Patients with other critical illness or injury have increased risk for ACS and frequently have atypical presentations. Definitive diagnosis of ACS often is not possible on initial evaluation and requires continuous observation, electrocardiographic monitoring, and/or laboratory confirmation. A brief history and physical examination may promote rapid triage, whereas a more detailed examination aids in the differential diagnosis and evaluation for possible complications. A brief physical examination should include vital signs and general observation, assessment of jugular venous distension, auscultation of the lungs and heart, evaluation of peripheral pulses, detection of neurologic deficits, and assessment for evidence of systemic hypoperfusion.

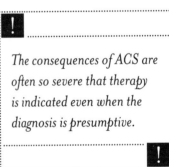

The consequences of ACS are often so severe that therapy is indicated even when the diagnosis is presumptive.

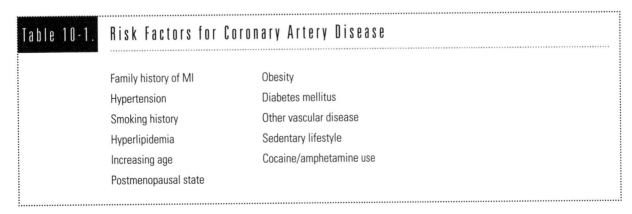

Table 10-1. Risk Factors for Coronary Artery Disease	
Family history of MI	Obesity
Hypertension	Diabetes mellitus
Smoking history	Other vascular disease
Hyperlipidemia	Sedentary lifestyle
Increasing age	Cocaine/amphetamine use
Postmenopausal state	

II. UNSTABLE ANGINA AND NON–ST-ELEVATION MYOCARDIAL INFARCTION

At presentation, patients with ischemic-type chest pain and an ECG without ST elevation are often presumed to have unstable angina. Other causes of prolonged chest pain, listed in **Table 10-2,** should also be considered. Unstable angina can present as rest angina, new-onset angina, or increasing angina (change in predictability of pain, such as pain that is more frequent, of longer duration, or induced by less effort). Based on serial ECGs and elevated levels of biochemical markers of cardiac injury, some patients with unstable angina subsequently are found to have an NSTEMI. The initial evaluation and management of patients with UA and NSTEMI are similar. Pathologic correlates include a partially or intermittently occluding thrombus and microemboli from the thrombus to the distal vasculature.

Table 10-2.	Differential Diagnosis of Prolonged Chest Pain
	Acute myocardial ischemia
	Aortic dissection/aortic aneurysm
	Pericarditis
	Pain associated with hypertrophic cardiomyopathy or esophageal and gastrointestinal disorders
	Pulmonary diseases such as pneumothorax, pulmonary embolism, or pleurisy
	Hyperventilation syndrome
	Aortic stenosis
	Musculoskeletal or chest wall diseases, costochondral pain
	Psychogenic pain

A. Diagnosis

The most important factors from a patient's history that suggest the likelihood of myocardial ischemia are the character of the pain, prior history of coronary artery disease, age, and number of risk factors. Results of physical examination are usually normal, although a fourth heart sound (S_4) may be heard during episodes of pain. A 12-lead ECG should be obtained and interpreted within 10 minutes of the patient's arrival. The ECG is most helpful if there is transient ST-segment depression (**Figure 10-2**) during anginal episodes. However, the ECG may be normal, or it may reveal nondiagnostic T-wave inversions or peaked T waves. The history, findings from physical examination, ECG interpretation, and cardiac markers should be used to assess the patient's short-term risk of an adverse outcome, such as death or nonfatal myocardial ischemia (**Table 10-3**). This risk assessment has implications for location of care, selection of medical therapy, and use of reperfusion interventions. Serial cardiac markers (MB fraction of creatine phosphokinase

> !
>
> *New-onset shortness of breath and/or new left branch bundle block should be considered evidence of ACS, particularly in women and diabetics, who may have atypical presentations.*
>
> !

[CK-MB], cardiac-specific troponins) along with serial ECGs should be obtained to determine if an NSTEMI is present. Cardiac-specific troponins (cTnT, cTnI) also provide useful prognostic information. Certain tests, such as hemoglobin/hematocrit, electrolytes, thyroid function, and arterial oxygen saturation, may be helpful in identifying a precipitating factor. Arterial puncture should be avoided, when possible, to minimize complications of anticoagulation.

Figure 10-2. Electrocardiogram of a Patient With Unstable Angina[a]

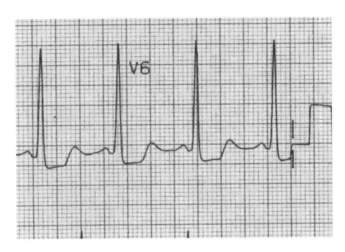

The ST-segment depression in lead V6 is characteristic of unstable angina.
[a] Reproduced with permission of Shih-Chung Lin, MD.

Table 10-3. Risk Factors for Death or Nonfatal Myocardial Ischemia[a]		
High Risk (1 or More of the Following)	**Intermediate Risk (No High Risks and 1 of the Following)**	**Low Risk (No High or Intermediate Risks and 1 of the Following)**
• Ongoing pain at rest (>20 min)	• Prolonged rest pain (>20 min) now resolved	• Increasing frequency, severity or duration of pain
• Pulmonary edema, S_3 or rales	• Rest pain <20 min or relieved with nitroglycerin	• Lower threshold for pain
• Hypotension	• Age >70 years	• Normal or unchanged ECG during pain
• Bradycardia, tachycardia	• T-wave inversions >0.2 mV	• Normal troponin
• Age >75 years	• Pathologic Q waves	
• Rest angina with dynamic ST-segment changes >0.05 mV	• Slightly elevated troponin (<0.1 ng/mL)	
• Elevated troponin (>0.1 ng/mL)		

[a] Adapted from Braunwald E, Mark DB, Jones RH, et al. *Unstable Angina: Diagnosis and Management*. Rockville, MD: Agency for Health Care Policy and Research and National Heart, Lung, and Blood Institute. US Public Health Service, US Department of Health and Human Services; 1994. AHCPR Publication 94-0602.

The use of transthoracic echocardiography, if equipment and expertise are available, allows bedside assessment of wall motion abnormalities as a marker for current or past ischemia and detection and follow-up of new abnormalities. This procedure also provides an estimate of left ventricular function and identification of valvular dysfunction and/or pericardial fluid. Echocardiography may allow assessment of other nonischemic causes of acute chest pain, such as myocarditis, heart failure, pulmonary embolism, and thoracic aortic dissection (although the window for visualization may be poor).

B. Management

Routine management of the patient with chest pain includes increasing myocardial oxygen supply and decreasing myocardial oxygen demand. Reversing myocardial ischemia and confirming the diagnosis of ACS is the essential priority. Patients with unstable angina should be admitted directly to a unit with cardiac monitoring (eg, telemetry unit, chest pain or observation unit) and placed at bed rest or reduced activity (see treatment algorithm in **Figure 10-3**). Oxygen (2-4 L/min by nasal cannula) should be administered to patients with respiratory distress or oxygen saturation as measured by pulse oximetry (SpO_2) <90% to 92%. Although oxygen is often administered to virtually all patients suspected of having acute myocardial ischemia, it is not known whether this therapy limits myocardial damage or reduces morbidity or mortality. If precipitating, reversible causes such as fever, anemia, hypoxemia, infection, hypertension, anxiety, hyperthyroidism, arrhythmias, or sympathomimetic drug ingestion (eg, cocaine, ephedrine) can be identified, they should be treated aggressively. Further management includes relief of pain and anti-ischemic therapy, therapy for platelet aggregation/thrombosis, as well as ongoing risk stratification and consideration of invasive reperfusion procedures.

Pain relief is an important element in the early management of the patient with ACS. Pain management should be directed toward acute relief of symptoms of ongoing myocardial ischemia and general relief of anxiety and apprehension. Control of ischemic pain is typically accomplished with a combination of nitrates, opiate agents, and β-adrenergic blockers. All categories of antianginal medications are effective in stabilizing patients with unstable angina (see list in **Table 10-4**). The goal is to reduce ischemia without causing hypotension or reflex tachycardia. Patients with ongoing ischemic discomfort should receive sublingual or spray nitroglycerin. If sublingual or spray nitroglycerin and the initiation of an intravenous β-blocker do not relieve pain, an assessment should be made about the need for intravenous nitroglycerin. Doses of intravenous nitroglycerin typically range from 25 to 350 μg/min. A reasonable initial infusion rate is 10 μg/min, with increases of 10 μg/min every 3 to 5 minutes as required to control pain. Excessive decreases in blood pressure with nitroglycerin are predominantly due to increased venous capacitance and can often be treated with careful intravenous crystalloid infusion. If the mean arterial pressure decreases by more than 25% when hypertension is present or if the systolic pressure decreases to <110 mm Hg in normotensive patients, nitroglycerin should not be increased. Instead, a second antianginal agent should be administered. Tolerance to the hemodynamic effects of nitroglycerin becomes important after 24 hours of continuous infusion, and efforts should be made to switch to other

> !
> *Since nitroglycerin reduces the efficacy of heparin, unfractionated heparin infusion rates require adjustment when intravenous nitroglycerin is used.*
> !

dosing regimens. The dose of intravenous nitrates should be reduced and changed to an oral regimen when ischemic manifestations have resolved for 12 to 24 hours. Nitrates should not be administered to patients with systolic blood pressure <90 mm Hg, severe bradycardia, significant tachycardia, or suspected right ventricle infarction. Nitrates are contraindicated in patients who have received a phosphodiesterase inhibitor for erectile dysfunction in the prior 24 hours (48 hours for tadalafil). Morphine sulfate is the analgesic of choice for management of pain associated with myocardial ischemia that is refractory to initial antianginal therapy.

Figure 10-3. Treatment Algorithm for Unstable Angina

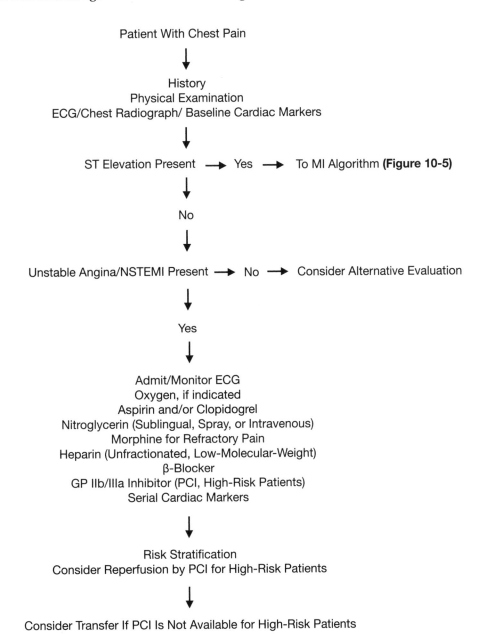

Abbreviations: ECG, electrocardiogram; MI, myocardial infarction; GP, glycoprotein; PCI, percutaneous coronary intervention

| Table 10-4 | Anti-ischemic Therapy |

Agent	Oral Dose	Spray Dose	Intravenous Dose
Nitroglycerin	0.3-0.4 mg tablet sublingually to a maximum of 3 doses; contraindicated when SBP <90 mm Hg	0.4 mg spray every 5 minutes to a maximum of 3 doses; contraindicated when SBP <90 mm Hg	10-25 μg/min initially; titrate to effect, drop in blood pressure, or maximum of 350 μg/min
Morphine			2-5 mg every 5-30 minutes as needed for pain
β-blockers			
Propranolol	20-40 mg every 6 hours		0.5-2 mg as single dose
Metoprolol	50-100 mg every 12 hours		5 mg every 5 minutes to a total dose of 15 mg
Atenolol	50-100 mg every 24 hours		5 mg every 10 minutes to a total dose of 10 mg
Diltiazem	30-60 mg every 8 hours		

β-Blockers, alone or in addition to intravenous nitroglycerin, should be initiated early in all patients without contraindications (**Table 10-5**). During the first few hours after the onset of ACS, β-blocking agents may diminish myocardial oxygen demand by reducing heart rate, systemic arterial pressure, and myocardial contractility. In addition, prolongation of diastole caused by a reduction in heart rate may augment perfusion to the ischemic myocardium, particularly the subendocardium. Intravenous administration of β-blockers facilitates rapid onset of action, and if a short-acting agent is used, hypotension can be rapidly reversed. In the presence of ongoing chest pain, a loading dose of β-blocker should be given intravenously and followed by oral administration.

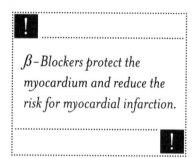

β-Blockers protect the myocardium and reduce the risk for myocardial infarction.

Nondihydropyridine calcium channel blockers (eg, diltiazem) do not reduce the risk of MI, and they may be considered (in the absence of contraindications) only if patients cannot tolerate a β-blocker or symptoms are not controlled with nitroglycerin and β-blockers together.

Table 10-5.	Contraindications to ß-Blockade in Acute Coronary Syndromes

Heart rate <50 beats/min

Moderate to severe left ventricular failure (uncompensated)

Shock

Marked first-degree atrioventricular block (with P-R interval >0.24 sec)

Second-degree or third-degree atrioventricular block

Systolic blood pressure <90 mm Hg

Peripheral hypoperfusion

Active bronchospastic disease (asthma or chronic obstructive pulmonary disease)

Antiplatelet and antithrombin agents (**Table 10-6**) are important interventions in UA and NSTEMI because of the contribution of platelet activation/aggregation and the coagulation system to platelet-rich thrombus formation. Three classes of antiplatelet drugs may be of benefit in myocardial ischemia: aspirin, adenosine diphosphate inhibitors (clopidogrel and ticlopidine), and glycoprotein (GP) IIb/IIIa inhibitors. The intensity of therapy with these agents is often tailored to the patient's risk assessment and to future plans for invasive procedures. Non–enteric-coated aspirin at a dose of 162 to 325 mg should be administered (by chewing) as soon as possible to all patients with UA/NSTEMI and be continued indefinitely. Clopidogrel should be considered as an alternative antiplatelet agent if aspirin is contraindicated. Clopidogrel is preferred over ticlopidine because it more rapidly inhibits platelet activation and lowers the risk of neutropenia. If a noninterventional approach is planned for the patient, clopidogrel added to aspirin has been found to decrease the risk of cardiovascular death, MI, and stroke. The addition of clopidogrel in patients undergoing percutaneous coronary interventions (PCIs) has also been found to be beneficial. Clopidogrel therapy is recommended for at least 1 month and up to 12 months, but the optimum duration has not been determined.

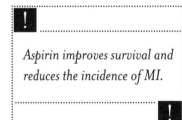

Aspirin improves survival and reduces the incidence of MI.

Table 10-6. Antiplatelet and Antithrombin Drugs Used in Acute Coronary Syndromes

Agents Administered Orally

Aspirin	162-325 mg chewed and swallowed initially, then
	75-325 mg as a minimum oral dose daily

Adenosine diphosphate inhibitors

Clopidogrel	75 mg orally daily; a loading dose of 300-600 mg
	can be used when rapid onset of action is needed
Ticlopidine	250 mg orally twice daily; a loading dose of 500 mg
	can be used when rapid onset of action is needed

Agents Administered Intravenously

Glycoprotein IIb/IIIa inhibitors

Abciximab	For planned PCI: 0.25 mg/kg intravenous bolus (10- 60 minutes before procedure),
	then 0.125 µg/kg/min intravenously (maximum 10 µg/min) for 12-24 hours
Eptifibatide	ACS: 180 µg/kg intravenous bolus, then 2 µg/kg/min intravenous infusion for 72-96 hours
	PCI: 135 µg/kg intravenous bolus; begin 0.5 µg/kg/min intravenous infusion,
	then repeat bolus in 10 minutes
Tirofiban	0.4 µg/kg intravenously for 30 minutes, then 0.1 µg/kg intravenous infusion for 48-96 hours

Abbreviations: PCI, percutaneous coronary intervention; ACS, acute coronary syndrome

High-risk patients (with continuing ischemia, elevated troponin levels) may be candidates for additional antiplatelet therapy with glycoprotein IIb/IIIa inhibitors. Several trials demonstrated a reduced rate of death or MI with use of GP IIb/IIIa inhibitors (tirofiban, eptifibatide) in combination with heparin. Use of GP IIb/IIIa inhibitors is associated with a slight increase in bleeding, primarily at vascular access sites. Glycoprotein IIb/IIIa inhibitors should also be utilized if a percutaneous coronary intervention (PCI) is planned, but they may be given just prior to intervention. The selection of a specific agent may depend on availability and the preferences of the interventional cardiologist. Coagulation and platelet baseline studies should be completed before the administration of GP IIb/IIIa inhibitors.

The combination of aspirin and heparin is more beneficial than aspirin alone in ACS. Heparin, unfractionated (**Appendix 13**) or low-molecular-weight, should be administered as an antithrombin agent unless the patient has significant contraindications. Low-molecular-weight heparin (particularly enoxaparin) is preferred over unfractionated heparin in UA/NSTEMI, unless surgical revascularization is planned within 24 hours. Serial platelet counts are required in order to monitor for heparin-induced thrombocytopenia. The role of direct thrombin inhibitors (hirudin [lepirudin] and bivalirudin) in ACS is continuing to be defined.

An angiotensin-converting enzyme inhibitor (ACE inhibitor) can be added to initial therapy of UA/NSTEMI when hypertension is refractory to nitroglycerin and β-block therapy. Thrombolytic agents have no proven efficacy in unstable angina or NSTEMI.

Most patients with unstable angina can be medically stabilized, and consultation can then be obtained for further risk stratification and/or invasive strategies (cardiac catheterization laboratory). An early invasive strategy is indicated for patients with UA/NSTEMI without serious comorbidity when there are high-risk indicators, as summarized in **Table 10-7.** Immediate expert consultation should be obtained for patients who cannot be medically stabilized or have serious comorbidity. Patients with UA/NSTEMI who have shock benefit from early reperfusion with PCI or coronary artery bypass graft (CABG) and should be triaged to the catheterization laboratory as soon as possible. Risk-factor modification, including the use of lipid-lowering agents (statins), weight reduction, and information about smoking cessation, is recommended in all cases of acute coronary syndromes.

Table 10-7.	High-Risk Indicators for an Early Invasive Strategy in UA/NSTEMI
	Recurrent angina at rest or with minimal exertion despite therapy
	Elevated troponin level
	New ST-segment depression
	Signs of heart failure
	Depressed left ventricular function (ejection fraction <40%)
	Hemodynamic instability
	High-risk findings on noninvasive stress testing
	Prior coronary artery bypass graft (CABG)
	Percutaneous coronary intervention within 6 months

III. ST-ELEVATION MYOCARDIAL INFARCTION

In patients with STEMI there is a high likelihood that a thrombus will totally occlude a coronary artery, resulting in a wave front of myocardial necrosis that begins at the endocardial surface within 15 minutes. The infarction progresses outward to the epicardium over a period of approximately 6 hours unless collateral flow, spontaneous reperfusion, or reperfusion via an intervention is established. The progression of infarction may be modulated by the extent of collateral flow and determinants of myocardial oxygen consumption, which affords an opportunity for myocardial salvage. As with the patient with UA/NSTEMI, prompt diagnosis and early treatment of the patient with STEMI have great influence on morbidity and mortality.

A. Diagnosis

Patients with STEMI typically present with prolonged chest pain and associated symptoms, but some patients have MIs that are painless (silent infarction/ ischemia) or have other related symptoms, such as dyspnea and fatigue. In the critically ill patient population, STEMIs may not be associated with classic symptoms and are often suspected when complications occur or ECG changes are noted. The findings from physical examination of patients with STEMI are nonspecific.

The most common finding in patients with normal sinus rhythm is the S_4 heart sound indicating decreased left ventricular compliance at the end of ventricular filling. Bibasilar crackles may be present and are helpful in defining the hemodynamic status. A brief, focused physical examination aids in the diagnosis and assessment of possible complications of STEMI. A limited neurological examination for evidence of prior stroke or cognitive deficits should also be conducted.

Within 10 minutes of the arrival of a patient with chest discomfort or symptoms suggestive of ACS, a 12-lead ECG should be performed and read. The ECG is diagnostic of STEMI in the absence of QRS confounders (ie, bundle branch block, pacing, left ventricular hypertrophy, Wolff-Parkinson-White syndrome) if it shows >1-millimeter ST elevation in ≥2 contiguous leads (**Figure 10-4**).

Figure 10-4. ECG Indicating an Anterolateral STEMI

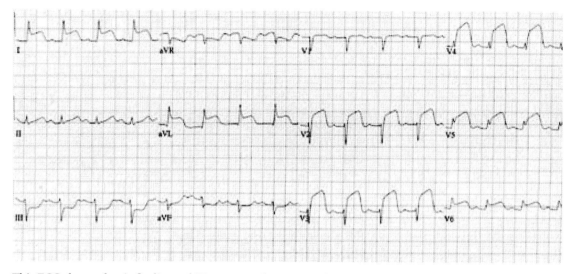

This ECG shows classic findings of ST-segment elevation in the anterior (V_2 through V_4) and lateral (I, aVL, V_5, V_6) leads, indicating an anterolateral STEMI. Reproduced with permission from Barbara McLean.

A right-sided ECG should be obtained in patients with an inferior STEMI to determine if ST elevation suggesting right ventricular infarction is present. Patients with ECG findings of new or undiagnosed left bundle branch block and chest pain compatible with myocardial ischemia are treated similarly to those with ST elevation. If the initial ECG is not diagnostic but the patient remains symptomatic and there is a high clinical suspicion for STEMI, serial ECGs at 5- to 10-minute intervals or continuous 12-lead ST-segment monitoring (if available) may be performed to detect the development of ST elevation.

If the diagnosis is in doubt, echocardiography may add helpful clarification. The diagnosis is confirmed by detecting elevated serum levels of CK-MB or cardiac-specific troponins. The delay in elevation of CK-MB and cardiac-specific troponins, however, prevents their use in initiating reperfusion therapy. Cardiac-specific troponins are the optimum cardiac markers for the evaluation of patients with STEMI who have coexistent skeletal muscle injury.

B. General Management

Once STEMI is suspected or diagnosed, the immediate concerns are to ensure the patient's stability and to intervene to limit infarct size by restoring blood flow to the infarct artery as soon as possible (see the treatment algorithm in **Figure 10-5**). Treatment of STEMI in the patient with other critical illness requires careful individualization. Absolute and relative contraindications to therapies must be considered and relative risk assessed. Choices may also be limited by the availability of specialized procedures, the need to transport the patient to another facility, or the unavailability of the oral route for administering medication.

Figure 10-5. Treatment Algorithm for Myocardial Infarction With ST Elevation

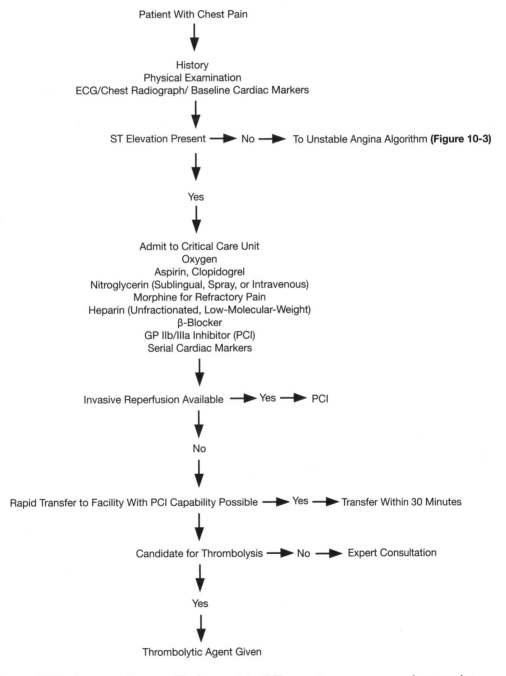

Abbreviations: ECG, electrocardiogram; GP, glycoprotein; PCI, percutaneous coronary intervention.

1. Early Therapy

Early therapy in STEMI is similar to the management of unstable angina and non–ST-elevation MI. Immediate 12-lead ECG, cardiac markers, and related laboratory tests should be completed. Immediate therapy includes the administration of supplemental oxygen for the first 6 hours and longer if indicated, the control of pain, and consideration of reperfusion therapy. Aspirin should be administered immediately. The addition of clopidogrel as part of antiplatelet therapy decreases mortality and major vascular events. Because of its multiple salutary effects on myocardial oxygen demand and supply, nitroglycerin is indicated for the first 48 hours for treatment of persistent ischemia, hypertension, or heart failure, unless systolic blood pressure is <90 mm Hg. Nitrates should not be used if hypotension limits the administration of β-blockers. It is reasonable to administer intravenous β-blockers promptly to patients with STEMI without contraindications, especially if a tachyarrhythmia or hypertension is present. β-blockers decrease the incidence of reinfarction and ventricular fibrillation but may increase the risk of cardiogenic shock, particularly in patients with hemodynamic instability. Arterial blood gases should generally be avoided, given the risk of bleeding in patients who have received or may receive anticoagulation or thrombolytic therapy.

2. Acute Reperfusion Therapy

Early reperfusion of the infarct-related coronary artery is associated with improved survival in patients with STEMI. Prompt restoration of flow in the infarct artery can be achieved by noninvasive pharmacological means (fibrinolysis), invasive primary PCI, or surgical intervention. A plan for early reperfusion of patients with STEMI should be developed by healthcare providers based on resources available in their facility and community.

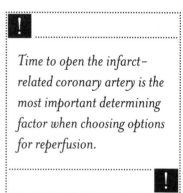

Time to open the infarct-related coronary artery is the most important determining factor when choosing options for reperfusion.

a. Percutaneous Coronary Intervention

Percutaneous coronary interventions include angioplasty with or without deployment of an intracoronary bare-metal or drug-eluting stent with support of pharmacologic measures to prevent thrombosis. Primary PCI is the preferred reperfusion technique if the procedure can be performed by experienced personnel within 12 hours of symptom onset. A goal of 90 minutes or less from hospital presentation to balloon inflation is optimum.

Primary PCI is particularly preferred over thrombolysis for patients with contraindications to thrombolysis or a high risk of bleeding, for patients with severe heart failure or cardiogenic shock (within 18 hours of onset), and for patients in whom the diagnosis of MI is in doubt. If primary PCI is not available, transfer to a facility with invasive reperfusion capability should be initiated as soon as possible (preferably within 30 minutes).

In other patients, the choice of reperfusion strategy depends on available resources, factors specific to the patient, and transport time to another facility for care. The higher the patient's mortality risk (as with large infarctions, heart failure or hemodynamic instability, previous infarctions, or acute left bundle branch block), the more primary PCI is preferred. Similarly, the higher the risk of thrombolysis, the more primary PCI is preferred. Conversely, the longer the time required for performance of PCI or transfer to another facility, the more thrombolysis is preferred. Patients presenting within 3 hours of the onset of symptoms appear to derive particular benefit from prompt reperfusion with thrombolytic therapy. Transfer for PCI is preferred over thrombolysis in patients who present 3 to 12 hours after onset of symptoms if transfer can be accomplished in a timely manner. In patients with clinical failure to reperfuse after thrombolytic therapy, rescue PCI, even if it requires transfer to another institution, is preferable.

Preprocedure management should include all of the strategies for ACS outlined previously. The use of heparin, clopidogrel, and GP IIb/IIIa inhibitors is warranted. Clopidogrel (300-600 mg orally) should be started as soon as the decision for PCI has been made. Potential complications of an invasive strategy for treating STEMI include problems with the arterial access site; adverse reactions to volume loading, contrast medium, and antithrombotic medications; technical complications; and reperfusion events.

Regardless of the reperfusion strategy chosen, timely implementation by experienced personnel is optimal. Routine, early use of PCI for patients who reperfuse with thrombolysis increases patient risk and is not recommended.

b. Fibrinolysis /Thrombolysis

Optimal limitation of infarct size when administering thrombolytics requires intervention within 6 hours of symptom onset, but thrombolytics may have some benefit as long as 12 hours after symptoms begin (**Table 10-8**). If the diagnosis is uncertain, the patient has contraindications to thrombolytic therapy, or the presentation is more than 3 hours after symptom onset, invasive reperfusion with PCI is preferred. The physician must weigh potential risks against benefits of thrombolysis for each patient. For patients with definite indications for thrombolysis and no absolute contraindications, intravenous thrombolytic therapy should be administered expeditiously. Several thrombolytic agents are now available, and all are effective (see list in **Table 10-9**). Findings that suggest reperfusion include relief of symptoms, maintenance or restoration of hemodynamic and/or electrical stability, reduction of at least 50% of the initial ST-segment elevation injury pattern on a follow-up ECG 60 to 90 minutes after initiation of therapy, and an early peak in the level of CK-MB (12-18 hours).

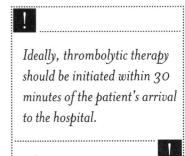

Ideally, thrombolytic therapy should be initiated within 30 minutes of the patient's arrival to the hospital.

Table 10-8.	Identification of Candidates for Thrombolytic Therapy

Definite Indications

Consistent clinical syndrome: chest pain, new arrhythmia, unexplained hypotension, or pulmonary edema

Diagnostic ECG: ST elevation of ≥1 mm in ≥2 contiguous precordial leads or ≥2 adjacent limb leads, or new or presumed to be new left bundle branch block

Time course: less than 12 hours since onset of pain

Relative Indications

Consistent clinical syndrome

Nondiagnostic ECG: left bundle branch block of unknown duration

Absolute Contraindications

Prior intracranial hemorrhage

Known cerebral vascular lesion

Ischemic stroke within past 3 months

Allergy to the agent

Significant head or facial trauma within past 3 months

Known intracranial neoplasm

Suspected aortic dissection

Active internal bleeding or bleeding diathesis (except menstruation)

Relative Contraindications

Severe uncontrolled hypertension on presentation (blood pressure >180/110 mm Hg)

History of chronic severe hypertension

Ischemic stroke >3 months ago or intracerebral pathology

Current use of anticoagulants

Traumatic or prolonged (>10 min) CPR or major surgery within past 3 weeks

Previous use of streptokinase/anistreplase: allergy or prior exposure (>5 days ago)

Active peptic ulcer disease

Recent internal bleeding (within past 2-4 weeks)

Bleeding diathesis (hepatic dysfunction, use of anticoagulants)

Noncompressible arterial or central venous puncture

Abbreviations: ECG, electrocardiogram; CPR, cardiopulmonary resuscitation.

Prehospital thrombolysis (full or reduced doses) may be administered to patients with STEMI in some communities. Most trials of prehospital thrombolysis do not demonstrate a reduction in mortality, but excellent results have been achieved when physicians or paramedics experienced in ECG interpretation and MI management are in the ambulance along with effective mechanisms for obtaining and transmitting ECGs. Prehospital thrombolysis may also be reasonable when transport times are >60 minutes, provided trained personnel are available.

Table 10-9.	Thrombolytic Agents Used in STEMI
Streptokinase	1.5 million units intravenously over 30-60 minutes
Alteplase	15 mg intravenous bolus, then 0.75 mg/kg (maximum 50 mg) intravenously over 30 minutes, then 0.50 mg/kg (maximum 35 mg) intravenously over 60 minutes
Anistreplase	30 units over 5 minutes
Reteplase	10 units intravenously over 2 minutes followed in 30 minutes by 10 units intravenously again over 2 minutes
Tenecteplase	Intravenous bolus adjusted for weight (30 mg if <60 kg, 35 mg if 60-70 kg, 40 mg if 70-80 kg, 45 mg if 80-90 kg, 50 mg if >90 kg)

3. Continuing Therapy

Patients who undergo PCI with angioplasty with or without stent placement should be treated with a GP IIb/IIIa inhibitor and clopidogrel. Clopidogrel administration should be discussed with the cardiologist because the optimum duration may vary with the type of stent used in PCI (bare metal vs drug-eluting). Anticoagulation with heparin is continued. After thrombolysis with a plasminogen activator, heparin should be used to maintain vessel patency for at least 48 hours. Infusion rates should be adjusted to keep the partial thromboplastin time at 1.5 to 2 times the control value. Heparin anticoagulation after use of streptokinase is not necessary. Patients with large anterior infarctions who do not receive thrombolysis or PCI and patients who have intramural thrombus detected or suspected on echocardiography should receive heparin. Aspirin in doses of 162 to 325 mg/day should be continued. Clopidogrel may also be beneficial in patients treated with thrombolytics who undergo delayed invasive reperfusion interventions. Intravenous nitroglycerin, if tolerated, is recommended for 48 hours post-MI in patients with hypertension, recurrent ischemia, or heart failure. In the absence of recurrent ischemia, heart failure, or arrhythmias, bed rest should not be continued beyond 12 to 24 hours.

Intravenous and oral β-blockers provide a mortality benefit by limiting infarct size, reducing recurrent ischemia, and decreasing arrhythmias in patients with STEMI who have no strong contraindications (**Table 10-8**). β-Blocker therapy is recommended with and without reperfusion therapy but is relatively contraindicated acutely in MI precipitated by cocaine because of the risk of coronary vasospasm. Long-term use of oral β-blockers is helpful in all patients who are at risk for recurrent cardiovascular events and who have no contraindications to their use.

Longer-acting calcium-channel blockers may be useful secondary therapy for recurrent myocardial ischemia but are not appropriate for first-line treatment. Immediate-release nifedipine is contraindicated in treatment of an acute MI. Diltiazem and verapamil are contraindicated in patients with STEMI and left ventricular dysfunction and heart failure.

Use of ACE inhibitors decreases mortality in all patients with STEMI. The greatest benefit is seen in patients with left ventricular dysfunction (ejection fraction <40%), anterior MI, or pulmonary congestion. Angiotensin-converting enzyme inhibition should be started within the first 24 hours after infarction with low doses of oral agents unless hypotension (systolic blood pressure <100 mm Hg) or other contraindications are present. An angiotensin receptor blocker (ARB) may be administered if the patient cannot tolerate an ACE inhibitor.

Expert consultation and/or transfer to another facility is indicated for patients who have persistent angina after MI, patients who develop cardiogenic shock, patients who have congestive heart failure despite aggressive therapy, or patients who have recurrent ventricular fibrillation or tachycardia despite aggressive antiarrhythmic therapy.

C. Risk Stratification for Patients With MI

It is crucial to identify high-risk patients with MI in whom severe or lethal complications may develop during the course of treatment. The following characteristics suggest high-risk patients who should be considered for aggressive therapy:

- Persistent ischemic symptoms after initial management

- Extensive infarction or ischemia

- Recurrent ischemia

- History of MI, CABG, or PCI

- Left ventricular dysfunction

- Angiographic findings compatible with high-risk coronary artery anatomy (eg, left main lesions)

D. Complications

Common early complications of MI are heart failure and cardiogenic shock, recurrent ischemia and/or infarction, and arrhythmias.

1. Heart Failure and Cardiogenic Shock

Bedside evaluation allows accurate determination of a patient's hemodynamic status (**Table 10-10**) and the need for hemodynamic monitoring and intervention. Patients with Killip classes I and II heart failure can be managed without invasive hemodynamic monitoring. Class III patients should be considered for hemodynamic monitoring if they do not respond promptly to medical therapy. Killip class IV patients generally require invasive monitoring with pulmonary artery catheterization and arterial blood pressure monitoring. Expert consultation should be sought and/or transfer arranged for patients with class III or IV findings. Invasive hemodynamic monitoring may also be warranted for patients with suspected mechanical complications of MI resulting in shock, such as papillary muscle rupture or dysfunction, ventricular septal defect, or cardiac tamponade.

Table 10-10. Killip-Kimball Hemodynamic Subsets	
Class	**Description**
I	No dyspnea; physical examination results are normal
II	No dyspnea; bibasilar crackles or S_3 on examination
III	Dyspnea present; bibasilar crackles or S_3 on examination; no hypotension
IV	Cardiogenic shock

Pharmacologic treatment for heart failure should be tailored to the patient's clinical and hemodynamic state. Patients with systolic arterial pressure >100 mm Hg, pulmonary artery occlusion pressure >15 mm Hg, and cardiac index <2.5 L/min/m² should be treated initially with a vasodilator, either intravenous nitroglycerin or intravenous nitroprusside in doses of 0.3 to 1 µg/kg/min, titrated up in increments of 0.5 µg/kg/min every 10 minutes. If arterial pressure decreases or the increase in cardiac output is inadequate, inotropic support with dobutamine should be initiated at 1 to 2 µg/kg/min and titrated to ≤15 µg/kg/min. Milrinone is an alternative inotropic agent. Loop diuretics, such as furosemide (20-40 mg intravenously or orally every 2-4 hours), should be used to reduce pulmonary congestion. Diuretics should be used with caution in hypotensive patients.

Patients with systolic arterial pressure <90 mm Hg, pulmonary arterial occlusion pressure >15 mm Hg, and cardiac index <2.5 L/min/m² have cardiogenic shock. These patients should be treated as soon as possible with intra-aortic balloon counterpulsation (IABC). Severely hypotensive patients (systolic arterial pressure <70 mm Hg) should be treated with norepinephrine to rapidly raise the systolic arterial pressure. If the systolic arterial pressure is 70 to 90 mm Hg with signs of shock, dopamine may be considered initially. Once the systolic blood pressure has stabilized to at least 90 mm Hg, dobutamine can be added to further increase cardiac output and reduce the dosage of vasopressor.

Interventional therapy with IABC may be indicated in patients with pump failure who do not respond promptly to medical therapy. Intra-aortic balloon counterpulsation has several potential benefits in these patients. During inflation, the balloon augments coronary blood flow and forward cardiac output. During deflation, it decreases afterload and preload as well. Intra-aortic balloon counterpulsation and other ventricular assist devices may stabilize the hemodynamic status sufficiently to allow PCI or coronary bypass surgery.

Evidence suggests that patients with STEMI who develop shock within 36 hours of MI benefit from early invasive reperfusion performed within 18 hours of onset of shock. In patients with 1- or 2-vessel disease, PCI is preferred. Patients who remain symptomatic and have 3-vessel disease or significant left main coronary artery disease should undergo urgent coronary bypass surgery. Percutaneous coronary intervention should also be performed in patients with severe heart failure and/or pulmonary edema and onset of symptoms within 12 hours.

a. Right Ventricular Infarction/Ischemia

Some patients have heart failure from ischemia of the right ventricle, which results in elevation of right atrial and right ventricular end-diastolic pressures to >10 mm Hg, cardiac index <2.5 L/min/m^2, and systolic arterial pressure <100 mm Hg. These patients generally have clear lung fields, no third heart sound, and distended internal jugular veins. The ECG usually reveals an inferior MI, and the ST segment in lead V1 may be elevated in the absence of elevation of any other standard precordial lead. An ECG tracing of the right precordial leads should be obtained and may reveal characteristic ST-segment elevation, especially in V4R. Initial therapy includes volume expansion until the blood pressure is stabilized, pulmonary arterial occlusion pressure is >20 mm Hg, or right atrial pressure is >20 mm Hg. Associated bradycardia or high-degree heart block may require chemical or electrical intervention. Agents such as nitrates and diuretics that reduce preload should be avoided. If volume expansion is inadequate to stabilize a patient, dobutamine can be administered. Intra-aortic balloon counterpulsation should be considered for refractory hypotension.

2. Recurrent Ischemia or Infarction

Recurrent ischemia or infarction occurs in ≤20% of patients treated with thrombolytic therapy for MI. Patients treated with primary PCI have a lower incidence of recurrent ischemia. Ischemia after MI can be caused by residual stenosis in the infarct-related artery or by disease in another coronary artery. An ECG taken during recurrent pain should be compared with ECGs from the index MI event. Reinfarction may present special diagnostic difficulties because cardiac troponin levels can be elevated for 5 to 14 days. If the first blood sample has an elevated cardiac troponin value when recurrent ischemia is suspected, then serial levels of a cardiac marker with a shorter time course of returning to normal, such as CK-MB or myoglobin, could be analyzed to clarify the possibility of recurrent infarction. No cardiac marker is reliable for diagnosis of reinfarction in the first 18 hours after onset of STEMI. Pericarditis should also be considered as a potential cause of recurrent chest pain after an MI.

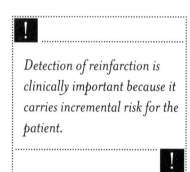

Detection of reinfarction is clinically important because it carries incremental risk for the patient.

Medical treatment of post-MI ischemia is similar to management of unstable angina but also includes cardiac catheterization and reperfusion, if possible and not recently accomplished. Recurrent infarction with ST elevation on ECG can be treated with repeat thrombolysis. Streptokinase-based drugs should not be used a second time because of the risk of allergic reactions. Plasminogen activator-based regimens can be repeated. Acute reperfusion with PCI or CABG may be required for stabilization.

3. Arrhythmias

Arrhythmias associated with ACS and reperfusion include atrial bradycardias, atrial tachyarrhythmias, atrioventricular (A-V) blocks, ventricular tachyarrhythmias, and asystole. Hemodynamically significant atrial bradycardia or A-V block can be initially treated with intravenous atropine in a dose of 0.5 mg every 3-5 minutes to a total dose of 3 mg while preparing for transcutaneous pacing. Atropine rarely corrects complete heart block or type II second-degree A-V block. Temporary transvenous pacing is indicated for complete heart block, bilateral bundle branch block, new or indeterminate-age bifascicular block with first-degree A-V block, type II second-degree A-V block, and symptomatic sinus bradycardia that is unresponsive to atropine. Transcutaneous pacing should be initiated for patients who have indications for emergent temporary pacing until transvenous pacing can be instituted (**Appendix 7**).

Atrial tachyarrhythmias, such as atrial fibrillation, may cause hemodynamic instability and precipitate myocardial ischemia, or may be clinically insignificant and transient. Immediate cardioversion is indicated in unstable patients. Depending upon the specific arrhythmia, intravenous adenosine, β-blockers, or diltiazem may be effective (**Appendix 4**). Careful attention must be given to contraindications for any of these agents.

Ventricular tachycardia and ventricular fibrillation should be treated according to current ACLS guidelines. After defibrillation, if indicated, amiodarone is the drug of choice in patients with an MI. Patients with new-onset, symptomatic ventricular ectopy may also benefit from treatment with amiodarone. Antiarrhythmic drugs are not recommended as prophylaxis for ventricular arrhythmias in the setting of acute MI.

E. Special Considerations

1. Perioperative Myocardial Infarction

Perioperative MI can occur prior to surgery, intraoperatively, and during the postoperative period. Postoperative MI is the most common, with the peak incidence on the third postoperative day. Perioperative MI is often associated with atypical presentations and is frequently painless. New-onset, or an increase in, ventricular arrhythmias is often the presenting finding, as is postoperative pulmonary edema. The diagnosis can be confirmed with serial ECG and cardiac marker determinations. Treatment is similar to standard treatment, except that thrombolytic therapy may be contraindicated depending on the type of surgery. Primary PCI should be considered for these patients. The mortality for perioperative MI is very high, 50% to 60% in some studies.

2. Effects of Coexisting Diseases

Many, if not most, critically ill patients suffer from more than one medical condition that may require significant alterations in the standard therapeutic approach. Many patients have relative or absolute contraindications to standard medications or procedures. Patients with stress ulceration or gastritis may not be candidates for aspirin therapy. Postoperative patients or patients with a bleeding diathesis may not be candidates for clopidogrel, heparin, thrombolytic therapy, GP IIb/IIIa inhibitors, or aspirin. β-Blockers should be avoided in patients with significant bronchospasm or decompensated heart failure. Because dopamine can significantly elevate pulmonary artery pressures or increase heart rate, lower doses or an alternative drug may be necessary in patients with respiratory failure or atrial tachyarrhythmias. Certain drugs will need dose adjustments for renal or hepatic dysfunction.

Acute Coronary Syndromes

■ The preliminary diagnosis of unstable angina/non–ST-elevation MI is based on the clinical symptoms, assessment of risk factors for coronary artery disease, and ECG interpretation.

■ A 12-lead ECG should be obtained and interpreted within 10 minutes in patients with possible myocardial ischemia.

■ Non–enteric-coated aspirin at a dose of 162 to 325 mg should be initially administered (by chewing) as soon as possible to all patients with suspected or diagnosed ACS.

■ High-risk patients (continuing ischemia, elevated troponin levels) with UA/NSTEMI may be candidates for additional therapy with glycoprotein (GP) IIb/IIIa inhibitors and an early invasive strategy.

■ The combination of aspirin and heparin is more beneficial in ACS than aspirin alone.

■ β-Blockers should be administered to all patients with ACS unless there are strong contraindications.

■ A plan for early reperfusion of patients with STEMI should be developed by healthcare providers based on resources available in their facility and community.

■ A goal of 90 minutes or less from hospital presentation to balloon inflation is optimum for primary PCI for STEMI.

■ Thrombolytic therapy for reperfusion in STEMI should ideally be initiated within 30 minutes of the patient's arrival to the hospital.

■ Patients who undergo PCI with angioplasty with or without stent placement should be treated with a GP IIb/IIIa inhibitor and an antiplatelet agent such as clopidogrel.

■ Use of angiotensin-converting enzyme (ACE) inhibitors decreases mortality in all patients with STEMI.

■ Evidence suggests that patients with STEMI who develop shock within 36 hours of MI benefit from early invasive reperfusion performed within 18 hours of onset of shock.

Suggested Readings

1. Antman EM, Anbe DT, Armstrong PW, et al; Committee to Revise the 1999 Guidelines for the Management of Patients With Acute Myocardial Infarction. ACC/AHA guidelines for the management of patients with ST-elevation myocardial infarction: a report of the American College of Cardiology/American Heart Association Task Force on Practice Guidelines [executive summary]. *J Am Coll Cardiol.* 2004;44:671. Full text available at http://www.acc.org/qualityandscience/clinical/guidelines/stemi/Guideline1/index.pdf.

2. Antman E, Bassand J-P, Klein W, et al. Myocardial infarction redefined: a consensus document of the Joint European Society of Cardiology/American College of Cardiology Committee for the Redefinition of Myocardial Infarction. *J Am Coll Cardiol.* 2000;36:959.

3. Bavry AA, Kumbhani DJ, Quiroz R, et al. Invasive therapy along with glycoprotein IIb/IIIa inhibitors and intracoronary stents improves survival in non–ST-segment-elevation acute coronary syndromes: a meta-analysis and review of the literature. *Am J Cardiol.* 2004;93:830.

4. Bhatt DL, Topol EJ. Current role of platelet glycoprotein IIb/IIIa inhibitors in acute coronary syndromes. *JAMA.* 2000;284:1549.

5. Braunwald E, Antman EM, Beasley JW, et al; Committee on Management of Patients with Unstable Angina. ACC/AHA guidelines for the management of patients with unstable angina and non–ST-segment elevation myocardial infarction: a report of the American College of Cardiology/American Heart Association Task Force on Practice Guidelines [executive summary]. *J Am Coll Cardiol.* 2002;40:1366. Full text available at http://www.acc.org/qualityandscience/clinical/guidelines/unstable/unstable.pdf.

6. Task Force on the Management of Acute Coronary Syndromes of the European Society of Cardiology. Management of acute coronary syndromes in patients presenting without persistent ST-segment elevation. *Eur Heart J.* 2002;23:1809. http://www.escardio.org.

7. Task Force on the Management of Acute Myocardial Infarction of the European Society of Cardiology. Management of acute myocardial infarction in patients presenting with ST-segment elevation. *Eur Heart J.* 2003;24:28. http://www.escardio.org.

8. Ting HH, Yang EH, *Rihal* CS. Narrative review: reperfusion strategies for ST-segment elevation myocardial infarction. *Ann Intern Med.* 2006;145:610.

Web Sites

1. American College of Cardiology. http://www.acc.org. Guidelines for management of acute coronary syndromes and related cardiovascular topics.

2. American Heart Association. http://www.americanheart.org. Guidelines for management of acute coronary syndromes and related cardiovascular topics.

3. European Society of Cardiology. http://www.escardio.org. Guidelines for management of acute coronary syndromes and additional cardiovascular information available in the section "Knowledge Centre."

Chapter 11:

Life-Threatening Infections: Diagnosis and Antimicrobial Therapy Selection

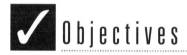

Objectives

- Understand and apply the terminology specific to life-threatening infections.

- List the risk factors for the development of infection.

- Identify systemic and site-specific clinical manifestations of life-threatening infections, and understand the use of clinical laboratory tests in the diagnosis of possible infections.

- Describe the different clinical and epidemiologic variables used to guide the selection of antimicrobial therapy.

- Outline antimicrobial treatment for empiric therapy and for specific infections.

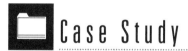

Case Study

A 75-year-old man presented to the emergency department with altered mental status. His family reported that the patient has had a productive cough for the last 2 days. His vital signs are blood pressure 110/70 mm Hg, heart rate 110/min, temperature 102.2°F (39°C), respiratory rate 20/min, and pulse oximetry 92% while receiving 2 L/min oxygen by nasal cannula. You are the patient's primary physician and are called to admit him to the hospital.

    – Does this patient have sepsis or severe sepsis?

    – What level of care is needed for this patient?

    – What initial interventions should be instituted immediately?

I. INTRODUCTION

Life-threatening infections are both a cause and a consequence of critical illness. The incidence of life-threatening infections or sepsis is increasing as a reflection of the growing population of patients at risk—the elderly; immunocompromised patients; those with malignancy, chronic illness, or multiple trauma; and so forth. Septic shock, the most severe form of systemic response to infection, is a common cause of mortality in critically ill adults and children. Early recognition and appropriate management of infections and their sequelae can decrease mortality.

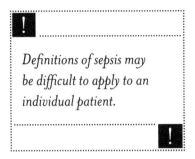

Definitions of sepsis may be difficult to apply to an individual patient.

Sepsis is defined as systemic manifestations of infection. *Severe sepsis* is sepsis associated with organ dysfunction, hypoperfusion, or hypotension. Abnormalities that suggest hypoperfusion and organ dysfunction may include, but are not limited to, lactic acidosis, oliguria, coagulation disorders, or an acute alteration in mental status. These abnormalities are not specific for sepsis and may be present in other conditions. *Septic shock* is sepsis with arterial hypotension, defined as a systolic blood pressure <90 mm Hg or a decrease of >40 mm Hg from the patient's baseline systolic blood pressure, despite adequate fluid resuscitation, with concomitant organ dysfunction. Patients receiving inotropic or vasopressor agents may not be hypotensive at the time that perfusion abnormalities are measured.

II. DIAGNOSIS OF INFECTION

The diagnosis of serious or life-threatening infection is based on a careful and complete assessment of the patient's history, including risk factors, and the presence of characteristic clinical manifestations. Atypical presentations that may occur, particularly in the elderly and in the immunocompromised patient, must also be considered. Laboratory, microbiologic, and imaging results also support the diagnosis of documented or suspected infection.

A. Epidemiologic Factors

Serious or life-threatening infections may occur in patients from the community, long-term care facilities (ie, nursing homes), or hospital settings. Serious or life-threatening community-acquired infections include bacterial pneumonia, central nervous system (CNS) infections or meningitis, urosepsis, intra-abdominal sepsis due to a ruptured or obstructed viscus, or sporadic uncommon infections, such as necrotizing fasciitis. Patients from long-term care facilities have a similar spectrum to community dwellers but often have infections with more resistant pathogens and may have different device-related infections. Finally, hospitalized patients are exposed to the most antimicrobial-resistant flora and to numerous invasive devices, and they have more comorbidities and greater severity of illness.

B. Predisposing Conditions

The presence of predisposing conditions should alert the care team to patients at higher risk of developing infections (**Table 11-1**). Permanent prosthetic implants such as heart valves, intravascular grafts, or orthopedic devices may become infected in either the early or the late postoperative period. Invasive procedures such as surgery, vascular catheterization, placement of urinary catheters, and endotracheal intubation breech the normal mucosal defense barriers and predispose patients to infection. The lack of predisposing conditions does not eliminate the possibility that a serious infection is present, particularly in patients admitted directly to the ICU from the community.

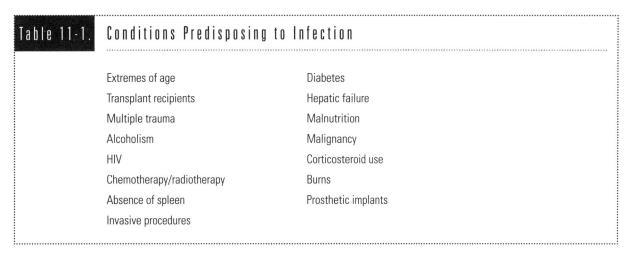

Table 11-1.	Conditions Predisposing to Infection	
	Extremes of age	Diabetes
	Transplant recipients	Hepatic failure
	Multiple trauma	Malnutrition
	Alcoholism	Malignancy
	HIV	Corticosteroid use
	Chemotherapy/radiotherapy	Burns
	Absence of spleen	Prosthetic implants
	Invasive procedures	

C. Clinical Manifestations

The clinical manifestations of life-threatening infections are diverse, and they may be subtle or overt and localized or systemic. An awareness of the signs and symptoms associated with specific infections allows early recognition and prompt institution of appropriate empiric antimicrobial and supportive management. However, most of the clinical manifestations are not specific.

1. Systemic Signs and Symptoms

Fever is the most frequent systemic manifestation of infection. However, patients with serious infection may be normothermic or even hypothermic, particularly if they are elderly, or in the presence of antipyretic medications, alcoholism, and renal or hepatic failure. Temperature probes on a urinary catheter or pulmonary artery catheter, when available, are the most reliable methods to measure the core temperature. Temperature measurement is most practically obtained via the oral or rectal routes, although the limitations of each method should be considered. Axillary temperatures are unreliable, and tympanic measurements have not been validated in the critically ill.

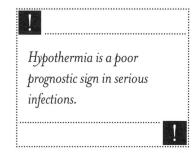

Hypothermia is a poor prognostic sign in serious infections.

Other systemic manifestations include chills, rigors, hypotension, tachypnea, dyspnea, tachycardia, and nausea and vomiting. Tachycardia is almost always present but may be absent in the presence of cardiac conduction disturbances, autonomic dysfunction, β-blockers or calcium-channel blockers, and drug fever. Hypotension may be due to dehydration and hypovolemia but may also indicate that septic shock is present, particularly if the blood pressure does not respond to volume resuscitation. Hypoperfusion of the kidneys may result in oliguria or anuria. Encephalopathy is a common clinical manifestation and ranges from lethargy/irritability to delirium and coma. Petechiae, ecchymosis, or both may be present, particularly on distal extremities.

2. Site-Specific Signs and Symptoms

Some signs and symptoms of infection could be associated with the specific source of infection:

- Infections of the central nervous system (CNS) may be associated with headache, seizures, meningismus, or focal neurologic findings. Altered mental status is often present but not specific for CNS infections.

- Diffuse or localized respiratory tract infections may be associated with dyspnea, tachypnea, cough, sputum production, or, rarely, hemoptysis. Chest auscultation findings, such as crackles, rhonchi, or tubular breath sounds, indicate whether the process is localized or diffuse. Diminished breath sounds and percussion dullness are suggestive of a pleural effusion.

- Intra-abdominal infections may cause abdominal pain, abdominal distension, nausea and/or vomiting, diarrhea, and anorexia. Diaphragmatic irritation can be perceived as pain in the side of the neck and proximal shoulder area or may cause hiccoughs. Findings on examination may include diffuse or local tenderness, rebound tenderness, ileus, or guaiac-positive stool. A wound infection with evidence of fascial disruption may signal an intra-abdominal infection below the fascia.

- Urinary tract infections may produce flank pain or abdominal pain, tenderness, dysuria, hematuria, and oliguria. Typically, a urinary catheter–associated infection does not produce localized symptoms.

- Cutaneous manifestations may result from a primary infection of the skin or skin structures (eg, pain, erythema, and induration due to cellulitis; wound margin erythema; tenderness or purulent discharge; vesicular lesions due to Herpes infection) or may result from disseminated systemic infection (eg, erythematous indurated papules or nodules of ecthyma gangrenosum due to bacteremia, septic emboli due to infective endocarditis, diffuse macular erythema due to toxic shock syndrome, distal symmetric purpura fulminans due to meningococcemia).

D. Laboratory Manifestations

Routine laboratory tests are not specific in the diagnosis of life-threatening infections but may be suggestive and allow assessment of organ function. The white blood cell (WBC) count is usually elevated with a shift to more immature forms (called a left shift). Leukocytosis is also commonly observed in noninfectious processes such as the early postoperative period, corticosteroid therapy, massive transfusions, and polytrauma. Conversely, a normal leukocyte count may be observed despite active infection in the elderly and in patients with hypersplenism or chronic myelosuppressive disorders. Neutropenia may result from overwhelming infection (especially in neonates and AIDS patients), severe viral infection, typhoid fever, brucellosis, and other infections. Toxic granulation within neutrophils may also be noted.

The most common coagulation abnormality in sepsis is isolated thrombocytopenia. A decline in platelet count may be a subtle, early clue to the presence of infection. Disseminated intravascular coagulation (DIC) is a less common finding but is a poor prognostic sign. Disseminated intravascular coagulation is characterized by an elevated prothrombin time, partial thromboplastin time, fibrin split products and/or D-dimer, and decreased fibrinogen.

Sepsis causes relative insulin resistance, usually resulting in hyperglycemia, whereas hypoglycemia is less frequent and often reflects low hepatic glycogen stores. Arterial blood gas measurements usually reflect metabolic acidosis, a low $PaCO_2$ due to respiratory compensation, and, often, hypoxemia. An elevated serum lactate level is a significant sign of compromised peripheral perfusion and oxygen balance due to severe sepsis or septic shock. Hepatic dysfunction is usually not severe but presents as a cholestatic picture with elevated bilirubin and mild elevation of transaminases. Renal insufficiency often occurs due to multiple factors such as hypotension and hypovolemia. Other possible nonspecific markers of inflammation/infection include procalcitonin and C-reactive protein.

E. Microbiologic Studies

Microbiologic studies are divided into those with results that will be immediately available (minutes to a few hours) and those requiring a period of incubation for growth or laboratory determinations. Among the studies with quickly available results is Gram stain of body fluids. Special stains (such as fungal and acid-fast stains), immunoassays (such as urine *Legionella* antigen and *Clostridium difficile* toxins), and counterimmunoelectrophoresis panels take more time to process.

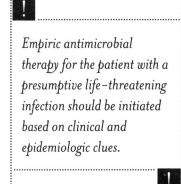

Empiric antimicrobial therapy for the patient with a presumptive life-threatening infection should be initiated based on clinical and epidemiologic clues.

Ideally, all cultures should be obtained before initiation or modification of antimicrobial therapy, but this may not be possible in the rapidly deteriorating patient. The selection of site(s) to culture should be guided by the clinical manifestations. Indiscriminately obtaining cultures from many sites not only may yield misleading results due to culture contamination or site colonization but is also not cost-effective and may pose additional risks to the patient. Repeat cultures may be appropriate to assess for changes in the type of organism or resistance patterns.

At least 2 sets of peripheral blood cultures (aerobic and anaerobic bottle) should be obtained either from different anatomic sites or from the same site but separated by 30 minutes. A blood volume of 10 to 15 milliliters per blood culture set is optimal in adults. Obtaining blood cultures from indwelling peripheral or central intravascular catheters may yield false-positive results because of microbial contamination of the catheter hub. Isolator blood cultures may improve the diagnostic yield for some organisms (eg, *Candida, Mycobacterium*) or for patients already receiving antimicrobial therapy.

Respiratory tract cultures require expectorated sputum from the nonintubated patient and tracheal suction or bronchoscopic specimens from an intubated patient. Many microbiology laboratories will screen the specimen for the number of epithelial cells and neutrophils to determine adequacy for culture. Quantitative cultures of lower respiratory tract secretions may discriminate between colonizing and pathogenic bacteria.

In the noncatheterized patient, urine cultures should be clean-catch voided specimens; in catheterized patients, specimens should be aspirated from the urinary catheter tubing. Semiquantitative culture is needed; however, thresholds for significance differ for clean-catch urine ($>10^5$ organisms/mL) and catheter-obtained urine ($>10^3$ organisms/mL). Urinalysis for the detection of pyuria will help to discriminate bacteriuria from cystitis or upper tract infection.

Intravascular catheters should be removed in aseptic fashion and the intradermal segment should be sent for semiquantitative culture. However, clinical correlation between the catheter culture result, blood culture(s), and appearance of the catheter exit site is required to discriminate between catheter-related bacteremia, local catheter-related infection, and simple colonization of the catheter itself. The best method for diagnosis of intravascular catheter-related bloodstream infections is the testing of paired cultures from peripheral and catheter blood samples.

F. Additional Studies

A complete description of additional studies for all infections is beyond the scope of this chapter. However, some of the additional studies specific for the chest, central nervous system, and abdomen/retroperitoneum are summarized in **Table 11-2.**

Table 11-2.	Selected Additional Studies for Infections

Chest

- An upright posterior-anterior (PA) and lateral chest radiograph
- A lateral decubitus chest radiograph or ultrasound to evaluate for possible pleural fluid
- Computed tomographic (CT) scan of chest to evaluate the mediastinum, lung parenchyma, and pleural-based lesions
- Thoracentesis if fluid is present
- Transthoracic and/or transesophageal echocardiogram

Central Nervous System

- Lumbar puncture for patients with possible CNS infection, including patients with evidence of meningismus and/or altered mental status for which no other cause is readily apparent. A lumbar puncture is mandatory in febrile neonates, because of the high incidence of sepsis with meningitis in these patients. Contraindications to lumbar puncture are severe thrombocytopenia and coagulopathy, suspected intracranial mass lesion, or severe respiratory compromise that precludes adequate positioning. If a significant delay of 1 hour or longer is anticipated before performing the lumbar puncture, empiric antimicrobials should be initiated immediately, prior to the procedure.
- CT or MRI of the head or spine
- Electroencephalography (EEG)

Abdomen/Retroperitoneum

- Supine, upright or supine decubitus films to assess for free air
- CT scan, usually with intravenous and oral contrast
- Hepatobiliary ultrasound
- Renal ultrasound

III. ANTIMICROBIAL THERAPY

 ## Case Study

A 23-year-old female who had been in a motor vehicle accident was transferred to the floor from the ICU. She had been intubated for 4 days due to pulmonary contusions. After 1 day on the floor, she develops fever, an elevated white blood cell count, and worsening hypoxemia. You are called to evaluate the patient.

- What is the likely source of this patient's infection?

- What factors would influence your choice of antimicrobial agent?

The first priority in managing a hemodynamically unstable patient with a severe or life-threatening infection is resuscitation (see **Chapters 6 and 7**). After evaluation of the patient by history, physical examination, and auxiliary tests (laboratory and imaging studies), antimicrobial agents should be instituted promptly.

Early use of appropriate empiric antimicrobial therapy reduces infection–associated mortality.

Early source control is paramount to favorable outcomes and is an essential adjunct to adequate antimicrobial therapy. Examples of source control include wound debridement, percutaneous or surgical drainage of a closed-space infection, foreign body removal, and surgery. It is important to understand that the antimicrobial therapy recommendations found in this chapter are general guidelines only. Antimicrobial choices must be individualized for each clinical scenario to match the clinical manifestations and the available epidemiologic information and microbiological data, including the patterns of microbial prevalence and resistance in your own institution or local community.

The selection of appropriate antimicrobial therapy depends on the following factors:

1. **The suspected microbial pathogen(s) and site of infection:** The most common sites for life-threatening infections in adult patients involve the lower respiratory tract, the intra-abdominal cavity, and the bloodstream. Rapidly progressive soft-tissue infections and central nervous system infections should also be considered and are often clinically obvious. Penetration of the selected antimicrobial to the site of infection should also be considered. The central nervous system and lungs are two sites that allow limited penetration of certain antimicrobials, therefore it is important to understand the pharmacokinetic characteristics of the selected agents to ensure maximal antimicrobial activity at those sites.

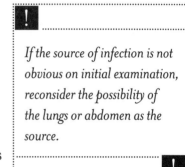

If the source of infection is not obvious on initial examination, reconsider the possibility of the lungs or abdomen as the source.

2. **Gram stain results of available specimens from the suspected site:** The description of early stain results directs the clinician to the broad categories of organism(s) that should be covered. Examples include Gram-positive cocci in clusters (*Staphylococci*) or pairs and chains (*Enterococci, Streptococci*), lancet-shaped diplococci (*pneumococcus*), Gram-positive bacilli (*Corynebacterium, Nocardia*), Gram-negative bacilli (*Escherichia coli, Klebsiella, Pseudomonas*), small pleomorphic Gram-negative bacilli (*Bacteroides* spp), Gram-negative coccobacilli (*Haemophilus* spp, *Moraxella, Acinetobacter*), and yeast (*Candida*). However, the clinician should wait for final culture results to make changes to initial antimicrobial therapy.

3. **Assessment for antimicrobial resistance:** Factors that predict that a particular bacterial pathogen may be resistant to a wider range of antimicrobials include the following:

   – Prior isolation of resistant strains from the same patient

   – Prior antimicrobial therapy (broad-spectrum antimicrobial therapy such as antipseudomonal penicillin/β-lactamase inhibitor combinations, third- and fourth-generation cephalosporins, fluoroquinolones, carbapenems, vancomycin, etc)

   – Longer hospital or ICU stay

- High endemic rate of multidrug-resistant bacteria in the institution or ICU (eg, methicillin-resistant *Staphylococcus aureus,* vancomycin-resistant *Enterococcus* (VRE), multidrug-resistant *Pseudomonas, Stenotrophomonas*)

- Ongoing epidemic outbreak in the hospital or ICU

- Chronic dialysis

- Residence in a nursing home or extended-care facility

- Immunosuppressive diseases or therapy

Certain common organisms have become increasingly resistant to formerly effective antimicrobials. This category includes *Streptococcus pneumoniae* with intermediate- and high-level resistance to penicillin and ceftriaxone, *Enterococcus faecium* strains resistant to ampicillin and vancomycin, *Staphylococcus aureus* resistant to oxacillin/methicillin (MRSA), Gram-negative bacilli (*E coli, K pneumoniae*) with extended-spectrum β-lactamase (ESBL) or chromosomal-mediated β-lactamase production observed in strains of *P aeruginosa,* or other mechanisms of multiple resistance to broad-spectrum antimicrobial therapy. It is vital to know and update the resistance pattern of the different bacterial pathogens in each institution and each ICU.

4. **Comorbid conditions:** Less nephrotoxic antimicrobials may be preferable in patients with diminished renal function or patients at risk for renal failure unless the benefit of use outweighs the risk of renal dysfunction. Other comorbidities to consider include bone marrow suppression, chronic or acute liver failure, prior hearing deficits, pregnancy, and a history of major hypersensitivity or other strong adverse reactions to a specific antimicrobial.

IV. RECOMMENDED ANTIMICROBIAL THERAPY

The use of the antimicrobial therapies recommended below is based on the suspected site of infection in the absence of culture results. The physician should always consider the dose, dose adjustments, possible interactions, and side effects of selected agents. Antimicrobial therapy should be given in maximum appropriate therapeutic doses, and in critically ill patients, intravenous administration is preferred to intramuscular or oral routes. Oral dosing of antimicrobials with similar bioequivalence (eg, quinolones) and adequate gastrointestinal absorption may be substituted after the patient becomes more stable. Dosage adjustments must be made for the elderly, neonates, children, and patients with renal or hepatic dysfunction. Antimicrobial de-escalation should be implemented in appropriate clinical situations once cultures are negative. In the treatment of infection, it is imperative that antimicrobial agents be used appropriately and responsibly.

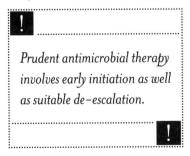

Prudent antimicrobial therapy involves early initiation as well as suitable de-escalation.

A. Central Nervous System

1. Meningitis

Of all infectious diseases, bacterial meningitis causes one of the most crucial emergencies. When bacterial meningitis is suspected clinically, antimicrobial therapy should be instituted immediately, without waiting for the results of lumbar puncture. Community-acquired acute bacterial meningitis in adults is most commonly caused by *S pneumoniae or N meningitidis*, and initial empiric therapy with a third-generation cephalosporin (ceftriaxone or cefotaxime) provides adequate empiric coverage, with vancomycin added if penicillin-resistant *S pneumoniae* is suspected or confirmed. If *S pneumoniae* is isolated, a third-generation cephalosporin should be continued until penicillin sensitivity is confirmed, at which point the patient should be switched to high-dose penicillin G. *N meningitidis* in CSF or blood culture should be treated with high-dose parenteral penicillin G. If *N meningitidis* is isolated, healthcare workers with significant exposure will require antimicrobial prophylaxis. In addition to antimicrobial therapy, adjunctive dexamethasone (0.15 mg/kg IV q 6 hours for 2-4 days) is also recommended to decrease morbidity and mortality, particularly in pneumococcal meningitis.

Special circumstances require different empiric antimicrobial coverage. *Listeria monocytogenes* may be a cause of bacterial meningitis in extremes of age (neonates, infants, and elderly people) and in patients with T lymphocyte defects, usually due to diabetes, corticosteroids, and immunosuppressive therapy (eg, organ recipients and patients with autoimmune disease). Patients with suspected *Listeria* meningitis should be covered with ampicillin (trimethoprim-sulfamethoxazole in the penicillin-allergic patient). Patients who have undergone recent neurosurgical procedures or placement of CSF shunts are at increased risk for *Staphylococcus aureus,* coagulase-negative staphylococci, and Gram-negative bacilli (*Pseudomonas, Klebsiella*). Therefore, such patients require initial empiric antimicrobial coverage with high-dose vancomycin and a third- or fourth-generation cephalosporin. If methicillin-susceptible *S aureus* is confirmed, nafcillin is the drug of choice.

Meningitis presenting in a subacute fashion over a period of several weeks or longer, with predominance of CSF lymphocytes, is more likely to occur in immunocompromised patients. Pathogens such as *Mycobacterium tuberculosis, Toxoplasma gondii,* and *Cryptococcus neoformans* should be considered in this setting.

2. Encephalitis or Meningoencephalitis

Many viral agents can cause encephalitis or meningoencephalitis, but only *Herpes simplex* (HSV) and cytomegalovirus (CMV) encephalitis are amenable to therapy. *Herpes simplex* encephalitis usually occurs in immunocompetent individuals presenting from the community. Fever, lethargy, confusion, and seizures are the most common presenting complaints. Hemorrhagic CSF and temporal lobe involvement in imaging studies (CT or MRI) or EEG are suggestive of HSV encephalitis. Polymerase chain reaction (PCR) testing of CSF is sensitive for diagnosis of this infection. If HSV encephalitis is suspected or confirmed, a 14- to 21-day course of parenteral acyclovir should be promptly initiated, pending further studies. Cytomegalovirus encephalitis usually occurs in patients with suppressed immune status (HIV and transplant patients) and could have the same clinical manifestations as HSV encephalitis. Polymerase chain reaction testing of CSF for CMV is also highly sensitive and therapy should include ganciclovir or foscarnet.

3. Brain Abscess

Brain abscess is an uncommon infection but should be suspected in patients with chronic infections of parameningeal structures, left-sided endocarditis, or congenital cyanotic heart disease. Brain abscesses have also been associated with immunosuppression, as in AIDS patients, intravenous drug abusers, or transplant recipients. Infections are often polymicrobial, and etiologic organisms include aerobic and anaerobic streptococci, staphylococci, Gram-negative bacteria, and anaerobes. Initial antimicrobial therapy should include penicillin, high-dose metronidazole, and a third-generation cephalosporin. Vancomycin can be substituted in patients who are allergic to penicillin or when there is a suspected or documented infection with methicillin-resistant *S aureus* or resistant pneumococcus. In patients at high risk for toxoplasmosis (eg, those with AIDS, cardiac transplant recipients), pyrimethamine/sulfadiazine should be part of the initial antimicrobial regimen. Less common causes of brain abscess include tuberculosis, nocardiosis, syphilis, amoeba, and other parasites. The diagnostic yield of CSF cultures for brain abscess is extremely low, and brain biopsy may be needed in patients who fail to respond to empiric therapy.

B. Respiratory Tract

1. Severe Community-Acquired Pneumonia (Immunocompetent Host)

The most common organism resulting in hospitalization for community-acquired pneumonia is *S pneumoniae*, but other causative organisms include *Legionella, Mycoplasma,* and *Chlamydia. Haemophilus influenzae* is an uncommon pathogen in the United States since the introduction of the vaccine against *H influenzae* type B in children. A β-lactam (ceftriaxone, cefotaxime, ampicillin-sulbactam) plus either a macrolide (azithromycin) or a respiratory fluoroquinolone are recommended in patients admitted to the ICU. If the patient is allergic to penicillin, a respiratory fluoroquinolone and aztreonam are recommended. If aspiration pneumonia is suspected (alcoholics, presence of poor dentition), then the addition of clindamycin is warranted unless a β-lactam/β-lactamase inhibitor combination is utilized. If *Pseudomonas* is a consideration, an antipneumococcal and antipseudomonal β-lactam (piperacillin-tazobactam, cefepime, imipenem, or meropenem) plus either ciprofloxacin or levofloxacin should be initiated. Alternatives to the fluoroquinolone in the suggested regimen include an aminoglycoside and azithromycin or an aminoglycoside and an antipneumococcal fluoroquinolone. Vancomycin or linezolid may be added if community-acquired MRSA is suspected.

2. Community-Acquired Pneumonia (Immunocompromised Host)

Immunocompromised patients with pneumonia may have the same pathogens as an immunocompetent host but with more severe infection. Radiographic evidence of interstitial pneumonia or a normal chest radiograph in a patient with prominent respiratory symptoms who has T cell deficiency (AIDS, chronic steroid use) should prompt the addition of trimethoprim-sulfamethoxazole in appropriate doses for possible *Pneumocystis carinii infection.* Consider the addition of steroids in *P carinii* pneumonia associated with significant hypoxemia. Focal lesions (eg, abscess, nodules) are suggestive of fungal infections, *M tuberculosis,* or *Nocardia.* Empiric coverage with antifungal agents, antimycobacterial agents, and trimethoprim-sulfamethoxazole may be warranted in these circumstances. Patients with suspected *M tuberculosis* infection also require respiratory isolation. Cytomegalovirus (CMV) or other viral infection should also be considered in the differential of an interstitial pneumonitis.

3. Nosocomial and Ventilator-Associated Pneumonia

Gram-negative organisms and *S aureus* are frequent causes of pneumonia in hospitalized patients or patients who require mechanical ventilation. Nosocomial organisms tend to be more resistant and are more likely to be present in patients with longer hospital stays, prior antimicrobial therapy, and more comorbidities. If possible, attempts should be made to obtain lower respiratory tract samples for quantitative microbiologic evaluation in mechanically ventilated patients. Adequate antimicrobial coverage can usually be provided with a third- or fourth-generation cephalosporin, β-lactam/β-lactamase inhibitor combinations, or a carbapenem, plus a fluoroquinolone or an aminoglycoside. If *Pseudomonas aeruginosa* is strongly suspected, 2 antipseudomonal antimicrobial therapies of different classes should be instituted and the possibility of multiresistant *Pseudomonas* should be ruled out. Therapy with trimethoprim-sulfamethoxazole should be included if the possibility of *Stenotrophomonas maltophilia* is suspected or confirmed. Vancomycin should be considered if methicillin-resistant *S aureus* is a possible pathogen. Pneumonia due to methicillin-sensitive strains of *S aureus* should be treated with an antistaphylococcal penicillin as these agents are superior to vancomycin. Patients with methicillin-resistant *S aureus* who are vancomycin-intolerant or are not responding to vancomycin may be treated with linezolid. If vancomycin is utilized, serum trough levels should be maintained no lower than 15 to 20 µg/mL since lung penetration of this agent is limited. Shorter courses (8 days) of therapy may be appropriate as long as non-lactose–fermenting organisms are not isolated.

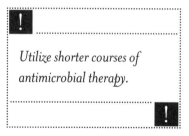

Utilize shorter courses of antimicrobial therapy.

C. Heart

Infections of the heart are usually severe and life-threatening and require coordinated medical care with a cardiologist and sometimes also with a cardiovascular surgeon. Microbiological studies and echocardiography (transthoracic or transesophageal) are the cornerstones for the diagnosis and management of any infection in the heart.

Infective endocarditis, or infection of the endocardial surface of the heart, most frequently involves the heart valves. Intravenous drug abuse, prosthetic valves, sclerosing of natural valves due to aging, hospital-acquired infections, and newly identified pathogens (*Bartonella* spp, *Coxiella burnetti, Tropheryma whipplei,* fungi) are the main risk factors of this condition. Demonstration of bloodstream infection and positive echocardiographic evidence of valvular vegetations are key to making the diagnosis, although peripheral embolic phenomena and other findings are strongly suggestive. Gram-positive cocci, mainly *Staphylococcus* and *Streptococcus*, but also *Enterococcus*, are the most common microorganisms isolated in infective endocarditis in the general population and in specific risk groups (intravenous drug users and prosthetic valve endocarditis), but Gram-negative, polymicrobial, fungal, and culture-negative endocarditis are becoming more common. Bactericidal antimicrobial therapy (such as penicillins/third-generation cephalosporins +/- an aminoglycoside, glycopeptides, linezolid, daptomycin, etc), high concentrations of the antimicrobial, the resistance pattern of the microorganism, and long-term therapy are the cornerstones of therapy.

D. Intravascular Catheters

In patients with confirmed or suspected intravascular catheter infection associated with organ dysfunction, systemic emboli, or cardiovascular instability, the intravascular catheter should be promptly removed. In addition, local changes at the catheter site (purulence, erythema) mandate catheter removal. In the absence of local changes or sepsis, an option is to insert a new catheter in the existing site over a guidewire. However this approach needs to be supported with negative blood cultures as well as negative culture of the intradermal portion of the removed catheter.

Coagulase-negative *Staphylococcus* and *S aureus* are the most common pathogens in catheter-related bloodstream infections. In the immunocompetent patient without systemic symptoms and with coagulase-negative staphylococcus line infection, the removal of the infected catheter line may be sufficient. Vancomycin is recommended in immunocompromised patients with coagulase-negative staphylococci line infection, patients with systemic manifestations, or patients with prosthetic devices at risk for becoming secondarily infected. If *S aureus* is the infecting organism, nafcillin is recommended; however, if there is a high rate of methicillin-resistant *S aureus* (MRSA) in the hospital or MRSA is confirmed, vancomycin should be used. A third- or fourth-generation cephalosporin or fluoroquinolone should be added if a nosocomial Gram-negative organism is suspected.

> **!**
>
> *With the increasing incidence of vancomycin-resistant organisms, attempts should be made to limit the indiscriminant use of vancomycin.*
>
> **!**

Candida is occasionally isolated from catheter tips and should increase the suspicion that occult candidemia may have been recently present. The treatment of choice is fluconazole, or if there is a possibility of resistant *Candida*, such as *T glabrata* or *C krusei*, caspofungin should be used. When a fungal microorganism is identified in an intravascular catheter-related bloodstream infection, a non-tunneled catheter should always be removed, whereas the removal of a tunneled catheter should be based on the likelihood of a catheter-related candidemia rather than candidemia from another source. The antimicrobial-impregnated catheters appear to have a lower rate of bloodstream infection. However, the maximum longevity of such catheters is still under investigation.

E. Abdomen

When an intra-abdominal infection is suspected, a surgeon must be promptly involved in the evaluation of the patient. Both the infecting flora and the antimicrobial therapy are related to whether the infection is community-acquired or healthcare-associated. For community-acquired infections, location of a possible perforation determines the probable organism, with Gram-positive, facultative, and aerobic Gram-negative bacteria beyond the proximal small bowel and anaerobes beyond the proximal ileum. Recommended therapies include β-lactam/β-lactamase inhibitor combinations and carbapenems as monotherapy or cephalosporins/fluoroquinolones with metronidazole. Antimicrobial therapy should be continued until clinical resolution, which typically occurs in 5 to 7 days. Further diagnostic workup should be pursued in patients with persistent or recurrent symptoms. Flora isolated from healthcare-associated intra-abdominal infections resembles that of other nosocomial infections. Antimicrobial therapy should be based on knowledge of the flora and antimicrobial susceptibilities of the particular institution. Anti-enterococcal therapy is indicated only when enterococci are isolated from patients with healthcare-associated infections. Antifungal therapy is indicated only in those who have isolated fungi and have comorbid conditions like recent immunosuppressive therapy for neoplasms, transplantation, and inflammatory disease or have postoperative or recurrent infections.

F. Urinary Tract

The most common pathogens in urinary tract infections are Gram-negative enteric bacteria. Hospitalized patients with urinary catheters commonly have bacteriuria yet exhibit no pyuria or localized symptoms. Such patients (in the absence of urologic obstruction) rarely develop sepsis or bacteremia arising from the urinary tract, and removal of the urinary catheter may allow resolution of the bacteriuria. Patients who develop upper urinary tract infection always merit antimicrobial therapy. More serious complications may be seen in diabetics or other immunocompromised patients, including those with emphysematous pyelonephritis, papillary necrosis, or perinephric abscess, which may require surgical intervention. Empiric antimicrobial options for Gram-negative urinary tract infections are dictated by susceptibility testing and include the following:

- Third-generation cephalosporins

- Fluoroquinolones

- Aminoglycosides

- Piperacillin/tazobactam

- Trimethoprim/sulfamethoxazole

Enterococcal infection in the urinary system should be suspected in patients who have long-term urinary catheters or who have had recent manipulation of the urinary tract, and therapy should include ampicillin, piperacillin, or vancomycin.

Candiduria is not uncommon and usually occurs in patients who have long-term urinary catheters and are receiving broad-spectrum antimicrobial therapy or patients with glycosuria. Therapeutic options include a short course of fluconazole (not effective against *T glabrata* or *C krusei*) or continuous amphotericin bladder irrigation. Relapse rates, however, are quite significant with either treatment. If candiduria is treated in a patient with an indwelling catheter, the catheter should be changed or removed during the treatment course.

G. Cutaneous Infection

Staphylococcus aureus or group A β-hemolytic streptococci are the most likely etiologic organisms in cellulitis or cutaneous abscess. *H influenzae* must also be considered in facial or orbital cellulitis. Onset of postoperative wound infections usually occurs 5 to 7 days after surgery. However, rapidly progressive wound infections occurring within 24 to 48 hours after surgery should prompt the consideration of *Clostridium perfringens* or group A β-hemolytic streptococci (*S pyogenes*). This type of infection warrants surgical debridement and prompt antimicrobial therapy directed by Gram stain and culture. Antimicrobial choices include the following:

■ Cefazolin or nafcillin if methicillin-resistant *S aureus* is unlikely

■ Vancomycin or linezolid if there is a possibility of methicillin-resistant *S aureus*

■ Penicillin G +/− clindamycin for wound infections developing within 48 hours to cover *C perfringens* and β-hemolytic streptococci

Wound toxic shock syndrome is a rare condition that can occur within 48 hours of a wound or surgical incision. The causes are toxin-producing *S aureus* or β-hemolytic streptococci, but often the wound does not appear infected. Presenting symptoms include fever, diarrhea, vomiting, hypotension, and uremia. Erythroderma and subsequent desquamation are characteristic but may be delayed for several days. Treatment involves opening the wound and prompt use of specific antimicrobial therapy.

H. Necrotizing Fasciitis

Infection of subcutaneous tissue and fascia can occur in any patient but may be more common in immunocompromised patients, especially diabetics. If gas is present in the tissue, cutaneous gangrene or bullae are noted, or the infection progresses rapidly, necrotizing fasciitis must be considered. Necrotizing fasciitis requires prompt surgical debridement in addition to broad-spectrum antimicrobial therapy. Such infections are usually polymicrobial, involving aerobic and anaerobic Gram-positive and Gram-negative organisms.

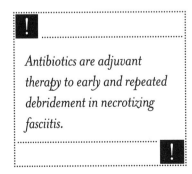

Antibiotics are adjuvant therapy to early and repeated debridement in necrotizing fasciitis.

Adequate empiric therapy should include vancomycin and a β-lactam/β-lactamase inhibitor, or a carbapenem and fluoroquinolone, or an aminoglycoside and clindamycin (the latter to reduce the amount of toxins).

I. Immunocompromised or Neutropenic Patients

In the absence of a specific source, pending culture results, broad-spectrum antimicrobial therapy is indicated in the immunocompromised or neutropenic patient with fever. Monotherapy can be effective, but combination therapy is indicated initially for more severely ill patients. To reduce the emergence of resistance, a third-generation cephalosporin as monotherapy should be avoided if *Pseudomonas* spp, *Acinetobacter* spp, *Enterobacter* spp, *Citrobacter* spp, or *Serratia* spp are prevalent.

Suggested antimicrobial regimens include the following:

- Third- or fourth-generation cephalosporin (ceftazidime or cefepime for *P aeruginosa* coverage) + aminoglycoside or fluoroquinolones

- Carbapenems

- Piperacillin/tazobactam

- Add vancomycin if gram positive organisms are likely

The use of white cell growth factors (ie, granulocyte colony-stimulating factor [G-CSF], granulocyte-macrophage colony-stimulating factor [GM-CSF]) may improve outcome by shortening the duration of neutropenia. These progenitor cell stimulants should be targeted for patients with an anticipated duration of neutropenia of 5 to 7 days and a high risk for serious infection.

J. Antibiotic-Associated Colitis

Antibiotic-associated diarrhea and colitis resulting from *Clostridium difficile* infection can complicate the course of treatment for many patients. Antimicrobials most commonly involved include clindamycin, penicillins, cephalosporins, and quinolones, although this infection has been described in association with almost all antimicrobials. Patients do not need to receive antimicrobial therapy to develop this condition.

Clostridium difficile is also recognized as an important nosocomial pathogen capable of cross-transmission to patients in adjacent areas. Diagnosis is usually done by identification of *C difficile* toxins and detection of cytotoxin activity in tissue culture. Treatment begins with discontinuation of the implicated antimicrobial therapy (if possible) and initiation of specific *C difficile* antimicrobial therapy if symptoms are moderate, severe or persistent. The preferred regimen is oral metronidazole 250 to 500 mg 3 times daily for 10 days. Oral vancomycin, 125 to 500 mg 4 times daily for 10 days is also effective, but its use is discouraged in an attempt to reduce development of resistant organisms. For patients who are unable to take oral medications intraluminal vancomycin with or without intravenous metronidazole is recommended. Fulminant colitis unresponsive to these measures or progressing to toxic megacolon may require total colectomy.

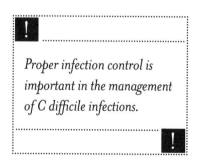

Proper infection control is important in the management of C difficile infections.

K. Fungal Diseases

Life-threatening infections due to fungi may be extremely difficult to diagnose by routine physical examination or routine cultures. *Candida albicans* is the most common etiologic organism in critically ill patients. Non-albicans species of *Candida* and other fungi have increased significantly in recent years. Fungal infection should be considered based on the geographic region and predisposing factors, such as HIV, malignancy, neutropenia, long-term use of steroids, broad-spectrum antimicrobial therapy, parenteral nutrition, severe burns or organ transplantation, or in the presence of central venous vascular catheters.

The polyenes (amphotericin B and lipid preparations of amphotericin B) have been the most commonly utilized antifungal agents for serious fungal infections. Newer antifungal agents (caspofungin, voriconazole) have shown comparable or superior clinical outcomes compared with the polyenes. All lipid formulations have less nephrotoxicity and their efficacy against *Candida* is equivalent to conventional amphotericin B. Fluconazole is still active against most *Candida* species and *Cryptococcus,* and itraconazole may be used for some of the mold infections. Both agents have an important role in primary or secondary prophylaxis. The newer agents, such as voriconazole, posaconazole, and caspofungin, have activity against resistant *Candida* strains and some of the mold infections resistant to other regimens. Recent studies suggest a role in the treatment of neutropenic fever and fungal infections in immunocompromised patients.

L. Other Therapy

In addition to antimicrobial therapy, surgical intervention must be considered in patients with life-threatening infections. Any abscess must be drained, and injured or ischemic organs must be repaired or removed. Vascular catheters that may be a source of infection should be removed. Early surgical consultation should be sought when considering the abdomen as a source of infection in the critically ill patient. Guidelines for tetanus prophylaxis are found in **Appendix 12.** Further management of the patient with septic shock is discussed in **Chapter 7.**

Life-threatening Infections

- Fever is the most frequent systemic manifestation that raises the suspicion of infection.

- Ideally, appropriate cultures should be obtained before initiation of antibiotics in patients with suspected infection.

- Selection of appropriate empiric antimicrobial therapy depends on the suspected microbial pathogen(s) and site of infection, Gram stain results of available specimens from the suspected site, assessment for antimicrobial resistance, and comorbid conditions.

- When bacterial meningitis is suspected clinically, antimicrobial therapy should be instituted immediately, without waiting for the results of lumbar puncture.

- The most common organism resulting in community-acquired, life-threatening pneumonia is *Streptococcus pneumoniae*.

- Resistant Gram-negative organisms and *S aureus* are frequent causes of pneumonia in hospitalized patients or patients who require mechanical ventilation.

- Bactericidal antimicrobial therapy, high concentrations of the antimicrobial agent, the resistance pattern of the microorganism, and long-term therapy are the cornerstones of therapy for infective endocarditis.

- Suspicion of intra-abdominal infection requires the prompt involvement of a surgeon in the evaluation of the patient.

- Necrotizing fasciitis requires prompt surgical debridement in addition to broad-spectrum antimicrobial therapy.

- In the absence of a specific source and pending culture results, broad-spectrum antimicrobial therapy is indicated in the immunocompromised or neutropenic patient with fever.

- Fungal infection should be considered in the presence of predisposing factors, such as malignancy, neutropenia, broad-spectrum antimicrobial therapy, parenteral nutrition, severe burns, or organ transplantation, or if central venous vascular catheters are in place.

Suggested Readings

1. American Thoracic Society, Infectious Disease Society of America. Guidelines for the management of hospital-acquired pneumonia, ventilator-associated pneumonia and healthcare-associated pneumonia. *Am J Resp Crit Care Med.* 2005;171:388.

2. Avecillas JF, Mazzone P, Arroliga AC. A rational approach to the evaluation and treatment of the infected patient in the intensive care unit. *Clin Chest Med.* 2003;24:645.

3. Calandra T, Cohen J. The International Sepsis Forum Consensus Conference on Definitions of Infection in the Intensive Care Unit. *Crit Care Med.* 2005;33:1538.

4. Dellinger RP, Carlet JM, Masur H, et al. Surviving Sepsis Campaign guidelines for management of severe sepsis and septic shock. *Crit Care Med.* 2004;32:858. Available online at http://www.survivingsepsis.org. http://www.survivingsepsis.org/files/surviving_sepsis_campaign_guidelines.pdf (This is the URL for the English version but there are several other language translations.)

5. Guerrant RL, Van Gilder T, Thielman N, et al. Practice guidelines for the management of infectious diarrhea. *Clin Infect Dis.* 2001;32:331. http://www.journals.uchicago.edu/CID/journal/issues/v32n3/001387/001387.html

6. Leone M, Bourgoin A, Combon S, et al. Empirical antimicrobial therapy of septic shock patients: Adequacy and impact on the outcomes. *Crit Care Med.* 2003;31:462.

7. Mandell LA, Wunderink RG, Anzueto A, et al. Infectious Diseases Society of America/American Thoracic Society consensus guidelines on the management of community-acquired pneumonia in adults. *Clin Infect Dis.* 2007;44:S27. Available at www.idsociety.org. http://www.journals.uchicago.edu/CID/journal/issues/v44nS2/41620/41620.html

8. Mermel LA, Farr BM, Sherertz RJ, et al. Guidelines for management of intravascular catheter-related infections. *Clin Infect Dis.* 2001;32:1249. Available at www.idsociety.org. http://www.journals.uchicago.edu/CID/journal/issues/v32n9/001689/001689.html

9. Pappas PG, Rex JH, Sobel JD, Willer SG, Dismukes WE, Walsh TJ, Edwards JE. Guidelines for treatment of candidiasis. *Clin Infect Dis.* 2004; 38:161. http://www.journals.uchicago.edu/CID/journal/issues/v38n2/32301/32301.html

10. Solomkin JS, Mazuski JE, Baron EJ, et al. Guidelines for the selection of anti-infective agents for complicated intra-abdominal infections. *Clin Infect Dis.* 2003; 37:997. http://www.journals.uchicago.edu/CID/journal/issues/v37n8/31800/31800.html

11. Tunkel AR, Hartman BJ, Kaplan SL, et al. Practice guidelines for the management of bacterial meningitis. *Clin Infect Dis.* 2004;39:1267. Available at www.idsociety.org (Guidelines) http://www.journals.uchicago.edu/CID/journal/issues/v39n9/34796/34796.html

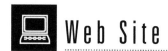 Web Site

Infectious Diseases Society of America. http://www.idsociety.org. This Web site contains regularly updated guidelines for management and prevention of specific infections. Some guidelines are available for PDA download.

Chapter 12

MANAGEMENT OF LIFE-THREATENING ELECTROLYTE AND METABOLIC DISTURBANCES

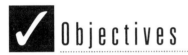

Objectives

- Review the emergent management of severe electrolyte disturbances.

- Recognize manifestations of acute adrenal insufficiency and initiate appropriate treatment.

- Describe the management of severe hyperglycemic syndromes.

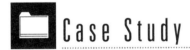

Case Study

An 80-year-old woman with hypertension, heart failure, and chronic renal insufficiency is admitted to the hospital with confusion, lethargy, poor oral intake, and weakness for the past 3 days. Her vital signs are blood pressure 108/70 mm Hg, heart rate 110/min, respiratory rate 18/min, and temperature 97.6°F (36.4°C). The ECG monitor shows nonsustained episodes of ventricular tachycardia.

- What risk factors does this patient have for electrolyte disturbances?

- Which electrolyte abnormalities might contribute to her presentation?

- How would you initiate the evaluation and treatment of this patient?

I. INTRODUCTION

Electrolyte and metabolic disturbances are common in critically ill and injured patients. These abnormalities alter physiologic function and contribute to morbidity and mortality. The most common life-threatening electrolyte and metabolic disorders in critically ill patients are disturbances in potassium, sodium, calcium, magnesium, and phosphate levels, adrenal function, and glucose regulation. With early recognition and treatment of these abnormalities, life-threatening complications might be avoided and outcomes improved.

II. ELECTROLYTE DISTURBANCES

Electrolyte disturbances result from an underlying disease process, and it is important to seek the cause of the abnormality as well as to treat the electrolyte change. Many clinical manifestations are not specific to a particular electrolyte change and may be due to multiple abnormalities. The urgency of treatment depends on the clinical circumstances rather than the absolute electrolyte concentration. All severe electrolyte abnormalities require frequent reassessment during correction.

A. Potassium

Potassium is primarily an intracellular ion that is essential for maintenance of the electrical membrane potential. Approximately 2% of the total body potassium is present in the extracellular compartment. Alterations in this ion primarily affect the cardiovascular, neuromuscular, and gastrointestinal systems.

1. Hypokalemia

Hypokalemia (potassium <3.5 mmol/L) results from renal or extrarenal losses, transcellular shifts, and decreased intake (**Table 12-1**). Life-threatening clinical manifestations of hypokalemia involve the cardiac and neuromuscular systems. Arrhythmias (ventricular and supraventricular, conduction delays, sinus bradycardia), electrocardiogram (ECG) abnormalities (U waves, QT interval prolongation, flat or inverted T waves), muscle weakness or paralysis, paresthesias, ileus, abdominal cramps, nausea, and vomiting are common manifestations.

Treatment of hypokalemia is aimed at correcting the underlying cause and administering potassium (**Figure 12-1**). Discontinue offending drugs (if possible), correct hypomagnesemia and other electrolyte disturbances, and correct alkalosis. Because potassium is primarily an intracellular ion, an estimated deficit cannot be calculated from serum values. Therefore, administration must be titrated against periodic reassessment of the serum levels. Infusion of 10 mmol potassium in 100 mL fluid over 20 minutes with additional doses administered sequentially is recommended

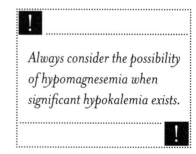

Always consider the possibility of hypomagnesemia when significant hypokalemia exists.

to avoid potential mishaps with more concentrated solutions. The infusion rate can be slowed after life-threatening symptoms resolve. Continuous ECG monitoring and close observation are necessary during parenteral administration of high concentrations of potassium chloride. Serum potassium levels must be monitored at frequent intervals during repletion (ie, every 1-2 hours during initial replacement). If acidemia is present, correct the potassium level before correcting pH, since potassium shifts intracellularly as the pH increases.

Table 12-1	Causes of Hypokalemia

Transcellular Shifts	Renal Losses	Extrarenal Losses	Decreased Intake
Acute alkalosis	Diuresis	Diarrhea	Malnutrition
Hyperventilation	Metabolic alkalosis	Profuse sweating	Alcoholism
Insulin	Renal tubular defects	Nasogastric suction	Anorexia nervosa
β-Adrenergic agonists	Diabetic ketoacidosis		
	Drugs (diuretics, aminoglycosides, amphotericin B)		
	Hypomagnesemia		
	Vomiting		
	Hyperaldosteronism		
	Cushing's syndrome		

Figure 12-1. Treatment of Hypokalemia

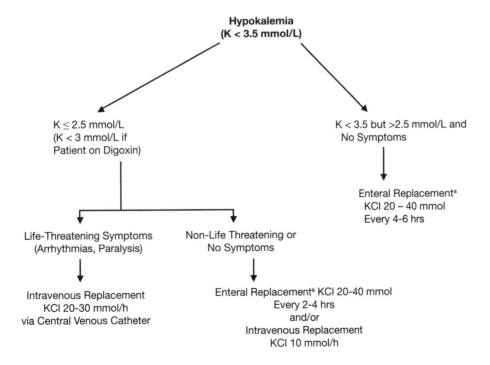

ᵃ Enteral replacement may be oral or via nasogastric tube; nausea and/or vomiting may preclude use of the enteral route

2. Hyperkalemia

Hyperkalemia (potassium >5.5 mmol/L) in critically ill patients most often results from renal dysfunction. Other causes are listed in **Table 12-2.** Pseudohyperkalemia may result from a white blood cell count >100,000/mm³ or platelet count >600,000/mm³. Hemolysis secondary to phlebotomy technique must also be considered.

Table 12-2.	Causes of Hyperkalemia
Renal dysfunction	Cell death
Acidemia	Rhabdomyolysis
Hypoaldosteronism	Tumor lysis
Drugs (potassium-sparing	Burns
diuretics, ACE inhibitors,	Hemolysis
succinylcholine, NSAIDs,	Excessive intake
trimethoprim-sulfamethoxazole, etc)	

Abbreviations: ACE, angiotensin-converting enzyme; NSAIDs, nonsteroidal anti-inflammatory drugs.

Clinical manifestations of hyperkalemia relate primarily to the heart and muscle (**Figure 12-2**). Arrhythmias, heart block, bradycardia, diminished conduction and contraction, ECG abnormalities (eg, diffuse peaked T waves, PR interval prolongation, QRS widening, diminished P waves, sine waves), muscle weakness, paralysis, paresthesias, and hypoactive reflexes are common manifestations.

Figure 12-2. Electrocardiographic Effects of Hyperkalemia

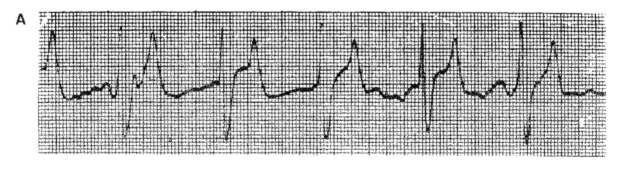

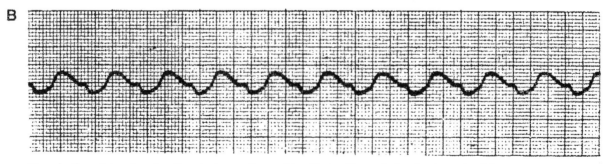

Two rhythm strips showing the electrocardiographic effects of hyperkalemia. A, peaked T waves and widened QRS complex. B, sine wave pattern.

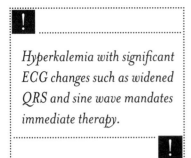

Hyperkalemia with significant ECG changes such as widened QRS and sine wave mandates immediate therapy.

Treatment of hyperkalemia involves the recognition and treatment of underlying diseases, the removal of offending drugs, the limitation of potassium intake, and the correction of acidemia or electrolyte abnormalities. Any serum potassium level >6 mmol/L should be addressed, but the urgency of treatment depends on clinical manifestations and ECG findings. Options for treating hyperkalemia are summarized in **Table 12-3.** Serum potassium levels, continuous cardiac monitoring, and serial ECG tracings should be monitored during evaluation and treatment.

Table 12-3. Options for Treating Hyperkalemia

If Significant ECG Abnormalities Are Present

Administer calcium chloride, 5-10 mL of a 10% solution, intravenously over 5-10 minutes to stabilize the myocardial cell membrane and decrease the potential for arrhythmias. If calcium gluconate is used, 10-20 mL of a 10% solution is needed for treatment because of the lower elemental calcium content. The effect lasts only 30-60 minutes and should be followed by additional treatment.

For Redistribution of Potassium

1. Administer insulin and glucose (10 units of regular insulin with 50 g of 50% dextrose over 5-10 minutes intravenously). Glucose monitoring is necessary to avoid hypoglycemia.

2. Administer sodium bicarbonate (1 mmol/kg intravenously over 5-10 minutes). Be aware of potential sodium overload with sodium bicarbonate. Sodium bicarbonate is less effective than glucose and insulin for decreasing the potassium level in patients with end-stage renal failure.

3. Administer inhaled β_2-agonists in high doses (albuterol [salbutamol], 10-20 mg), which can decrease serum potassium by approximately 0.5 mmol/L.

For Removal of Potassium From the Body

1. Increase urine output with a loop diuretic and isotonic fluids.

2. Increase gastrointestinal potassium loss with sodium polystyrene sulfonate 25-50 g in sorbitol, enterally or by enema. (Be aware of potential sodium overload.)

3. Initiate dialysis.

B. Sodium

Sodium functions as the primary determinant of blood osmolality in the body and is involved in the regulation of extracellular volume. Abnormalities in circulating sodium primarily affect neuronal and neuromuscular function.

1. Hyponatremia

The most common cause of hyponatremia (sodium <135 mmol/L) associated with a low serum osmolality (hypo-osmolar hyponatremia) is excess secretion of antidiuretic hormone (ie, euvolemic hyponatremia). Hypo-osmolar hyponatremia or dilutional hyponatremia can also be associated with hypovolemic and hypervolemic conditions. A common defect is impaired ability to excrete free water through the kidneys. Hyponatremia can also result less frequently from the presence of a nonsodium solute, such as glucose and mannitol. These causes are characterized by a normal or elevated serum osmolality. Pseudohyponatremia, a spurious form of iso-osmolar hyponatremia, may occur in the presence of severe hyperlipidemia, hyperproteinemia, or hyperglycemia when the sodium concentration is measured by flame photometry. **Figure 12-3** outlines a diagnostic approach to determining the etiology of hyponatremia.

Figure 12-3. Diagnostic Approach to the Etiology of Hyponatremia

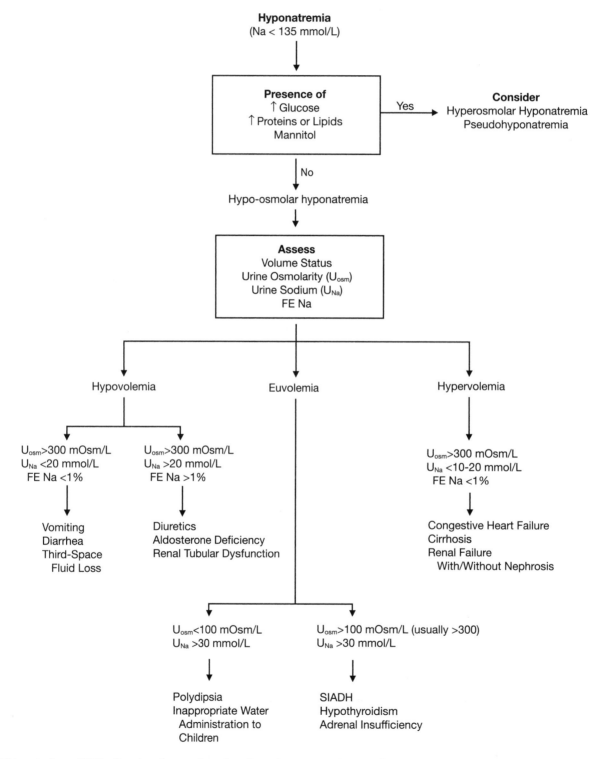

Abbreviations: FE Na, fractional excretion of sodium; SIADH, syndrome of inappropriate antidiuretic hormone.

Clinical manifestations of hyponatremia involve the central nervous system (CNS) and muscular system and include disorientation, decreased mentation, irritability, seizures, lethargy, coma, nausea/vomiting, weakness, and respiratory arrest. Treatment requires identifying the type of hyponatremia, treating the underlying disease, removing offending drugs, and improving the circulating sodium level. Hypovolemic hyponatremia usually responds to intravascular volume repletion (ie, with normal saline). As volume is replaced, antidiuretic hormone is suppressed and the kidneys begin to excrete free water. Hypervolemic hyponatremia is usually not severe and improves with successful treatment of the underlying condition.

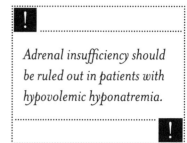

Adrenal insufficiency should be ruled out in patients with hypovolemic hyponatremia.

Euvolemic hyponatremia is almost always secondary to elevated levels of antidiuretic hormone. Diagnosis is facilitated by determining urine osmolality (U_{osm}) before treatment (especially with diuretics) to compare with a calculated serum osmolality [(2 × serum sodium) + glucose/18 + BUN/2.8]. The urine osmolality is inappropriately higher than serum osmolality (usually >300 mOsm). If the hyponatremia is acute or the patient is symptomatic, the serum sodium level should be increased by restricting free-water intake, increasing free-water clearance with loop diuretics, and replacing intravascular volume with normal saline (154 mmol/L) or hypertonic 3% saline (513 mmol/L). Hypertonic saline is indicated for treatment of patients with severe symptoms, such as seizures, coma, or impending respiratory arrest. The goal of therapy in this situation is to remove free water and not sodium. The increase in serum sodium should be controlled, and although the precise rate of increase is controversial, the serum sodium increase should be limited to approximately 8 to 12 mmol/L in the first 24 hours. One option is to accelerate the rate of serum sodium elevation early in the treatment course in the presence of life-threatening symptoms, such as seizures, and to slow the rate of increase after resolution of the symptoms. If hypertonic saline is used, 1 mmol/kg sodium chloride should be infused initially (3% saline contains ~0.5 mmol/mL). The same amount can be administered in incremental doses to a maximum of 3 to 5 mmol/kg or until symptoms resolve. Alternatively, the change in serum sodium expected after administering 1 liter of fluid can be estimated by using the following formulas:

$$\text{Change in Serum Sodium} = \frac{\text{Infusate Sodium} - \text{Serum Sodium}}{\text{Total Body Water} + 1}$$

$$\text{Change in Serum Sodium} = \frac{(\text{Infusate Sodium} + \text{Infusate Potassium}) - \text{Serum Sodium}}{\text{Total Body Water} + 1}$$

Total Body Water = 0.6 × Weight (kg) for men; 0.5 × Weight (kg) for women

The sodium concentrations of various infusates are listed in **Table 12-4.** The formulas presented above do not take into account other fluid gains and losses (eg, urine output) and therefore should serve only as guides to intervention. Serum sodium levels should be monitored at frequent intervals during therapy for hyponatremia. When serum sodium is ≥125 to 130 mmol/L, restriction of free water alone allows for slower return of the sodium level to normal. Correction of the serum sodium level that is too rapid may result in CNS injury (ie, osmotic demyelinating syndrome), especially in chronic hyponatremia. If the hyponatremia is chronic and asymptomatic, regardless of the magnitude of hyponatremia, free-water restriction alone may be sufficient to allow for slow return of serum sodium to normal.

Table 12-4. Sodium Concentrations of Selected Infusates

Infusate	Sodium Concentration (mmol/L)
5% sodium chloride	855
3% sodium chloride	513
0.9% sodium chloride	154
Ringer's lactate	130
0.45% sodium chloride	77
5% dextrose in water	0

2. Hypernatremia

Hypernatremia (sodium >145 mmol/L) indicates intracellular volume depletion with a loss of free water that exceeds sodium loss. Causes of hypernatremia are listed in **Table 12-5.**

Table 12-5. Causes of Hypernatremia

Water Loss	Reduced Water Intake	Excessive Sodium Intake
Diarrhea	Altered thirst	Salt tablets
Vomiting	Impaired access	Hypertonic saline
Excessive sweating		Sodium bicarbonate
Diuresis		
Diabetes insipidus		

The clinical manifestations of hypernatremia relate to CNS and muscle function. Manifestations of hypernatremia include altered mentation, lethargy, seizures, coma, and muscle weakness. Polyuria suggests the presence of diabetes insipidus or excess salt and water intake.

Treatment focuses on correcting the underlying cause of hypernatremia. Nearly all patients with hypernatremia require free-water repletion. The water deficit can be estimated by using the following equation:

Water Deficit (L) = 0.6 (0.5 for women) × weight (kg) [(measured Na/normal Na) – 1]

Example: Water deficit of a 70-kg man with Na of 160 mmol/L
0.6 × 70 [(160/140) – 1]
42 [1.14 – 1]
42 × 0.14 = 5.88 L water deficit

A portion of free water should be replaced initially at a speed commensurate with the severity of symptoms, and the patient should be reevaluated for subsequent replacement. If the patient is hemodynamically unstable (hypotensive, orthostatic, or with significant tachycardia), administer normal saline until intravascular volume is corrected. When the patient is hemodynamically stable, replace water with 5% dextrose in water, 0.45% NaCl, or 0.2% NaCl with 5% dextrose. To estimate the change in serum sodium expected after administering 1 liter of fluid, use the same formulas as for hyponatremia:

$$\text{Change in Serum Sodium} = \frac{\text{Infusate Sodium} - \text{Serum Sodium}}{\text{Total Body Water} + 1}$$

$$\text{Change in Serum Sodium} = \frac{(\text{Infusate Sodium} + \text{Infusate Potassium}) - \text{Serum Sodium}}{\text{Total Body Water} + 1}$$

In stable patients, water may be replaced via the enteral route (ie, nasogastric tube). In the rare patient with sodium overload, sodium may be removed with loop diuretics or dialysis (provided intravascular volume is adequate). Administration of aqueous vasopressin or desmopressin should be considered for patients with central diabetes insipidus.

Sodium concentration should be measured frequently during treatment, and therapy should be adjusted for optimal correction of the sodium level. If hypernatremia developed over a period of hours, reducing the serum sodium by 1 mmol/L/h is appropriate. In hypernatremia of longer or unknown duration, a slower rate of correction (0.5 mmol/L/h) is recommended. Increasing free-water intake in maintenance fluids allows for a slow return of sodium levels to normal.

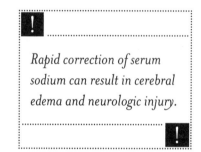

Rapid correction of serum sodium can result in cerebral edema and neurologic injury.

C. Other Electrolyte Abnormalities

1. Calcium

Calcium is required for muscle contraction, nerve impulse transmission, hormone secretion, blood clotting, cell division, cell motility, and wound healing. Effective calcium levels in a seriously ill patient are best assessed by using ionized calcium measurements, if available. If treatment decisions are based on total serum calcium, the albumin concentration must be considered. In general, for each increase or decrease in serum albumin of 1 g/dL, the serum calcium increases or decreases by 0.8 mg/dL (0.2 mmol/L). However, the relationship between albumin and serum calcium is less reliable in critically ill patients.

a. Hypocalcemia

Hypocalcemia (total calcium <8.5 mg/dL [<2.12 mmol/L], ionized calcium <1 mmol/L) is common in critically ill patients and results from impairment of the parathyroid and/or vitamin D systems **(Table 12-6).** Cardiovascular abnormalities, the most common clinical manifestations of hypocalcemia in critically ill patients, include hypotension, bradycardia, arrhythmias, heart failure, cardiac arrest, digitalis insensitivity, and QT-interval and ST-segment prolongation. Neuromuscular manifestations include weakness, muscle spasm, laryngospasm, hyperreflexia, seizures, tetany, and paresthesias.

Table 12-6.	Causes of Hypocalcemia
Hypoparathyroidism	Liver disease
Sepsis	Renal disease
Burns	Calcium chelators
Rhabdomyolysis	Hypomagnesemia
Pancreatitis	Massive transfusion
Malabsorption	

Treatment is aimed at correcting the underlying disease process and any concomitant electrolyte abnormalities, and administering calcium. Mild hypocalcemia is well tolerated, and aggressive treatment may result in tissue injury (especially during ischemic and septic states). If the hypocalcemia is severe or if the patient is symptomatic, administer 100 mg calcium intravenously over 5 to 10 minutes (3-4 mL of 10% calcium chloride or 10 mL of 10% calcium gluconate), followed by calcium in the amount of 0.3 to 2 mg/kg/h. Calcium preparations vary in their content of elemental calcium: 1 g of 10% calcium chloride contained in 10 mL has 272 mg of calcium; 1 g of 10% calcium gluconate contained in 10 mL has 90 mg of calcium. When the circulating calcium concentration is stable, calcium may be replaced via the enteral route (ie, 500-1,000 mg every 6 hours).

Monitor ionized or total calcium levels frequently during treatment, and adjust repletion to maintain calcium in the lower normal range so as not to suppress parathyroid gland function. If calcium replacement alone fails to maintain the circulating calcium level, consider administration of vitamin D and magnesium. Adverse effects of calcium administration include hypercalcemia, bradycardia, nausea/vomiting, flushing, tissue calcium precipitation, and digitalis toxicity.

b. Hypercalcemia

The most common causes of hypercalcemia (total calcium >11 mg/dL [>2.75 mmol/L], ionized calcium >1.3 mmol/L) are the result of calcium release from bone (**Table 12-7**). The clinical manifestations of hypercalcemia relate primarily to the cardiovascular and neuromuscular systems and include hypertension, cardiac ischemia, arrhythmias, bradycardia, conduction abnormalities, digitalis toxicity, dehydration, hypotension, weakness, depressed mentation, coma, seizures, and sudden death. Gastrointestinal manifestations include nausea/vomiting, anorexia, abdominal pain, constipation, pancreatitis, and ulcer disease. Nephrogenic diabetes insipidus with polyuria may occur and contribute to volume depletion. Renal stones, nephrocalcinosis, and renal failure are also encountered.

Table 12-7.	Causes of Hypercalcemia

Hyperparathyroidism	Excess intake of vitamin A or vitamin D
Malignancy	Thyrotoxicosis
Immobilization	Granulomatous disease

Treatment of hypercalcemia is aimed at controlling the underlying disease, rehydrating the patient, and lowering the calcium level. The circulating calcium level frequently needs to be lowered while the primary disease is being evaluated and treated. Intravascular volume should be restored with normal saline to ensure adequate tissue perfusion and renal blood flow (urine output 2-3 mL/kg/h). Saline also decreases renal tubular calcium reabsorption. Diuresis with a loop diuretic, once adequate hydration is ensured, further increases renal calcium loss. Serum potassium and magnesium levels should be monitored and low levels corrected. In patients with renal failure, pulmonary edema, or life-threatening hypercalcemia, calcium levels may be lowered with dialysis. After initial stabilization, therapy with calcitonin and bisphosphonates can be considered.

2. Hypophosphatemia

Phosphate is important in cellular energy metabolism. Hypophosphatemia (phosphate <2.5 mg/dL [0.81 mmol/L]) results from transcellular shifts, renal loss, gastrointestinal loss, or inadequate intake **(Table 12-8).** Phosphate depletion primarily affects the neuromuscular and central nervous systems. Clinical manifestations include muscle weakness, respiratory failure, rhabdomyolysis, paresthesias, lethargy, disorientation, obtundation, coma, and seizures. Other manifestations include impaired renal tubular function, impaired pressor responses, hepatic dysfunction, immune dysfunction, impaired protein synthesis, hemolysis, impaired platelet function, and impaired oxygen off-loading from hemoglobin.

Table 12-8	Causes of Hypophosphatemia

Transcellular Shift	Renal Loss	Gastrointestinal Loss	Decreased Intake
Acute alkalosis	Hyperparathyroidism	Malabsorption	Malnutrition
Carbohydrate administration	Diuretic use	Diarrhea	Parenteral nutrition
Drugs (insulin, epinephrine)	Hypokalemia	Intestinal fistulas	
	Hypomagnesemia	Antacids	
	Steroids		

Treatment of hypophosphatemia consists of controlling the underlying disease, removing offending drugs, correcting electrolyte abnormalities, and replacing phosphate. Phosphate levels <1 mg/dL (<0.32 mmol/L) associated with symptoms are considered life-threatening and require immediate treatment. For emergency treatment, administer phosphate at 0.6 to 0.9 mg/kg/daily intravenously. When circulating phosphate levels are stable, maintenance replacement of phosphate is 1,000 mg/day intravenously plus excess losses (ie, in urine or stool). Phosphate may be administered as potassium phosphate (93 mg phosphate/mL, 1.1 mmol/mL potassium) or sodium phosphate (93 mg phosphate/mL). Enteral administration of phosphate is preferred in patients with serum phosphate levels >1 to 1.5 mg/dL (>0.32-0.48 mmol/L).

Serum phosphate should be monitored during repletion and therapy adjusted to achieve a circulating level of 3 to 4 mg/dL (0.97-1.29 mmol/L). Adverse effects of phosphate administration include hyperphosphatemia, hypocalcemia, tissue calcium precipitation, renal injury, and diarrhea (enteral phosphate).

3. Hypomagnesemia

Magnesium is important to the body for energy transfer and electrical stability. Causes of hypomagnesemia (magnesium <1.8 mg/dL or 1.5 mEq/dL [<0.75 mmol/L]) are listed in **Table 12-9.**

Clinical manifestations of hypomagnesemia overlap those of hypokalemia and hypocalcemia. These manifestations include cardiovascular abnormalities (eg, QT interval prolongation, arrhythmias, vasospasm, myocardial ischemia), neuromuscular abnormalities (ie, weakness, tremor, seizures, tetany, obtundation, coma), and electrolyte abnormalities (eg, hypokalemia, hypocalcemia).

Table 12-9	Causes of Hypomagnesemia		
Renal Loss	**Gastrointestinal Loss**	**Transcellular Shift**	**Decreased Intake**
Renal tubular dysfunction	Malabsorption	Refeeding	Malnutrition
Diuresis	Diarrhea	Recovery from hypothermia	Alcoholism
Hypokalemia	Nasogastric suction		Parenteral nutrition
Drugs (amino-glycosides, amphotericin, etc)			

Treatment of hypomagnesemia consists of treating the underlying disease, discontinuing problematic drugs, correcting concomitant electrolyte abnormalities, and replenishing magnesium. For emergency treatment of hypomagnesemia (eg, arrhythmias), administer 1 to 2 g magnesium sulfate intravenously over 5 to 10 minutes. Magnesium sulfate can be administered over a longer interval (10-60 minutes) in less urgent situations. Depending on the clinical situation, subsequent intravenous replacement ranges from 1 to 2 g magnesium sulfate every 4 to 6 hours. Once serum magnesium levels stabilize, intravenous maintenance doses are 0.1 to 0.2 mmol/kg daily (1 g magnesium sulfate = 8 mmol). Maintenance magnesium may also be administered enterally. The dose of magnesium should be reduced if renal failure is present. Magnesium levels should be monitored during repletion. Deep tendon reflexes can be used to assess for hypermagnesemia during replacement (ie, decreased at serum level 4-5 mg/dL [1.65-2.06 mmol/L]).

III. METABOLIC DISTURBANCES

Case Study

A 34-year-old male presented to the emergency department with nonspecific complaints of a flu-like syndrome. His vital signs include respiratory rate 24/min, heart rate 126/min, blood pressure 96/48 mm Hg, and temperature 103.2°F (39.5°C). His laboratory results are remarkable for a white blood cell count 18,000/mm³ with 14% bands. After blood cultures, antibiotics, and volume resuscitation, he feels better and is admitted to the floor. Two hours later, he is found to be lethargic with a palpable systolic blood pressure of 60 mm Hg. After transfer to the ICU, aggressive fluid resuscitation (40 mL/kg) and 10 mg/min of norepinephrine, he remains hypotensive.

- What metabolic disorders may contribute to the refractory hypotension?

- What testing is needed?

- What interventions should be considered?

A. Acute Adrenal Insufficiency

Acute adrenal insufficiency in the critically ill patient may result from preexisting or previously undiagnosed chronic disease of the adrenal glands or hypothalamic-pituitary axis or acute conditions affecting these endocrine organs (**Table 12-10**). Patients with chronic disease may develop acute adrenal failure precipitated by infection or other stressors. In addition, functional impairment during a serious illness may result in a relative or absolute insufficiency of glucocorticoids that usually reverses with recovery from the illness. Relative adrenal insufficiency occurs when the cortisol response is normal or high, but it is reduced in relation to the severity of illness.

Table 12-10. Etiologies of Adrenal Insufficiency

Chronic Conditions

Adrenal glands

      Autoimmune destruction

      Granulomatous disease (tuberculosis)

      HIV infection

      Other infection (CMV, fungal)

      Primary or metastatic malignancy

      Drug effects (ie, ketoconazole)

Hypothalamic/pituitary axis

      Withdrawal from exogenous glucocorticoid therapy

      Hypopituitarism (tumors, infarction, radiation)

      Sarcoidosis, histiocytosis

      Head trauma

Acute Conditions

Critical illness (affects adrenal glands and hypothalamic-pituitary axis)

      Hypoperfusion

      Cytokine effects (alter cortisol metabolism, receptor affinity)

Acute adrenal hemorrhage

      Meningococcemia

      Disseminated intravascular coagulation

      Anticoagulation (warfarin, heparin, etc)

Drug effects

      Increased cortisol metabolism (phenytoin, phenobarbital, rifampin)

      Interference with glucocorticoid synthesis (ketoconazole, etomidate)

Lack of specific signs and symptoms makes early recognition of acute adrenal insufficiency difficult in the critically ill patient. Clinical manifestations suggestive of acute adrenal insufficiency include weakness, nausea/vomiting, abdominal pain, tachycardia, orthostatic hypotension, hypotension refractory to volume or vasopressor agents, and fever. Suggestive laboratory findings may include eosinophilia, hyponatremia, hyperkalemia, acidosis, hypoglycemia, and prerenal azotemia. Acute adrenal hemorrhage may cause abdominal, flank, or back pain. These clinical and laboratory manifestations overlap significantly with manifestations of other common critical illnesses such as sepsis. Important clues for possible adrenal insufficiency in seriously ill patients are vasopressor dependency and/or failure to respond to adequate fluids, fever without an apparent source or unresponsive to antibiotics, and a discrepancy between the expected disease severity and the condition of the patient.

> **!**
>
> *Electrolyte abnormalities are less likely with acute adrenal insufficiency compared to chronic adrenal insufficiency.*
>
> **!**

The value of testing the hypothalamic-pituitary-adrenal axis using baseline cortisol levels and/ or the short adrenocorticotropic hormone (ACTH) stimulation test is limited in the seriously ill patient due to variation in testing methodology, delayed reporting of results, and lack of consensus criteria for absolute or relative adrenal insufficiency. Proposed definitions of adrenal insufficiency in critical illness include a random cortisol level <15 µg/dL (others suggest ≤20 or 25 µg/dL) and/or a cortisol increment ≤9 µg/dL after ACTH administration. Prompt improvement in hemodynamic status after administration of hydrocortisone may be an important physiologic indicator. If chronic adrenal insufficiency is suspected, a short ACTH stimulation test may be useful in diagnosis. However, retesting after resolution of the acute illness may be warranted. For more information about the short ACTH stimulation test, see **Appendix 14.**

> **!** *Hydrocortisone also provides some mineralocorticoid effects.* **!**

Emergent treatment is indicated in critically ill patients, even if the diagnosis is not firmly established. The treatment steps for acute adrenal insufficiency are presented in **Table 12-11.**

Table 12-11. Emergent Treatment for Acute Adrenal Insufficiency

1. Obtain baseline blood samples for cortisol (if indicated), electrolytes, glucose, etc.

2. Infuse normal saline or D5 normal saline (large volumes may be required) and vasopressor agent to support blood pressure as needed.

3. Treat precipitating conditions.

4. Perform a short ACTH stimulation test, if desired, for diagnosis and management. An ACTH test is not recommended in septic shock to identify patients who should receive hydrocortisone.

5. Administer a glucocorticoid. If the diagnosis of adrenal insufficiency is known or a short ACTH stimulation test will not be used to guide therapy, hydrocortisone 200-300 mg every 24 hours can be administered intravenously in divided doses every 6-8 hours or as a continuous infusion. Dexamethasone 4 mg intravenously can be used initially if a short ACTH stimulation test is to be performed.

6. The addition of daily fludrocortisone (50 µg orally) may be considered if the administered glucocorticoid has no significant mineralocorticoid activity.

If a clinical response to glucocorticoid administration is observed and relative adrenal insufficiency is suspected, treatment should be continued until resolution of the critical illness (7 days is recommended in septic shock). Although recommendations vary, tapering of the glucocorticoid may avoid rebound effects associated with abrupt discontinuation. Patients with persistent adrenal insufficiency (chronic or newly diagnosed) should be converted to oral steroid therapy.

B. Hyperglycemic Syndromes

1. Diabetic Emergencies

Serious metabolic complications of diabetes result from a relative or absolute lack of insulin coupled with increased production of counterregulatory hormones such as glucagon, catecholamines, cortisol, epinephrine, and others. Life-threatening hyperglycemic syndromes include diabetic ketoacidosis (DKA) and hyperglycemic hyperosmolar state (HHS). These hyperglycemic syndromes differ in the severity of dehydration and degree of acidosis (ketosis) but share many clinical manifestations and therapeutic interventions. In addition, patients may manifest components of both syndromes. **Table 12-12** lists characteristics that may distinguish the syndromes, but considerable variability is possible. Although DKA and HHS may be the initial presentation of diabetes, the most common precipitating factors are infection and medication noncompliance. Other precipitants include corticosteroid use, myocardial infarction, stroke, alcohol abuse, pancreatitis, trauma, and pregnancy.

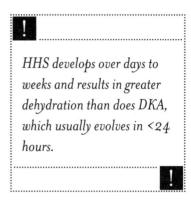

HHS develops over days to weeks and results in greater dehydration than does DKA, which usually evolves in <24 hours.

Table 12-12. Characteristics of Hyperglycemic Syndromes		
	DKA	**HHS**
Glucose	>250 mg/dL	>600 mg/dL
Arterial/venous pH	≤7.3	>7.3
Anion gap	Increased	Variable
Serum/urine ketones	Positive	Negative or small
Serum osmolality	Normal	Increased

Clinical manifestations result from hyperglycemia in both syndromes and from excess ketone production in DKA. Hyperglycemia causes hyperosmolality, osmotic diuresis, fluid and electrolyte loss, dehydration, and volume depletion. Ketones cause acidosis and also contribute to the osmotic diuresis. Clinical features of both hyperglycemic syndromes may include weakness, dehydration, polyuria, polydipsia, tachycardia, hypotension, anorexia, nausea/vomiting, and ileus. Abdominal pain, hyperpnea (Kussmaul respirations), and fruity odor to the breath are more characteristic of DKA, whereas altered mental status (ranging from lethargy to coma) and arrhythmias are more common in HHS. Laboratory investigation may reveal hyperglycemia, hyperosmolality (more common in HHS), glucosuria, ketonemia/ketonuria (DKA), anion gap metabolic acidosis (DKA), hypokalemia or hyperkalemia, hypophosphatemia, hypomagnesemia, leukocytosis, and azotemia. Serum sodium concentrations may be decreased due to translocation of water to the extracellular space. An elevated serum sodium concentration suggests severe dehydration.

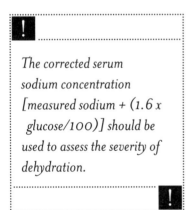

The corrected serum sodium concentration [measured sodium + (1.6 x glucose/100)] should be used to assess the severity of dehydration.

An initial rapid evaluation of the patient with possible hyperglycemic condition should include assessment of mental status, degree of dehydration (vital signs, orthostatic changes, urine output), and presence of infection. Laboratory studies should include complete blood count, electrolytes, renal function, glucose (plasma or fingerstick), urine or serum ketones, and arterial blood gas (or venous pH in hemodynamically stable patients). An electrocardiogram should be obtained to evaluate for ischemia and changes due to electrolyte abnormalities. If infection is suspected, appropriate cultures should be obtained.

The goals for treatment of hyperglycemic syndromes are to restore the fluid and electrolyte balance, provide insulin, and identify precipitating factors. The initial management of DKA and HHS is outlined in **Table 12-13.** Volume deficits correlate with the severity of hyperglycemia and are usually greater in HHS. Urine output should be maintained at 1 to 3 mL/kg/h to ensure adequate tissue perfusion and clearance of glucose. Invasive hemodynamic monitoring (eg, arterial catheter, pulmonary artery catheter) may be required in patients with underlying cardiovascular disease.

Table 12-13. Initial Management of Hyperglycemic Syndromes

Fluids

1. Assess severity of dehydration.

2. Institute crystalloid resuscitation, initially with normal saline at approximately 15-20 mL/kg/h in the first hour in the absence of cardiac dysfunction to restore hemodynamic stability and renal perfusion. Subsequent fluid infusion rates should be guided by assessment of hydration and urine output and 250-500 mL/h is often adequate.

3. After stabilization of the hemodynamic status, fluids with less chloride (eg, 0.45% saline) should be considered to avoid or minimize the development of hyperchloremic metabolic acidosis. The corrected serum sodium should also be used to guide fluid selection.

4. Add glucose to fluids when glucose is 250-300 mg/dL (13.9-16.7 mmol/L) in DKA. Administer 10% dextrose if necessary to maintain glucose >150 mg/dL (>8.3 mmol/L). In HHS, add glucose to fluids when glucose is 300 mg/dL (16.7 mmol/L) to maintain the glucose concentration between 250-300 mg/dL (13.9-16.7 mmol/L).

Insulin

1. Administer a regular insulin loading dose as an intravenous bolus (0.1-0.15 units/kg) followed by an infusion at 0.1 units/kg/h. Hold insulin if potassium concentration is <3.3 mmol/L until potassium is replaced.

2. If the glucose concentration does not fall by 50 mg/dL (2.8 mmol/L) in the first hour, consider increasing the insulin infusion rate or administering additional insulin boluses (10 units regular insulin hourly). Lack of response may also be due to inadequate volume resuscitation or serious infection.

3. In DKA, continue insulin infusion or decrease by 50% when the glucose reaches 250 mg/dL (13.9 mmol/L). Maintain the glucose concentration between 150 and 200 mg/dL (8.3 and 11.1 mmol/L) until acidosis and ketosis are resolved.

4. In HHS, decrease insulin infusion when the glucose concentration reaches 300 mg/dL (16.7 mmol/L) to maintain the glucose at 250-300 mg/dL (13.9-16.7 mmol/L) until the plasma osmolality is ≤315 mOsm/kg and the patient is alert.

Electrolytes

1. If serum potassium is <3.3 mmol/L, hold insulin and administer potassium 40 mmol/h as potassium chloride or potassium phosphate (or combination) until potassium is >3.3 mmol/L in order to avoid arrhythmias or severe weakness.

2. If serum potassium is >3.3 mmol/L but <5 mmol/L and urine output is adequate, administer potassium 20-30 mmol in each liter of fluids in order to maintain the potassium 4-5 mmol/L.

3. If serum potassium is >5 mmol/L, do not administer potassium in fluids until <5 mmol/L.

4. Consider phosphate replacement with potassium phosphate if serum levels are low (<1 mg/dL, 0.32 mmol/L) or severe symptoms are present.

! *Glucose concentrations should be monitored every 1-2 hours.* !

The intravenous route for insulin administration is the most reliable and easiest to titrate. Because of the short half-life of intravenous insulin, a continuous infusion is necessary with serial monitoring of the glucose and electrolyte concentrations. Smaller doses of insulin may be adequate in HHS.

Glucose-containing fluids may be started earlier than recommended if blood glucose cannot be monitored frequently. When glucose and/or serum osmolality are controlled, acidosis has cleared, and the patient is stable, the patient may be advanced to subcutaneous insulin. An insulin sliding scale with subcutaneous administration of regular and longer-acting preparations can be started and should overlap for 1 to 2 hours with discontinuation of the insulin infusion.

Insulin and correction of acidosis shifts potassium intracellularly and may lead to precipitous drops in serum potassium levels. Oral potassium replacement can be considered if nausea and vomiting are not present. Potassium and other electrolyte levels should be monitored frequently (especially in the first 6 hours) until levels stabilize and acidosis is resolved.

Acidosis is well tolerated by patients with DKA, and bicarbonate therapy is controversial in DKA. No benefit has been found when bicarbonate is administered to DKA patients with pH 6.9 to 7.1, and fluid and insulin therapy result in rapid improvement in pH. Bicarbonate administration may be considered if the arterial pH is <6.9 (give 100 mmol bicarbonate over 1 hour to increase pH >7). Do not attempt to normalize blood pH with bicarbonate, since acidosis resolves as ketones are metabolized.

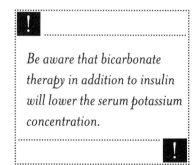

Be aware that bicarbonate therapy in addition to insulin will lower the serum potassium concentration.

2. Hyperglycemia in Critical Illness

Hyperglycemia is common in diabetic and nondiabetic patients with a critical illness and may be due to increased stress hormones, inflammatory mediators, glucocorticoid therapy, excessive nutritional calories, decreased activity, and other mechanisms. Significant hyperglycemia may be associated with poor wound healing, impaired immune function, increased inflammation, endothelial dysfunction, and other adverse effects leading to increased morbidity and mortality. Tight glucose control (80-110 mg/dL, 4.4-6.1 mmol/L) achieved with continuous insulin infusion has been demonstrated to improve mortality in mechanically ventilated surgical patients, primarily those patients with an ICU length of stay greater than 5 days. A sliding scale of subcutaneous regular insulin is not useful in achieving these goals because the insulin dose is determined after the glucose has increased. Mortality benefits have not been consistently achieved with tight glucose control (80-110 mg/dL, 4.4-6.1 mmol/L) in medical ICU patients in other studies, and the incidence of hypoglycemia has been higher.

The exact target range for glucose control in the critically ill patient continues to be debated. Recommendations have included 80 to 110 mg/dL (4.4-6.1 mmol/L), 140 to 180 mg/dL (7.8-10 mmol/L), and <150 mg/dL (8.3 mmol/L). The ability to provide adequate nursing support and monitoring may affect the goals chosen. In addition, different types of blood sampling and glucose measurement methods may yield different results. A protocol of blood sampling, insulin infusion, and target glucose should be chosen to achieve consistency and minimize hypoglycemia. Continuing investigations of glucose control should provide further guidance for the clinician.

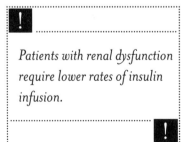

Patients with renal dysfunction require lower rates of insulin infusion.

C. Additional Metabolic Disturbances

1. Thyroid Storm

Thyroid storm occurs most often in patients with Graves' disease or toxic nodular goiter. Precipitating factors include infection, surgery, labor/delivery, acute medical illness, trauma, or emotional stress. Thyroid storm is characterized by exaggerated classic manifestations of hyperthyroidism plus fever, CNS dysfunction (apathy, agitation, coma, etc), congestive heart failure, arrhythmias, and gastrointestinal symptoms (vomiting, diarrhea, jaundice).

Therapy should be initiated immediately, without awaiting results of thyroid hormone tests. An endocrinologist or critical care specialist should be consulted as soon as possible. Supportive and specific measures are presented in **Table 12-14.**

Table 12-14. **Measures for Treating Thyroid Storm**

Supportive Measures

1. Cool with acetaminophen and cooling blankets. (Salicylates should be avoided since they affect binding of thyroxine [T_4] and triiodothyronine [T_3] to their binding proteins.)

2. Hydrate using glucose-containing fluids.

3. Identify and treat the precipitating cause.

Specific Measures

1. Inhibit T_4 synthesis with propylthiouracil 800-1200 mg orally initially, then 200-300 mg orally every 6 hours; or with methimazole 80-120 mg orally or rectally initially, then 20-30 mg orally or rectally every 6 hours.

2. Inhibit adrenergic effects with propranolol 1-10 mg intravenously (titrated) or 40-120 mg orally every 6 hours.

3. Inhibit T_4 release by administering saturated solution of potassium iodide (SSKI) 5 drops orally every 6-8 hours; or sodium iodine 0.5 g intravenously every 12 hours. Initiate 1 hour after propylthiouracil or methimazole is given.

4. Inhibit T_4 to T_3 conversion by administering dexamethasone 2 mg intravenously or orally every 6 hours or sodium ipodate 0.5-1 g orally every day.

---

2. Myxedema Coma

Myxedema coma (life-threatening hypothyroidism) is a rare manifestation of chronic hypothyroidism that occurs most frequently in elderly patients during winter months. Precipitating factors include infection, drugs (eg, sedatives, hypnotics), surgery, neurologic disorders (eg, cerebrovascular accident, seizures), acute medical illness, trauma, and exposure to cold. Clinical manifestations are an exaggeration of less severe hypothyroidism and result in widespread organ dysfunction. Features of life-threatening hypothyroidism include hypothermia, obtundation/coma, bradycardia, heart failure, hypoventilation, hyporeflexia, hyponatremia, hypoglycemia, anemia, and decreased ECG voltage.

The diagnosis of myxedema coma is clinical, and treatment should not be delayed pending laboratory results. Treatment with T4 is unlikely to cause harm if the diagnosis is in error, but delay in therapy can be fatal. An endocrinologist or critical care specialist should be consulted as soon as possible. In addition to obtaining blood for thyroid function tests, the measures presented in **Table 12-15** should be instituted.

Table 12-15. Emergent Treatment of Myxedema Coma

1. Secure airway and ventilate, if necessary.
2. Treat hypotension with fluids.
3. Treat precipitating cause.
4. Provide passive warming (eg, blankets).
5. Provide glucose.
6. Treat significant hyponatremia with diuresis (eg, loop diuretic).
7. Give hydrocortisone 100 mg intravenously every 8 hours, or assess adrenal function (**Appendix 14**).
8. Administer thyroxine (T_4) intravenously, 300-500 µg initially, followed by 50-100 µg daily until oral T_4 can be administered.

Key Points

Life-threatening Electrolyte and Metabolic Disturbances

■ In the presence of life-threatening arrhythmias or paralysis associated with hypokalemia, give potassium chloride 20 to 30 mmol/h through a central venous catheter.

■ If hyperkalemia-associated ECG abnormalities are present, administer calcium chloride or calcium gluconate intravenously over 5 to 10 minutes. Then consider shifting potassium intracellularly with 50% dextrose and regular insulin intravenously, inhaled β-agonists, and/or sodium bicarbonate.

■ In symptomatic euvolemic hyponatremia, limit the increase in serum sodium to approximately 8 to 12 mmol/L in the first 24 hours. Too rapid a correction of serum sodium may result in CNS injury.

■ Patients with hypernatremia and hemodynamic instability should have normal saline administered until intravascular volume is corrected. Subsequently, replace water with 5% dextrose in water, 0.45% NaCl, or 0.2% NaCl with 5% dextrose.

■ Emergent treatment with a glucocorticoid is indicated in critically ill patients with possible adrenal insufficiency, even if the diagnosis is not established.

■ The goals of treatment of hyperglycemic syndromes are to restore the fluid and electrolyte balance, provide insulin, and identify precipitating factors.

■ In diabetic ketoacidosis, insulin infusion should be continued until the ketosis and acidosis have resolved. Glucose-containing fluids should be administered to prevent hypoglycemia during insulin infusion.

■ Maintain the glucose between 250 and 300 mg/dL (13.9-16.7 mmol/L) in hyperglycemic hyperosmolar syndrome until the plasma osmolality is ≤315 mOsm/kg and the patient is alert.

■ Potassium should be added to the fluid therapy of hyperglycemic syndromes as soon as serum potassium is recognized to be <5 mmol/L and urine output is adequate.

■ A protocol of blood sampling, insulin infusion, and target glucose should be chosen to avoid hyperglycemia and minimize hypoglycemia in critically ill patients.

Suggested Readings

1. Adrogué HJ, Madias NE. Hypernatremia. *N Engl J Med.* 2000;342:1493.

2. Adrogué HJ, Madias NE. Hyponatremia. *N Engl J Med.* 2000;342:1581.

3. American Diabetes Association. Hyperglycemic crises in diabetes. *Diabetes Care.* 2004;27(suppl 1):S94. Also available at www.diabetes.org.

4. Cooper MS, Stewart PM. Corticosteroid insufficiency in acutely ill patients. *N Engl J Med.* 2003;348:727.

5. Gennari JF. Disorders of potassium homeostasis: hypokalemia and hyperkalemia. *Crit Care Clin.* 2002;18:273.

6. Marik PE, Zaloga GP. Adrenal insufficiency in the critically ill. *Chest.* 2002;122:1784.

7. Sarlis NJ, Gourgiotis L. Thyroid emergencies. *Rev Endocr Metab Disord.* 2003;4:129.

8. Touyz RM. Magnesium in clinical medicine. *Front Biosci.* 2004;9:1278.

Chapter 13

SPECIAL CONSIDERATIONS

✓ Objectives

- Outline the diagnosis and management of pulmonary embolism.

- Describe appropriate prophylactic therapy for venous thromboembolism.

- List general management principles of severe gastrointestinal hemorrhage.

- Describe appropriate prophylactic therapy for the prevention of stress-related gastritis.

- List principles of poisoning management.

- Identify principles of management for temperature-related illness and injury.

Case Study

An obese female with chronic tobacco abuse and congestive heart failure arrives at the emergency department complaining of shortness of breath and right pleuritic chest pain for the past 2 days. She has a heart rate of 110/min with clear lung fields and mild bilateral pretibial edema. When she arrived, her SpO_2 on room air was 89%; that has increased to 94% on 3 L/min oxygen by nasal cannula. A chest radiograph did not show any infiltrates. As her primary care physician, you are called for assistance in her management.

- What risk factors and clinical findings suggest the possibility of a pulmonary embolism?

- What tests are indicated to establish a diagnosis of pulmonary embolism?

I. INTRODUCTION

In addition to the medical conditions discussed in previous chapters, the clinician may be called on to care for patients with other severe and/or life-threatening problems. The management and prevention of some of these commonly encountered conditions are reviewed in this chapter.

II. PULMONARY EMBOLISM

A. Diagnosis

A patient's history and clinical findings may be unreliable for diagnosis of a pulmonary embolism (PE). Risk factors for PE and other venous thromboembolic disease, shown in **Table 13-1,** often contribute to a high index of suspicion. Predisposing factors include any condition that may cause venous stasis, injury to the vascular endothelium, or hypercoagulability (Virchow's triad).

Table 13-1.	Risk Factors for Pulmonary Embolism/Venous Thromboembolism	
Family history	Central venous catheterization	
Advanced age	Recent surgery	
Obesity (body mass index >30)	Immobility, paralysis	
Prior history of deep vein thrombosis/PE	Stroke with partial or full paralysis	
Venous insufficiency	Trauma	
Venous injury or repair	Malignancy (past or current)	
Inherited hypercoagulable disorders (protein C or S deficiency, lupus anticoagulant, etc)	Cancer therapy	
	Selective estrogen receptor modulators	
Acute medical illness, ICU admission	Pregnancy and postpartum period	
Heart or respiratory failure	Estrogen therapy	
Nephrotic syndrome	Smoking	

The classic combination of dyspnea, pleuritic chest pain, and hemoptysis occurs in a minority of patients with PE. Routine blood studies are nondiagnostic. Chest radiographs are frequently unremarkable but may show nonspecific findings of atelectasis, pleural effusion, elevated hemidiaphragm, and/or infiltrates. The ECG may show nonspecific ST-T wave changes, an $S_1Q_3T_3$ pattern, or right bundle branch block, but a pattern of acute cor pulmonale is infrequently present.

Sinus tachycardia and premature atrial contractions are the most frequently encountered arrhythmias. Often the most significant information provided by the ECG is the exclusion of other potential sources of chest pain, such as acute ischemia or pericarditis. Hypoxemia, a nonspecific finding in cardiopulmonary disease, is commonly present, but a normal PaO_2 value or normal alveolar-arterial oxygen tension difference [$P(A - a)O_2$] does not rule out PE. Signs and symptoms of PE are shown in **Table 13-2.**

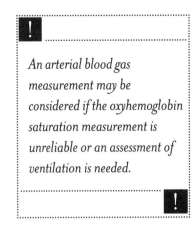

An arterial blood gas measurement may be considered if the oxyhemoglobin saturation measurement is unreliable or an assessment of ventilation is needed.

Table 13-2.	Clinical Manifestations of Pulmonary Embolism	
Dyspnea	Fever (usually low-grade)	
Chest pain	Hypoxemia	
Cough	Cyanosis	
Tachypnea	Apprehension	
Tachycardia	Syncope	
Diaphoresis	Previously noted leg swelling	
Hemoptysis		

A correct diagnosis of PE is essential because appropriate therapy decreases mortality. The current diagnostic strategy recommends that the clinician formulate a clinical likelihood of low, moderate, or high clinical suspicion of pulmonary embolus (**Figure 13-1**). One scoring system used to determine pretest probability of PE is presented in **Table 13-3.** D-dimer assays with high sensitivity and high negative predictive value are frequently used as an initial step in algorithms for the diagnosis of PE in outpatients. A negative D-dimer result in a patient with low clinical probability of PE may reliably exclude the diagnosis. Patients with a positive D-dimer result or with a moderate or high clinical probability assessment require further diagnostic evaluation. D-dimer measurements have limited utility for the evaluation of PE in hospitalized patients because of the high proportion of positive results.

Figure 13-1. A Diagnostic Approach to Pulmonary Embolism

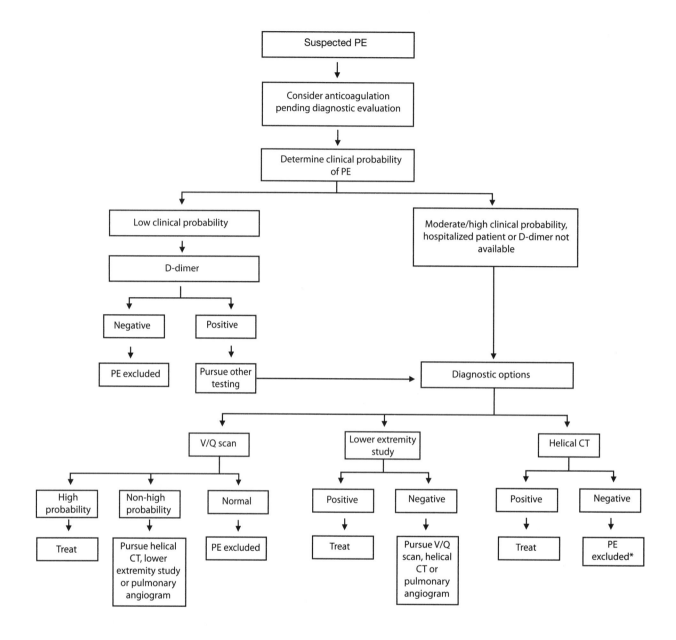

*Consider pulmonary angiogram if clinical suspicion is high; negative predictive value is increased by a negative lower extremity study

Table 13-3.	Clinical Probability Assessment for PE[a]	
Clinical signs and symptoms of DVT (objective leg swelling and pain with palpation)		3
PE as likely, or more likely, than an alternative diagnosis		3
Immobilization (bed rest, except to access bathroom, for ≥3 consecutive days or surgery in previous 4 weeks)		1.5
Previous objective diagnosis of DVT or PE		1.5
Previous objective diagnosis of DVT or PE		1.5
Heart rate >100 beats/min		1.5
Hemoptysis		1
Active cancer (treatment ongoing or within previous 6 months or palliative treatment)		1
0-<2: Low probability		
2-6: Moderate probability		
>6: High probability		

[a] Adapted from Wells PS, Anderson DR, Rodger M, et al. Excluding pulmonary embolism at the bedside without diagnostic imaging: management of patients with suspected pulmonary embolism presenting to the emergency department by using a simple clinical model and D-dimer. *Ann Intern Med.* 2001;135:99.

B. Therapy

The treatment of pulmonary embolism can usually be limited to anticoagulation. (**Appendix 13** for recommended intravenous unfractionated heparin therapy for full anticoagulation.) Low-molecular-weight heparin (LMWH) can be effective in treating PE and is often preferred due to its convenient dosing, absence of need for laboratory monitoring, and lower incidence of heparin-induced thrombocytopenia. In patients with suspected PE and no contraindications to anticoagulation, baseline activated partial thromboplastin time (APTT), prothrombin time (PT), and complete blood cell count (CBC) should be obtained, and heparin therapy should be initiated while waiting for test results. Contraindications to heparin therapy include recent major trauma with hemorrhage, recent central nervous system (CNS) hemorrhage or infarction, active gastrointestinal (GI) bleed, and clinically significant heparin-induced thrombocytopenia. When unfractionated heparin is used, the APTT should be monitored to achieve a value 1.5 to 2.5 times the mean normal value. Oral warfarin therapy is started on day 1 and adjusted to achieve an INR of 2 to 3. Heparin therapy can be discontinued after 5 days if the INR with warfarin has been therapeutic for 2 days. In massive PE, a longer period of intravenous heparin (~10 days) is often recommended. Oral anticoagulation should continue for at least 3 to 6 months, but some patients may have indications for longer therapy.

The use of thrombolytic agents in the treatment of PE should be individualized, and clinicians have some latitude in using these agents. In general, patients with acute massive PE with hemodynamic instability who are at low risk of bleeding are the best candidates for thrombolytic therapy. In hemodynamically stable patients, including those with a large PE, the risk of major bleeding still seems to outweigh the benefit of thrombolysis. Tissue plasminogen activator (t-PA) is preferred at a dose of 100 milligrams infused over a 2-hour period, but none of the thrombolytic agents has been shown to improve mortality in this clinical situation. Streptokinase has also been used with a loading dose of 250,000 international units followed by 100,000 international units per hour for 24 hours. Local administration of a thrombolytic agent via a catheter is not recommended. Surgical embolectomy or extraction/fragmentation of the embolus by transvenous catheters requires specialized expertise not commonly available, and associated mortality is high.

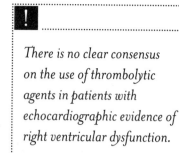

There is no clear consensus on the use of thrombolytic agents in patients with echocardiographic evidence of right ventricular dysfunction.

An inferior vena cava filter should be considered in patients at high risk of recurrent emboli when

- There is a strong contraindication to anticoagulation
- Emboli recur during anticoagulation
- Bleeding occurs during anticoagulation

Retrievable filters may be an option in some centers. If possible, anticoagulation for treatment of the embolus should be resumed as soon as possible after insertion of a filter.

C. Prevention of Venous Thromboembolism

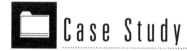 Case Study

A middle-aged man presents with an acute ischemic stroke and right hemiparesis. He received tissue plasminogen activator (t-PA) and there was improvement in the neurologic deficits.

- Should this patient receive prophylaxis for venous thromboembolism?
- What type of venous thromboembolism prophylaxis would be appropriate for this patient if the decision is made to treat?

Many critically ill or injured patients are at risk of developing venous thromboembolism (VTE), either PE or deep venous thrombosis (DVT). The development of thrombosis can lead to longer hospital stays, increased resource utilization, venous abnormalities, and death. Thromboprophylaxis is cost effective and highly efficacious in preventing venous thromboembolism. Both pharmacologic (heparins, direct thrombin inhibitors such as fondaparinux) and mechanical interventions (intermittent pneumatic compression device [IPC], graduated compression stockings [CS]) may be used for prophylaxis in hospitalized patients (**Appendix 15**). Mechanical methods for prophylaxis are generally less effective but are acceptable options for patients at high risk of bleeding and when combined with anticoagulants.

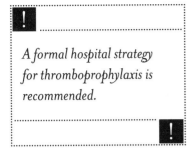

A formal hospital strategy for thromboprophylaxis is recommended.

Recommendations are based on specific patient groups, level of risk for VTE, and risk of bleeding. Clinicians should follow manufacturers' instructions for dosing of LMWH, especially in the setting of renal failure and obesity. Caution must be used when instituting anticoagulant therapy in patients with recent or ongoing hemorrhage, renal failure, or concomitant use of antiplatelet therapy.

III. SEVERE GASTROINTESTINAL HEMORRHAGE

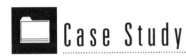

Case Study

A 64-year-old man with arthritic pain had been taking ibuprofen 4 times a day for months without significant relief. He started to complain of fatigue and progressive weakness. Today he developed nausea and started vomiting bright red blood. He called an ambulance and was brought to the emergency department. He is pale, tachycardiac, and dizzy. His blood pressure is 95/60 mm Hg and his hematocrit is 28%.

– What additional clinical and laboratory assessments are indicated?

– How would you prioritize interventions?

A. General Management Principles

Medications for ulcer prophylaxis and treatment have reduced the incidence of stress gastritis and severe upper gastrointestinal (GI) bleeding. However, when present, such bleeding can be life-threatening and requires early surgical consultation as well as rapid assessment, diagnosis, and intervention. The distinction between upper GI and lower GI sources of hemorrhage is important in determining the appropriate diagnostic/therapeutic approach. The ligament of Treitz is the anatomic marker that separates the upper GI tract from the lower GI tract when discussing hemorrhage.

An ECG should be obtained in patients with GI bleeding and heart disease or advanced age to assess for myocardial ischemia.

Typically, patients with life-threatening GI hemorrhage are older and have other chronic organ system disease(s). Therefore, the critical consequences of hemorrhage, hypotension, and anemia may be poorly tolerated and may lead to other systemic manifestations of poor oxygen delivery, such as myocardial ischemia. Prompt assessment, resuscitation, and early diagnosis (even during resuscitation) and intervention are needed to prevent these secondary consequences.

A general approach to managing GI bleeding is outlined in **Table 13-4.** Obtain blood for typing and crossmatching as soon as possible. An appropriate hemoglobin level should be maintained based on patient condition and coexisting disease. If a reserve of blood products (eg, 4 units packed red cells) cannot be immediately available, early patient transfer should be planned.

Table 13-4.	Management of Gastrointestinal Bleeding

Assessment	Airway
	Protective reflexes
	Level of consciousness
	Volume status
	Vital signs, orthostatic changes
	Central venous pressure
	Urine output
	Severity of condition
	Visible blood loss
	Hemoglobin, hematocrit, platelet count
	Coagulation status (APTT, PT)
	Protective reflexes
	Hypoperfusion abnormalities (ie, cardiac ischemia)
	Nasogastric or orogastric tube
	Confirm or rule out upper-GI source
	Lavage stomach for upper endoscopy
Resuscitation	Consider intubation
	Altered mental status
	Inability to protect airway
	Copious hematemesis
	Need for sedation/endoscopy
	Intravenous access
	Large-bore (≥16 gauge) peripheral catheter(s) or
	central venous catheter
	Fluid administration
	Normal saline or lactated Ringer's
	Transfusion of red blood cells
Diagnostic/Therapeutic Interventions	Endoscopy with directed therapy
	Surgical assessment/intervention
	Correct coagulopathy
	Fresh frozen plasma for factor deficiency
	Platelet transfusion if <50,000/mm^3
	Pharmacologic therapy for variceal bleeding
	Transfer to facility with diagnostic and/or therapeutic capability
Continuing Care	Monitored environment
	Adequate blood bank resources
	Frequent assessment
	Volume status
	Hypoperfusion abnormalities
	Laboratory parameters

B. Severe Upper Gastrointestinal Hemorrhage

Severe upper GI hemorrhage is diagnosed by hematemesis or the presence of blood in the gastric aspirate, although 10% to 15% of patients with duodenal ulcer may have little or no blood in the gastric aspirate due to bleeding below the level of the stomach. When obtaining a patient's history and physical examination, it is important to note previous upper GI bleeding, the presence of ulcerative disease, alcohol consumption, stigmata of cirrhosis, coagulation disorders, and use of aspirin, nonsteroidal anti-inflammatory agents, or anticoagulants. Common causes of upper GI hemorrhage include duodenal and gastric ulcers, esophageal and gastric varices, Mallory-Weiss tear, malignancy, and gastritis.

Endoscopy is needed to establish the diagnosis, and endoscopic therapy may control hemorrhage and reduce rebleeding. If endoscopy is not quickly available, consider transfer to a facility with endoscopic capabilities.

When uncontrolled variceal bleeding is suspected prior to endoscopic diagnosis, intravenous pharmacologic therapy with the following agents may be considered:

- Somatostatin 250 µg bolus followed by 250 µg/h

- Octreotide 25 to 100 µg bolus followed by 25 to 50 µg/h

- Vasopressin 20 units over 20 minutes followed by 0.1 to 0.4 units/min

- Terlipressin 1 to 2 mg every 4 hours (not available in the United States)

Somatostatin or a somatostatin analogue such as octreotide are the agents of choice because of their favorable side-effect profile. Nausea and abdominal pain are sometimes associated with bolus doses, but significant adverse effects are uncommon. Maintenance infusions continued for a minimum of 24 to 48 hours may be effective in both stopping acute variceal bleeding and preventing early rebleeding from varices. Vasopressin is an alternative choice but may cause coronary artery vasospasm, angina, or hypertension. Concomitant nitroglycerin may prevent the deleterious effects of vasopressin on the coronary circulation. Terlipressin is a synthetic vasopressin analogue with fewer side effects and a longer half-life. None of the above agents are recommended in the routine management of nonvariceal bleeding.

Following endoscopy with successful therapeutic intervention, an intravenous bolus of a proton pump inhibitor followed by continuous infusion for 72 hours is effective in decreasing nonvariceal rebleeding. If endoscopy is unsuccessful in controlling the bleeding, surgical intervention may be needed for control.

C. Severe Lower Gastrointestinal Hemorrhage

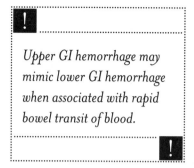

Upper GI hemorrhage may mimic lower GI hemorrhage when associated with rapid bowel transit of blood.

Frequent causes of lower GI hemorrhage are diverticular disease, angiodysplasia, large hemorrhoids, colonic polyps, inflammatory bowel disease, rectal ulcer/tear, upper GI source, and malignancy. Evaluation should include special attention to a history of diverticular disease, inflammatory bowel disease, previous abdominal aortic aneurysm repair (may suggest life-threatening aortic-enteric fistula), or the presence of a coagulation disorder. Physical examination must include inspection and a careful rectal examination to identify hemorrhoids or rectal carcinoma.

Gastric aspiration should be performed to eliminate an upper GI source of hemorrhage. A guaiac-negative nasogastric aspirate that contains bile makes an upper GI bleeding source unlikely. Upper GI endoscopy may be considered based on assessment of the most likely bleeding source. Lower GI endoscopy is important for diagnosis, treatment, anticipation of rebleeding, and planning other diagnostic interventions or surgery. If endoscopy is unavailable, transfer to another facility or direct surgical intervention will be dictated by the patient's condition. Angiography with embolization therapy may be considered for unstable patients or those who are poor surgical risks.

D. Prevention of Stress-Related Gastritis

Identification and treatment of patients at risk for stress-related gastritis will reduce complications, length of stay, and costs. To minimize the potential complications of pharmacologic prophylaxis for stress ulceration (ie, nosocomial pneumonia), routine use of such therapy should be limited to patients with known risk factors for stress gastritis. The risk of stress ulceration and GI bleeding depends on a patient's underlying illness, its severity, and related comorbidities. Significant risk factors include mechanical ventilation for longer than 48 hours, coagulopathy, severe infection, hypotension, severe head trauma (GCS <10), severe burns or trauma, renal or hepatic failure, major surgery, and prolonged ICU stay. Appropriate therapeutic agents include histamine receptor blocking agents (H_2 receptor antagonists) and sucralfate, a mucosal protecting agent. Proton pump inhibitors may also be considered, although less evidence is available to support their beneficial effects.

IV. POISONING AND DRUG TOXICITY

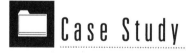

Case Study

A young woman was found by her parents on the bathroom floor the morning after a party. She was difficult to arouse, and when she was stimulated, she became agitated and violent. Her parents transported her to the emergency department.

– What are the immediate priorities and interventions in caring for this patient?

– What are the likely toxins, based on the patient's history and clinical presentation?

Patients who have ingested prescription, over-the-counter, or recreational drugs present in a number of ways. General categories of patient presentation and possible responsible agents are listed in **Table 13-5.** Reliable information about the substance(s), amount(s) ingested, and time of ingestion is often not available. Similarly, although qualitative urine toxicology screens and quantitative blood tests may be available, they cannot identify all agents that could have been ingested. Therefore, the initial evaluation and treatment for such patients are often symptom-based. Specific antidotes, treatments, and/or precautions based upon historical or laboratory evidence of particular ingestants can be utilized when applicable. In some countries, specialized resource centers are available to assist in the treatment of poisoning. The overall mortality from acute poisoning is low, but the treating clinician must quickly evaluate critical issues and attempt to identify patients at highest risk.

Table 13-5. Clinical Characteristics That Aid Diagnosis of Poisoning/Overdose

Clinical Presentation	Possible Agents
Coma, lethargy	Alcohols, antidepressants, barbiturates, benzodiazepines, cocaine (CNS bleed),gamma hydroxybutyrate, lithium, opiates, salicylates, selective serotonin reuptake inhibitors (SSRIs)
Agitation, confusion, bizarre behavior	Cocaine, amphetamines, antidepressants, phencyclidine, hallucinogens
Ventilatory compromise (respiratory acidosis)	Opiates, alcohols, antidepressants, barbiturates, benzodiazepines, gamma hydroxybutyrate
Metabolic acidosis	Salicylates, methanol/ethylene glycol, iron, isoniazid, carbon monoxide, cyanide
Hyperadrenergic, hyperthermia	Amphetamines, anticholinergics, cocaine, theophylline
Rhabdomyolysis	Amphetamines, cocaine, phencyclidine
Hypotension	Antidepressants, antihypertensives, opiates, organophosphates/carbamates, sedatives/hypnotics
Bradycardia/hypotension	ß-Blockers, calcium-channel blockers, digoxin, sedatives/hypnotics
Seizures	Amphetamines, antidepressants, cocaine, cyanide, isoniazid, lithium, organophosphates/carbamates, salicylates, SSRIs, theophylline
Hypothermia	Ethanol, hypoglycemic agents, opiates, sedatives/hypnotics
Nystagmus	Alcohols, carbamazepine, phenytoin, phencyclidine, sedative/hypnotics
Nausea/vomiting	Acetaminophen, alcohols, iron, salicylates, theophylline
Tachyarrhythmias	Amphetamines, antidepressants, cocaine, digoxin, theophylline

A. General Management

1. Initiate airway support as required. A careful assessment of the patient to ensure adequate ventilation, oxygenation, and protective airway reflexes is critical.

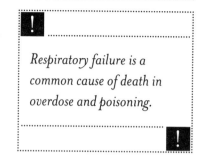

Respiratory failure is a common cause of death in overdose and poisoning.

2. Initiate management of cardiovascular compromise as indicated. Obtain adequate venous access and establish monitoring (eg, pulse oximeter, ECG, automated blood pressure device). Address initial concerns in monitored variables (eg, isotonic fluid administration, supplemental oxygen, seizure control or prophylaxis, cooling or warming the patient, vasopressors, or inotropes).

3. Consider the following interventions for a patient with altered mental status:

   a. Fifty mL 50% dextrose (50 g) intravenously, preferably after a blood glucose test is done.

   b. Naloxone 0.2 to 2 mg, intravenous, intramuscular, or via an endotracheal tube. Larger doses (6-10 mg), redosing, or an infusion may be required, especially when synthetic and long-acting opiates are involved.

   c. Thiamine 100 mg slow intravenous administration. (Administer prior to concentrated dextrose solutions to reduce the risk of Wernicke's encephalopathy.)

4. Develop a patient database with further history, physical examination, laboratory studies, and other information (eg, chest radiograph, ECG).

5. Little evidence exists for use of gastric-emptying procedures. Ipecac is not used in poisoned patients, and gastric lavage may be considered only in life-threatening overdoses within 1 hour of ingestion.

6. Activated charcoal should be administered to patients with significant toxic ingestions at an initial dose of 1 g/kg. The effectiveness of activated charcoal decreases with time from ingestion, so early administration is indicated.

7. Although cathartics are often routinely used in overdoses, there is no evidence of efficacy. Caution is warranted in the very young and elderly because of potential fluid losses.

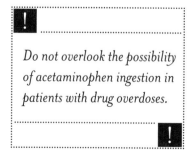

Do not overlook the possibility of acetaminophen ingestion in patients with drug overdoses.

B. Specific Management

After the patient is stabilized, more specific therapy may be warranted. Specific antidotes and/or interventions that may be considered are listed in **Table 13-6.** The use of more advanced interventions, such as hemodialysis or hemoperfusion, should be individualized to each patient and may require consultation or transfer.

Table 13-6. Antidotes and Interventions for Specific Toxins

Toxin	Antidote or Intervention
Acetaminophen	N-acetylcysteine
Alcohols (methanol, ethylene glycol)	Ethanol, fomepizole, hemodialysis
Amphetamines	Benzodiazepines
Benzodiazepines	Flumazenil[a]
ß-Blockers	Glucagon, calcium chloride, pacing, catecholamines
Calcium-channel blockers	Calcium chloride, glucagon, pacing, catecholamines
Carbon monoxide	100% oxygen, hyperbaric oxygen
Cocaine	Benzodiazepines
Cyanide	Nitrites and thiosulfate, hydroxocobalamin
Cyclic antidepressants	Blood alkalinization (pH 7.5-7.55), hypertonic saline, magnesium, α-agonist for hypotension
Digoxin	Digoxin-specific Fab fragments, atropine, lidocaine, pacing
Heparin	Protamine sulfate
Hypoglycemic agents	50% dextrose, somatostatin or octreotide
Iron	Deferoxamine
Isoniazid	Pyridoxine (vitamin B_6)
Lithium	Hemodialysis
Nitrites	Methylene blue
Opiates	Naloxone, intubation/ventilation
Organophosphates, carbamates, nerve gases	Atropine, pralidoxime or obidoxime
Salicylates	Urine alkalinization, hemodialysis
Theophylline	Multiple-dose charcoal, hemoperfusion
Warfarins	Vitamin K_1

[a] Flumazenil should not be administered to patients who chronically ingest benzodiazepines or have overdosed on cyclic antidepressants.

V. TEMPERATURE-RELATED ILLNESS

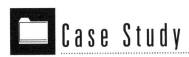 Case Study

Upon arrival at work one morning in the middle of the summer, an Arizona road construction crew found one of their coworkers in a ditch. He was obtunded and minimally responsive. His skin was sunburned and he had no signs of sweating. He was hypotensive and tachycardic. In the emergency department, his core temperature was >42.2°C (108°F).

– How would you manage this patient's hypotension?

– Which method of cooling would you institute?

A. Heat Stroke

Heat stroke, characterized by dysfunction of the hypothalamic temperature-regulating mechanism, altered mental status, and elevated core body temperature, is the most common cause of life-threatening hyperthermia. In addition to environmental heat and humidity, predisposing factors include cardiovascular disease, strenuous exertion, obesity, increased age, diabetes, skin or sweat gland abnormalities, and drugs (eg, alcohol, anticholinergics, diuretics, sympathomimetics, β-adrenergic blockers) that limit a patient's ability to dissipate body heat. The patient's core temperature is usually >40°C (>104°F). Clinical manifestations in heat stroke include major CNS dysfunction (eg, confusion, seizures, coma), tachypnea, tachycardia, dizziness, nausea, and diarrhea. Hypotension is common, skin is hot and flushed, and sweating may be absent or present.

Treatment of heat stroke is directed toward hemodynamic stabilization with replacement of intravascular volume, immediate reduction of the core body temperature, and reversal or prevention of complications. The following resuscitation measures should be instituted:

- Maintain adequate airway, oxygenation, and ventilatory assistance (if needed).

- Maintain blood pressure and urine output. Administer intravenous fluids; the type and amount depend on assessment of electrolytes, volume status, vital signs, and cardiac function. Hypokalemia or hyperkalemia, hypernatremia, hypocalcemia, and hypophosphatemia may occur.

- Cool the patient immediately. (Monitor with a rectal or esophageal thermistor capable of recording high temperatures.)

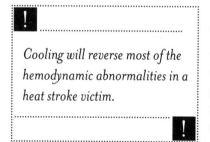

Cooling will reverse most of the hemodynamic abnormalities in a heat stroke victim.

In most environments it is easy to perform evaporative cooling by misting the unclothed patient with tepid (not cold) water and circulating air with a fan. An ice water bath is another option for cooling, but it may induce shivering and vasoconstriction, thus generating more body heat and slowing the heat's dissipation. It is also possible to apply ice packs or ice water soaks to the axillae and groin. Antipyretics and cooling blankets are ineffective.

Seizures and hypotension are complications that usually respond to cooling. Other potential complications of heat stroke include rhabdomyolysis, acute renal failure, metabolic acidosis, coagulopathy, hepatic failure, cardiac arrhythmias, and coma.

B. Hypothermia

Hypothermia is usually due to cold exposure or immersion and is defined as a core temperature <35°C to 36°C (<95°F -96.8°F). Predisposing factors include extremes of age, diabetes, malnutrition, chronic illness, trauma, erythrodermas, and drugs such as alcohol, barbiturates, phenothiazines, and benzodiazepines. Clinical manifestations vary with the severity of hypothermia. Neurologic changes range from impaired judgment to coma. Muscle tone is increased, and shivering may be present at core temperatures from 32°C to 36°C (89.6°-96.8°F). Among the cardiorespiratory findings are arrhythmias (including ventricular fibrillation), hypotension, and hypoventilation. Osborn or J waves may be seen on the ECG (**Figure 13-2**).

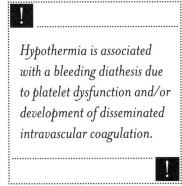

Hypothermia is associated with a bleeding diathesis due to platelet dysfunction and/or development of disseminated intravascular coagulation.

Figure 13-2. Electrocardiogram From a Patient With Hypothermia

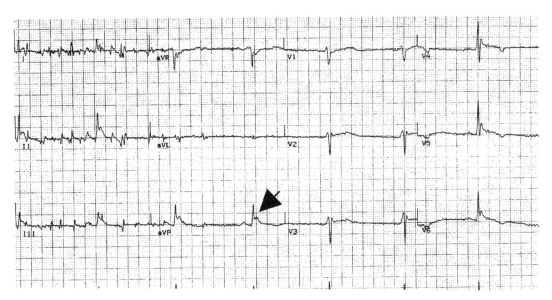

ECG of hypothermic patient showing J wave (arrow).
Reproduced with permission from Zimmerman JL. Hyperthermia, hypothermia, and rhabdomyolysis.
In: Hall JB, Fried EB, eds. SCCM/ACCP 4th Combined Critical Care Course. 4th ed. Des Plaines, IL: Society of Critical Care Medicine; 2007: 457.

The following resuscitation measures should be instituted and continued until rewarming occurs:

■ Remove wet clothes and apply blankets.

■ Protect the airway.

■ Institute cardiopulmonary resuscitation if there is no evidence of perfusion.

■ Monitor cardiac rhythms.

■ Avoid excessive patient manipulation or stimulation that may precipitate arrhythmias. Special care is needed when inserting central venous catheters in the chest so that the wire or catheter does not enter the heart. Pulmonary artery catheters are relatively contraindicated.

■ Administer warm intravenous fluids (crystalloids). The patient is often hypovolemic because of a cold diuresis.

- Correct electrolyte abnormalities.

- Monitor core temperature by inserting a rectal or esophageal temperature probe capable of recording low temperatures.

- Insert an orogastric tube.

- Initiate rewarming.

The choice of a rewarming technique depends on the patient's temperature and response to simple measures. Passive external rewarming blankets or insulating material as well as active external rewarming with heating blankets, radiant heat, or warm water baths are useful in mild hypothermia (34°C-36°C [93.2°F-96.8°F]) and as an adjunct in more severe hypothermia. Active, external rewarming with heat lamps, convective heaters to increase room temperature, or forced-air rewarming devices may be considered in moderate hypothermia (30° to 34°C [86° to 93.2°F]) when advanced facilities are unavailable. Active core rewarming is preferred in severe hypothermia (<30°C [<86°F]), loss of cardiac activity, or failure to elevate temperature by 1°C to 2°C (1.8°F-3.6°F) per hour with other methods. Intubation and inhalation of heated, humidified oxygen as well as administration of warm IV fluids are effective and readily available. Irrigation of the stomach and/or bladder with warm isotonic fluids is only marginally effective and may distract from more effective therapy. Consultation should be considered to institute peritoneal lavage, pleural lavage, or warming via a hemodialysis machine or cardiopulmonary bypass in the most unstable patients.

> **!**
>
> *The intramuscular and subcutaneous routes of medication administration should be avoided in hypothermia because of erratic absorption.*
>
> **!**

With extreme hypothermia, the blood pressure and pulse may be very difficult to record. Electrocardiographic monitoring and careful attention for other signs of life (eg, movement, respirations) may demonstrate a stable physiology in a patient with a profound reduction in oxygen consumption. Vasoactive drugs should be used cautiously because of their arrhythmogenic potential. If cardiopulmonary resuscitation is required, recall the following:

- Defibrillation should be attempted but may be ineffective until core temperature is above 28°C to 30°C (82.4°F-86°F).

- Adrenergic drugs may be ineffective below 30°C (86°F).

- Full resuscitative efforts should generally be continued until the core temperature is >30°C to 32°C (>86°F-90°F).

- The decision to terminate resuscitation is individualized on the basis of the circumstances causing the hypothermia and other factors.

VI. AORTIC DISSECTION

A. Clinical Presentation

Aortic dissection typically occurs after trauma or in hypertensive patients in the fifth and sixth decades of life, but it can occur in younger adults with Marfan or Ehlers-Danlos syndrome. Symptoms are often severe and usually include unrelenting chest pain, frequently associated with back or epigastric pain. A patient with moderate to severe hypertension, severe chest pain, and an enlarged mediastinum on chest radiograph has an aortic dissection until proven otherwise. Involvement of major branches of the aorta can lead to coma, hemiplegia, extremity ischemia, spinal cord infarction, or paraplegia. Aortic dissection is frequently misdiagnosed as acute myocardial infarction, pulmonary embolism, stroke, esophagitis, pancreatitis, peptic ulcer disease, biliary colic, and ureteral colic.

New-onset limb ischemia or aortic valve insufficiency may also suggest aortic dissection. Physical examination should therefore include careful auscultation for a new murmur of aortic insufficiency, assessment for asymmetric blood pressure or pulses in upper extremities, and careful palpation of pulses in all extremities for significant asymmetry. The diagnostic standard is angiography, if available. Computed tomographic scanning with rapid-sequence contrast and transesophageal echocardiography may also be used for diagnosis.

B. Management

Control of blood pressure and heart rate is critical. As immediate surgical consultation is obtained or plans are initiated for transfer, treatment with parenteral antihypertensive agents should be initiated. The combination of intravenous propranolol and sodium nitroprusside or intravenous labetalol as a single agent is the treatment of choice. Intravenous esmolol is an alternative to propranolol. If sodium nitroprusside is necessary to lower blood pressure, concomitant β-blockade is required to reduce the rate of rise of systolic blood pressure (shear force), and intra-arterial pressure monitoring is usually necessary. The clinical goals are to relieve pain and achieve a low normal blood pressure (systolic pressure 100-120 mm Hg) while maintaining a mean arterial pressure of 60 to 70 mm Hg. Medical management is always a temporizing measure until complete diagnostic studies and surgical evaluation have been finalized.

Special Considerations

■ A negative result with a high-sensitivity D-dimer assay in outpatients with low clinical probability of pulmonary embolism can exclude the diagnosis. Patients with moderate or high clinical probability of PE and hospitalized patients require further diagnostic testing.

■ In patients with suspected PE and no contraindications to anticoagulation, unfractionated or low-molecular-weight heparin therapy should be initiated while diagnostic tests are being obtained.

■ Patients at risk for venous thromboembolism should receive appropriate pharmacologic and/or mechanical prophylaxis.

■ In facilities that are unable to maintain 4 units of blood in reserve for potential transfusion, consideration should be given to transferring patients with serious GI bleeding to a facility with a higher level of care.

■ Endoscopy is needed to establish the etiology of upper GI hemorrhage and to institute potentially definitive therapy.

■ Lower GI endoscopy is important for diagnosing, treating, and planning interventions for patients with severe lower GI hemorrhage.

■ Patients at risk for stress-related gastritis should be started on an H_2 receptor antagonist or sucralfate.

■ In the treatment of patients with known or suspected poisoning/overdose, airway adequacy and circulatory stabilization are initial priorities.

■ Treatment of heat stroke is aimed at immediate cooling by means of evaporative techniques or ice-water bath/packs, along with hemodynamic stabilization.

■ Active core rewarming is indicated in cases of severe hypothermia, loss of cardiac activity, or failure to warm adequately with other methods.

■ Control of blood pressure and heart rate is critical in the management of patients with aortic dissection.

Suggested Readings

1. American Heart Association. Hypothermia. *Circulation.* 2005;112:iv-136.

2. American Heart Association. Toxicology in ECC. *Circulation.* 2005;112:iv-126.

3. Barkun AB, Bardou M, Marshall JK. Consensus recommendations for managing patients with nonvariceal upper gastrointestinal bleeding. *Ann Intern Med.* 2003;139:843. http://www.annals.org/cgi/reprint/139/10/843.pdf.

4. Bouchama A, Knochel JP. Heat stroke. *N Engl J Med.* 2002;346:1978.

5. Büller HR, Agnelli G, Hull RD, et al. Antithrombotic therapy for venous thromboembolic disease: The Seventh ACCP Conference on Antithrombotic and Thrombolytic Therapy. *Chest.* 2004;126(suppl):401S.

6. Geerts WH, Pineo GF, Heit JA, et al. Prevention of venous thromboembolism: The Seventh ACCP Conference on Antithrombotic and Thrombolytic Therapy. *Chest.* 2004;126(suppl):338S.

7. Kahn IA, Nair CK. Clinical, diagnostic, and management perspectives of aortic dissection. *Chest.* 2002;122:311.

8. Sharara AI, Rockey DC. Gastroesophageal variceal hemorrhage. *N Engl J Med.* 2001;345:669.

9. Wells PS, Anderson DR, Rodger M, et al. Excluding pulmonary embolism at the bedside without diagnostic imaging: management of patients with suspected pulmonary embolism presenting to the emergency department by using a simple clinical model and D-dimer. *Ann Intern Med.* 2001;135:98.

10. Zimmerman JL, Rudis M. Poisonings. In: Parrillo JE, Dellinger RP, eds. *Critical Care Medicine.* 2nd ed. St. Louis, MO: Mosby; 2001:1501.

Web Sites

1. American Orthopaedic Society for Sports Medicine. Exertional heat illnesses consensus statement. http://www.sportsmed.org/sml/document.asp?did=68.

2. Institute for Clinical Systems Improvement. http://www.icsi.org. The Web site contains guidelines and order sets for venous thromboembolism management and prophylaxis.

Chapter 14:

CRITICAL CARE IN PREGNANCY

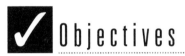

Objectives

- Describe the physiologic and metabolic alterations unique to pregnancy.

- Discuss the diagnosis and management of hypertensive disorders of pregnancy.

- Identify clinical manifestations and treatment of the HELLP syndrome.

- Outline the approaches to managing peripartum cardiomyopathy, thromboembolic disease, and other conditions in pregnancy.

- List priorities for managing the traumatized pregnant patient.

Case Study

You are called to assess a 25-year-old primigravid woman at 34 weeks gestation in labor who has an increased blood pressure of 180/110 mm Hg, heart rate 120/min, SpO$_2$ 90% while receiving room air, and severe respiratory distress. A chest radiograph shows pulmonary edema.

 – What are possible diagnoses?

 – What immediate interventions are needed?

 – What additional evaluations are indicated?

I. INTRODUCTION

A pregnant woman may present for critical care support in 2 main ways: either with a disease state that is unique to pregnancy or with critical illness that is not unique to pregnancy. Diseases specific to pregnancy include preeclampsia, eclampsia, HELLP syndrome (hemolysis, elevated liver enzymes, and a low platelet count), and amniotic fluid embolism syndrome, all of which usually require immediate therapy that may be lifesaving. Some critical illnesses not unique to pregnancy, such as preexisting maternal hypertension, thromboembolic disease, cardiac disease, and trauma, can be precipitated or aggravated by pregnancy. The normal physiologic, metabolic, and hormonal changes of pregnancy may alter the presentation of disease processes and add a level of complexity to diagnosis and treatment.

II. PHYSIOLOGIC ALTERATIONS

A. Cardiovascular Alterations

Changes in blood volume and cardiovascular status are among the most dramatic changes that occur in pregnancy. These are adaptive mechanisms that accommodate the increased metabolic needs of both the mother and the fetus during pregnancy, labor, and delivery. Blood volume increases in each trimester and reaches 30% to 50% above prepartum values by the end of gestation. Cardiac output also increases up to 50% above prepartum values by the 24th week of gestation and then plateaus until labor and delivery. Cardiac output increases primarily as a result of increased stroke volume during the first and second trimesters and by increasing the heart rate by 15 to 20 beats/min during the third trimester until term. Improved myocardial contractility may account in part for an increase in cardiac output. A significant decrease (25%-30%) in cardiac output may occur during the third trimester if the patient is placed in the supine position, owing to compression of the aorta and inferior vena cava by the gravid uterus, increasing afterload and restricting venous return to the heart. The decrease in cardiac output is exaggerated in women with poorly developed venous collaterals who exhibit significant hypotension and bradycardia in the supine position, described as the supine hypotensive syndrome of pregnancy. Filling pressures (central venous and pulmonary artery pressures) typically do not change during pregnancy. A decrease in blood pressure (BP) is seen in the second trimester as a result of diminished systemic vascular resistance (SVR) secondary to the vasodilating effects of progesterone. Peak reduction in BP occurs at 24 weeks; systolic pressures are reduced by 5 to 10 mm Hg and diastolic pressures by 10 to 15 mm Hg. By term, the BP should increase to prepartum values.

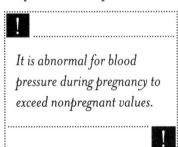

It is abnormal for blood pressure during pregnancy to exceed nonpregnant values.

Another normal cardiovascular change that occurs during pregnancy that may cause or exacerbate illness is remodeling of the heart with enlargement of all 4 chambers. In particular, left atrial enlargement may precipitate supraventricular and atrial arrhythmias. Systolic ejection murmurs and a third heart sound are commonly heard during pregnancy, but diastolic, pansystolic, and late systolic murmurs suggest a more serious underlying cardiac disorder.

In addition to being structurally remodeled with chamber enlargement, the heart is rotated upward and to the left as the uterus enlarges and the diaphragm elevates. Because of this displacement of the heart, cardiomegaly and increased vascular markings may be seen on the chest radiograph. These changes have no clinical significance if the patient has no other evidence of cardiac disease.

Healthy pregnant women tolerate the cardiovascular and hemodynamic effects associated with pregnancy, as do patients with mild to moderate cardiac disease, although the incidence of heart failure and arrhythmias is higher in patients with cardiac disease. Maternal mortality is less than 1% for patients with cardiac disease. However, patients with either primary or secondary pulmonary hypertension (often a result of occult mitral stenosis) or right-to-left shunts have maternal mortality rates as high as 50% and poor fetal outcomes. Concurrent hemodynamic and fetal monitoring is often necessary for pregnant patients with New York Heart Association (NYHA) functional class III or class IV heart disease.

B. Pulmonary Alterations

Pulmonary changes in pregnancy include an increase in tidal volume of approximately 40%, a decrease in functional residual capacity (FRC) of 25%, and an increase in oxygen consumption as a result of the increased metabolic needs of the mother and the fetus. During pregnancy, metabolic demands can increase up to 32% above nonpregnant values by term. The increases in metabolic demands are due to the increase in uterine mass and the size of the fetus. Only 4% of this increase is attributed to maternal metabolic demands during pregnancy. The combination of decreased FRC and increased oxygen consumption during pregnancy diminishes the oxygen reserves of the mother and subsequently increases the hypoxic risk to both the mother and the fetus in the event of maternal hypoventilation or apnea.

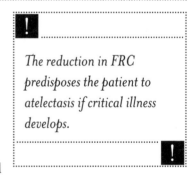

The reduction in FRC predisposes the patient to atelectasis if critical illness develops.

Oxygen requirements increase by approximately 30 to 40 mL/min in pregnancy and are met by an increase in minute ventilation, primarily as a result of increased tidal volume. The increase in minute ventilation results in a mild compensated respiratory alkalosis with a decline in the $PaCO_2$ to ~30 mm Hg (4.0 kPa). The pH does not change due to renal compensation that results in a decrease in serum bicarbonate concentration. Pregnant women who present with a "normal" $PaCO_2$ level of 40 mm Hg (5.3 kPa) should prompt the clinician to look for a cause of impending ventilatory failure.

C. Gastrointestinal Alterations

Hormonal and anatomic changes in pregnancy affect the gastrointestinal tract. Starting at the end of the first trimester, a reduction in lower esophageal sphincter tone due to high progesterone levels contributes to an increased risk for aspiration. Alterations in gastric motor function may cause nausea, vomiting, and dyspepsia.

D. Hematologic Alterations

The 40% to 60% increase in plasma volume that occurs by the third trimester is associated with an increase of only 25% in red cell mass at term. The disproportionate rise in plasma volume results in dilutional anemia (the physiologic anemia of pregnancy); hemoglobin concentration is ~11 g/dL (110 g/L) at 24 weeks. The hematocrit stabilizes at this time but may slightly increase later in the pregnancy, when there is less discrepancy between the increases in blood volume and red cell mass. The white blood cell count climbs to 10,000 cells/mm^3 at term, with a slight reduction in platelet count. Plasma concentrations of all clotting factors except XI, XIII, and antithrombin III increase in pregnancy. Fibrinogen levels may be as high as 600 mg/dL (6.0 g/L) at term. Fibrinogen levels <150 mg/dL (<1.5 g/L) are considered abnormal. Although coagulation test results and bleeding times do not change, these compositional changes result in a hypercoagulable state that, in association with venous stasis and vessel wall trauma, increases the risk for thromboembolic disease. An increase in the circulating levels of numerous endogenous procoagulant proteins contributes to the hypercoagulable state.

III. HYPERTENSIVE DISORDERS

De novo hypertensive disorders associated with pregnancy are not uncommon, but pregnancy can also precipitate or unmask underlying maternal essential hypertension. Patients with a preexisting history of diabetes mellitus, renal disease, or vascular disease, or with a family history of hypertension are more predisposed to developing hypertension during pregnancy.

A. Diagnosis of Hypertensive Disorders

1. Pregnancy-Induced Hypertension

Pregnancy-induced hypertension is defined as gestational hypertension without the presence of proteinuria. It usually manifests as diastolic hypertension that resolves 1 to 2 months after delivery, although many women will later develop chronic hypertension. There is also a relatively high rate of recurrence of diastolic hypertension with subsequent pregnancies.

2. Essential Hypertension

Essential hypertension accounts for approximately one third of all causes of hypertension during pregnancy. It may present at any time during gestation. If it occurs in the last trimester, it is differentiated from preeclampsia by the lack of proteinuria. It should be considered in older multiparous women who present with hypertension. Echocardiography can reveal left ventricular hypertrophy, which suggests chronic disease. Other causes of hypertension that are not pregnancy related, such as renal artery stenosis, pheochromocytomas, and Cushing's syndrome, may need to be considered. If blood pressure is well controlled, there is no significant increase in maternal or fetal complications such as placenta previa, abruption, or preeclampsia.

3. Preeclampsia

Preeclampsia is a multisystem disease that occurs during pregnancy. The diagnosis of preeclampsia is defined by the development of hypertension with proteinuria, usually with generalized peripheral edema, after 20 weeks of gestation. It often presents after the 32nd week of gestation and may present up to 1 week after delivery.

Preeclampsia is classified as severe if at least 1 of the following signs is present:

■ Resting BP ≥160 mm Hg systolic or 110 mm Hg diastolic at any time, or 140 mm Hg systolic or 90 mm Hg diastolic associated with any of the complications listed below. Diastolic hypertension, rather than isolated systolic hypertension, is more commonly observed in preeclampsia.

■ Proteinuria ≥5 g/24 h or 3+/4+ on urine dipstick.

■ Oliguria (urine output <30 mL/h for 3 consecutive hours).

■ A wide spectrum of systemic symptoms including, but not limited to, pulmonary edema, right upper quadrant pain, impaired liver function, headache, visual changes, and thrombocytopenia.

4. Eclampsia

Eclampsia is defined as preeclampsia with generalized tonic-clonic seizures. In some cases, severe preeclampsia may present initially with eclamptic seizures. Although seizures are the most dramatic manifestation of eclampsia, other intracranial catastrophes, such as hemorrhage or stroke, are more likely to cause death.

Eclampsia usually occurs after 20 weeks of gestation or within 48 hours after delivery but should be considered in the differential diagnosis of seizures up to 14 days after delivery. Eclampsia that occurs >48 hours after delivery is more likely to be misdiagnosed.

B. Management of Hypertensive Disorders

1. General Guidelines

Patients with eclampsia or severe preeclampsia require hospital admission. Administration of magnesium sulfate for the prevention of seizures, judicious control of blood pressure, and maternal and fetal monitoring should be initiated early. Issues such as ICU admission, management, and delivery of the fetus should be discussed with an obstetrician and the critical care physician as soon as possible. Preventing maternal injury, ensuring maternal and fetal oxygenation, and initiating seizure prophylaxis are the most important aspects of therapy. The therapy of choice is delivery, but the maturity of the fetus must be considered. In most cases of severe preeclampsia that occur after 32 weeks of gestation, the baby should be delivered. Consultation with a maternal–fetal medicine specialist is recommended

2. Seizure Prophylaxis

Magnesium sulfate (20% solution) is used prophylactically in preeclampsia to avoid progression to eclampsia and to treat eclamptic seizures. This drug is not thought to jeopardize the fetus. Magnesium sulfate therapy is usually initiated when the diastolic BP is >100 mm Hg and signs of impending seizure, such as visual blurring, scotomata, or hyperreflexia, or signs of severe preeclampsia are present. Clinical studies are under way to better define the appropriate use of magnesium sulfate.

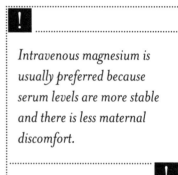

Intravenous magnesium is usually preferred because serum levels are more stable and there is less maternal discomfort.

Magnesium can be administered intravenously and intramuscularly. A loading dose of 4 to 6 g in 200 to 250 mL normal saline over 10 to 15 minutes is followed by an intravenous infusion of 1 to 2 g/h. Magnesium levels are checked 2 to 4 hours later and should be 2 to 3.5 mmol/L (4-7 mEq/L). Maternal respiratory rate, deep tendon reflexes, level of consciousness, and urine output are monitored regularly and correlate well with serum levels. Respiratory depression, somnolence, or loss of patellar reflexes suggest magnesium levels in excess of the therapeutic range (>3.5 mmol/L, or 7 mEq/L). Since magnesium is excreted renally, the infusion rate should be decreased if urine output drops. The maintenance infusion should be decreased or withheld on the basis of the serum creatinine level. The antidote for magnesium toxicity is 1 g calcium chloride (10 mL of 10% solution) given intravenously over several minutes.

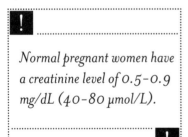

Normal pregnant women have a creatinine level of 0.5-0.9 mg/dL (40-80 μmol/L).

3. Blood Pressure Control

The goal of antihypertensive therapy is prevention of maternal complications such as stroke, intracranial hemorrhage, and acute heart failure. There are no convincing data to determine the optimal BP that should be reached with antihypertensive medications. Although it is not necessary to lower BP to normal levels, diastolic BP (DBP) should be reduced to 90 to 100 mm Hg. In patients with extremely elevated BP, the mean arterial pressure should be lowered gradually in increments of 10% to 15%. Aggressive antihypertensive therapy that results in precipitous drops in BP could further compromise an already stressed fetus by shunting blood away from the placental circulation. There is consensus that therapy is necessary if the systolic BP (SBP) is >160 mm Hg or the DBP is >110 mm Hg, or if the SBP is >30 mm Hg or the DBP is >15 mm Hg from the patient's baseline BP. Lower BP levels may need to be treated if associated with evidence of end-organ damage. Admission to the hospital for acute antihypertensive therapy is recommended for marked elevations in BP or if the patient has end-organ involvement. Treatment in these instances includes immediate delivery of the fetus and antihypertensive management. Intravenous therapy is the standard method of delivering antihypertensive therapies for life-threatening conditions. If intravenous access is not obtainable or available, intramuscular injections may be used.

Drugs that are generally used to treat hypertension associated with severe preeclampsia are parenteral hydralazine (2.5-5 mg administered as a slow intravenous push every 15-20 minutes) and labetalol (20 mg intravenously initially, and titrated every 10-15 minutes). If the initial 20 mg dose of labetalol is not effective, 40 mg should be given. If the 40 mg dose does not lower the BP to the desired level, it should be followed by an 80-mg dose. Historically, hydralazine has been the first-line therapy for hypertension associated with preeclampsia. However, the use of labetalol has increased substantially because of concern about the precipitous drops in BP that can occur with hydralazine therapy, particularly in the volume-depleted preeclamptic patient. Diuretics should usually be avoided because most preeclamptic patients have a significantly decreased plasma volume. Nitroprusside has also been used, despite reports of cyanide toxicity in animal models. Nitroglycerin (because of its primary venodilator effect) may be effective when used to treat pulmonary edema associated with severe preeclampsia but is less effective in preeclamptic hypertension. Intravenous calcium-channel blockers such as diltiazem and nicardipine may also be useful for treating severe hypertension. Although not used in the United States, oral nifedipine therapy for hypertension in preeclampsia has been effective.

> **!**
>
> *Angiotensin–converting enzyme (ACE) inhibitors are contraindicated in pregnancy because of associated fetal and neonatal complications.*
>
> **!**

4. Supportive Measures

Cardiogenic and noncardiogenic pulmonary edema often occurs during severe preeclampsia. Treatment includes supplemental oxygen to maintain maternal PaO_2 >70 mm Hg (>9.3 kPa) with oxygen saturations (SpO_2) ≥94% to prevent fetal hypoxia and acidosis. The indications for tracheal intubation and mechanical ventilation are the same as those for the nonpregnant patient. It is important to remember that because of increased maternal oxygen consumption and a decrease in the functional lung surface area, the mother is at greater risk for hypoventilation and apnea. Intubation should be approached cautiously in the pregnant woman due to the potential for hypoxemia during induction, the increased risk of aspiration, and the possibility of oropharyngeal edema. Usually, smaller endotracheal tubes (6.5 or 7 mm) are necessary. A pregnant woman who requires intubation should be approached as a full-stomach intubation. Ventilation with a bag-mask device and intubation should proceed with cricoid pressure throughout the procedure due to the increased risk of aspiration. In cardiogenic pulmonary edema, fluid restriction and diuretics are often the initial primary treatment. However, since preeclamptic and eclamptic patients frequently have intravascular volume depletion, continuous invasive hemodynamic monitoring with a PAC (pulmonary artery catheter) or CVP (central venous pressure) may be required to optimize management. Central venous pressure values have not been shown to correlate with pulmonary artery filling pressures during pregnancy but may guide volume resuscitation.

The vasoconstriction of the renal vasculature in severe preeclampsia frequently leads to oliguria. Intravenous fluid challenges should be instituted cautiously. The empiric use of diuretics in the absence of invasive hemodynamic monitoring to assess intravascular volume is discouraged. Noninvasive techniques such as echocardiography may be used to assess the cardiac output, volume status, and ejection fraction. Repeated fluid boluses will usually be tolerated by preeclamptic patients with a good ejection fraction and cardiac output. Most preeclamptic women with oliguria will respond to 1 to 2 liters of crystalloid without the need for invasive monitoring. Failure of the patient to respond to repeated fluid challenges, or the presence of cardiac or respiratory failure, should prompt consideration of invasive hemodynamic monitoring and critical care consultation. Vasodilator therapy may be beneficial if intravascular volume is adequate.

5. Monitoring

All patients should have their blood pressure monitored regularly, and those who are hypertensive require more frequent measures. When magnesium sulfate is used, monitoring includes checking patellar reflexes, respiratory rate, and periodic magnesium levels. Invasive hemodynamic monitoring of preeclamptic patients is infrequently required, although it is recommended for patients with significant cardiac, respiratory, or renal abnormalities.

IV. HELLP SYNDROME

The HELLP syndrome is a life-threatening condition that can occur during or after pregnancy. Recent studies have suggested that HELLP is a unique entity with an incidence of 1 in 1,000 pregnancies. It is seen in 4% to 12% of preeclamptic patients. The HELLP syndrome is characterized by the following:

- Hemolysis: hemolytic microangiopathic anemia with an abnormal peripheral smear, a total bilirubin >1.2 mg/dL (21 µmol/L), or serum lactate dehydrogenase (LDH) level >600 U/L.

- Elevated liver enzymes: aspartate aminotransferase (AST) >70 U/L or LDH >600 U/L

- Low platelet count: <150,000/mm³

Variations of the syndrome do not necessarily include all manifestations. The HELLP syndrome can present with a variety of nonspecific clinical signs and symptoms, including epigastric or right upper quadrant pain, gum or nose bleeds, petechiae, malaise, nausea, and vomiting. Most HELLP syndrome cases occur at a gestational age of 27 to 36 weeks. Postpartum presentations occur in 20% of cases, usually within 1 to 2 days after delivery. One third of patients with HELLP syndrome have no evidence of preeclampsia (edma, proteinuria, hypertension) during the pregnancy.

Sometimes, HELLP syndrome can be confused with acute fatty liver of pregnancy, thrombotic thrombocytopenic purpura (TTP), or adult hemolytic-uremic syndrome (HUS), and it may mimic or mask severe sepsis. Laboratory tests that are helpful in differentiating acute fatty liver and HELLP are listed in **Table 14-1**. HELLP syndrome almost always indicates a need for urgent delivery because of its relation to increased fetal and maternal morbidity and mortality.

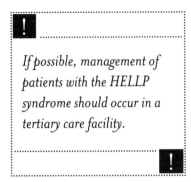

If possible, management of patients with the HELLP syndrome should occur in a tertiary care facility.

Treatment of HELLP syndrome includes supportive care, intravenous magnesium sulfate, and antihypertensive therapy (see section above). Dexamethasone for postpartum onset HELLP (10-12 mg every 12 hours) may improve maternal outcomes, although there is insufficient evidence of any beneficial effect on maternal or fetal mortality. Early plasmapheresis has also been performed when symptomatic and severe thrombocytopenia continues after aggressive platelet replacement, especially when the possibility of thrombotic thrombocytopenic purpura is being considered. Patients complaining of persistent, severe, or worsening epigastric or right upper quadrant pain should be carefully examined for spontaneous rupture of the liver. Computed tomography or MRI can be useful in diagnosing intrahepatic bleeding. Other complications may include intracerebral hemorrhage, acute renal failure, and fulminant hepatic failure.

Table 14-1. Laboratory Differentiation of Acute Fatty Liver and HELLP Syndrome

Test	Acute Fatty Liver	HELLP	Eclampsia/Preeclampsia
Fibrinogen	↓	Normal or ↑	Normal or ↑
Glucose	↓	Normal	Normal
Ammonia	↑	Normal	Normal
ALT (usual range)	300 U/L	150 U/L	60 U/L
Bilirubin	↑	Normal, mild ↑	Normal, mild ↑
DIC	75%	20%-40%	Rare

Abbreviations: ALT, alanine aminotransferase; DIC, dissemintated intravascular coagulation

V. PERIPARTUM CARDIOMYOPATHY

A. Clinical Manifestations

Peripartum cardiomyopathy is defined as congestive heart failure that occurs during the last month of pregnancy or in the first 5 months postpartum. Clinical symptoms include severe progressive dyspnea, progressive orthopnea, paroxysmal nocturnal dyspnea, or syncope with exertion. Signs include evidence of right and left heart failure, generalized or chamber-specific cardiomegaly seen on a chest radiograph, evidence of pulmonary hypertension, murmurs, prominent jugular vein distension, cyanosis, clubbing, or dysrhythmias. Most patients present with dramatic symptoms soon after delivery. Peripartum cardiomyopathy is associated with maternal age >30 years, first pregnancy, twin pregnancies, gestational hypertension, and pregnant women who receive tocolytic agents. The course tends to be more severe in older patients of higher parity with later onset of symptoms after delivery.

B. Management

Initial evaluation of the patient with possible peripartum cardiomyopathy includes a chest radiograph, electrocardiogram (ECG), and echocardiogram. Initial therapy includes bed rest, sodium restriction, diuretics, and possibly vasodilators. Patients who present with pulmonary edema and cardiac decompensation often require invasive hemodynamic monitoring for careful and judicious fluid management, intravenous inotropic support, and afterload reduction. Useful drugs include digoxin, dobutamine, and milrinone as inotropic agents and ACE inhibitors for afterload reduction (ACE inhibitors are contraindicated prior to delivery). Although loop diuretics can be used for symptomatic relief of systemic and pulmonary congestion, they should be used cautiously in the last month of gestation due to their effect on uteroplacental perfusion. If symptoms develop in the antepartum period, consultation between the obstetrician, critical care physician, and anesthesiologist can guide decisions regarding early delivery. Early delivery is not usually recommended since many patients experience worsening of symptoms postpartum. Urgent delivery may be considered in pregnant women with advanced heart failure or hemodynamic instability. Critical patients who require inotropic and mechanical support should undergo cesarean section. Anticoagulation should be considered in the pregnant woman with peripartum cardiomyopathy, enlarged cardiac chambers, ejection fraction <35%, and atrial fibrillation since systemic and pulmonary emboli are significantly more common in comparison to other cardiomyopathies. Cardiac function returns to normal in approximately 50% of patients. The 50% of patients who continue to have symptoms have a mean survival time of ≤5 years. Right and left ventricular-assist devices may serve as a bridge for patients who may eventually recover or who require cardiac transplantation as the definitive treatment because of failure of pharmacological therapy. Subsequent pregnancies are discouraged in women who have no resolution of the signs and symptoms of heart failure 6 months after delivery.

VI. THROMBOEMBOLIC DISEASE

The incidence of thromboembolic disease in pregnant women and the immediate postpartum period is 5 times the incidence in nonpregnant women. A higher risk occurs with increased parity, cesarean section, operative vaginal delivery, previous deep venous thrombosis, and increased maternal age.

Although manifestations of pulmonary embolism in pregnant women are similar to those in nonpregnant women (**Chapter 13**), the physiologic changes of pregnancy complicate evaluation. Lower-extremity edema, leg pain, and dyspnea are common findings in pregnancy and create a diagnostic dilemma for the clinician. If a chest radiograph is obtained to rule out other pulmonary problems, such as pneumonia, the fetus must be shielded. After 16 weeks of gestation, D-dimer values are elevated above the usual normal range and are therefore of little diagnostic utility. Doppler scanning of the lower extremities (compression ultrasound) is usually the first test for diagnosing deep vein thrombosis (DVT) in pregnancy when available, but it is less accurate for calf DVT and isolated iliac thrombosis. For diagnosing pulmonary embolism, ventilation/perfusion ($\dot{V}/\dot{Q}$) scanning is reliable in a pregnant woman, and it may be beneficial to initially perform perfusion scanning alone. If there are no perfusion defects, the scan can be considered negative. Spiral CT is an alternative method to visualize pulmonary embolism; it is more sensitive for emboli in the central arteries and less sensitive for subsegmental emboli. Pulmonary angiography remains the gold standard for the diagnosis of acute pulmonary embolism because the fetal radiation exposure is less than that of spiral CT, but it is invasive and its performance and interpretation require expertise. The teratogenic and oncogenic risks to the fetus from these diagnostic tests are not significant, and the risk of maternal death from undiagnosed thromboembolic disease outweighs the risk of radiation exposure. An appropriate diagnostic evaluation should always be performed when indicated. Heparin therapy should be immediately initiated when the diagnosis of pulmonary embolism is suspected and should be continued if the diagnosis is confirmed.

The treatment of stable pulmonary embolism in the pregnant patient parallels that in the nonpregnant patient, except that warfarin is relatively contraindicated in pregnancy and absolutely contraindicated during the first trimester, when the risk of teratogenicity is greatest. Instead, unfractionated heparin can be administered intravenously by a weight-adjusted dose regimen to achieve an activated partial thromboplastin time (APTT) of 1.5 to 2.5 times control. Treatment is then converted to subcutaneous administration, starting at 5,000 IU of unfractionated heparin every 12 hours and aiming for the same APTT goal measured 6 hours after

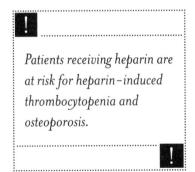

Patients receiving heparin are at risk for heparin-induced thrombocytopenia and osteoporosis.

administration. Low-molecular-weight heparins (LMWH) are safe for the fetus and can be used for the treatment of thromboembolic disease. Due to the decreased half-life of LMWH in pregnancy, twice-daily dosing is preferred, and either the dose must be adjusted proportionately for weight change or antifactor Xa levels must be monitored weekly.

After delivery, warfarin can be substituted for 3 to 6 months of total therapy, depending upon maternal risk factors. Intrapartum management requires that unfractionated heparin be discontinued at least 4 to 6 hours before delivery and that LMWH be discontinued 24 hours before elective delivery. Heparin can usually be resumed 6 to 24 hours after delivery. The risks with intrapartum use of heparin include a significantly increased likelihood of hemorrhage with cesarean delivery, bleeding and hematoma formation if a regional or epidural anesthetic is used, and increased bleeding if an episiotomy or operative vaginal delivery is performed. Patients with massive pulmonary embolism and/or hemodynamic instability should be managed much like nonpregnant patients, with careful consideration of risks (**Chapter 13**).

VII. SEVERE ASTHMA

Asthma is the most common pulmonary condition in pregnancy. Among asthmatic patients, 50% have no change in symptoms, 30% improve, and 20% worsen. Pharmacologic treatment of asthma usually does not require modification during pregnancy (**Chapter 4**). Supplemental oxygen should be administered, if necessary, during acute exacerbations. Noninvasive positive-pressure ventilation should be used cautiously during pregnancy because of the increased risk of aspiration. During asthmatic attacks, management with inhaled β-agonists and systemic steroids is preferred. Parenteral corticosteroids should be administered early in the course of moderate to severe asthma exacerbations. If there is evidence of a concurrent respiratory infection, appropriate antibiotics should be added to the treatment regimen. Hypercapnia, especially in a pregnant woman who normally has a mild respiratory alkalosis, indicates impending respiratory failure.

Patients with severe asthma who require intubation and mechanical ventilation should have the minute ventilation adjusted to avoid hyperventilation and respiratory alkalosis. An alkalotic pH may lead to reduction of uteroplacental blood flow, impairing fetal oxygenation. Occasionally, life-threatening asthma can be refractory despite mechanical ventilation and intensive medical therapy. In such cases, termination of pregnancy via cesarean section may be considered as an option.

VIII. SEPTIC PELVIC THROMBOPHLEBITIS

Septic pelvic thrombophlebitis, characterized by infected clot(s) in the pelvic veins, can occur in the peripartum period after vaginal and cesarean deliveries as well as after both spontaneous and therapeutic abortions. Physical findings are nonspecific. Fever that fails to respond to empiric antibiotics in a postpartum patient should prompt consideration of septic pelvic thrombophlebitis. Evidence of systemic septic emboli (eg, sepsis, metastatic abscesses, and septic pulmonary emboli) may be present. Ultrasonography or CT studies are not diagnostic but may occasionally show evidence of a clot. Patients are typically treated on the basis of clinical suspicion and as a diagnosis of exclusion. Heparin, as outlined above, is used in addition to antibiotics for management. A reduction in fever usually occurs within 24 hours. Anticoagulant therapy is continued for 3 to 6 months postpartum.

IX. POSTPARTUM HEMORRHAGE

Primary postpartum hemorrhage (PPH) is defined as excessive bleeding within 24 hours of a vaginal or cesarean delivery. It is the leading cause of postpartum death worldwide. The usual signs of tachycardia and hypotension associated with severe bleeding may occur late because of the hypervolemia associated with pregnancy. Concealed pelvic hematomas with ongoing blood loss may also be masked initially. The most frequent cause of PPH is uterine atony, which occurs in 5% of deliveries. Risk factors for uterine atony include overdistension of the uterus, retained placental products, uterine muscle fatigue, and the use of halogenated anesthetic agents. The diagnosis is made clinically by palpation of a large and boggy uterus. The second most frequent cause of PPH is lacerations of the lower genital tract that occur spontaneously or as a result of traumatic labor. Disseminated intravascular coagulation (DIC) resulting from placental abnormalities, HELLP syndrome, and amniotic fluid embolism syndrome may also cause hemodynamically significant postpartum hemorrhage.

General treatment measures include aggressive and early fluid resuscitation and attempts to locate the source of the bleeding. Higher maternal mortality occurs when treatment is delayed and blood loss is underestimated. Patients with ongoing blood loss, any amount of blood loss resulting in hemodynamic instability, or a total blood loss exceeding 2,000 mL require packed red blood cell transfusions in addition to fluid administration. Depending upon the amount of blood loss and the presence of coagulopathy, additional blood products may be needed. Angiographic embolization and surgical therapy, including hysterectomy, may be required for severe uterine hemorrhage not responsive to uterotonic drug therapy.

X. AMNIOTIC FLUID EMBOLISM

Amniotic fluid embolism is a catastrophic syndrome with significant morbidity and mortality that occurs during pregnancy or in the immediate postpartum period. The presentation includes typical findings of hypoxia, shock, altered mental status, and disseminated intravascular coagulation; seizure activity, agitation, fetal distress, fever, chills, nausea, and vomiting may also be present. The diagnosis of amniotic fluid embolism is clinical and a diagnosis of exclusion. It is considered in pregnant or postpartum women who abruptly and dramatically present with profound shock and cardiovascular collapse associated with severe respiratory distress. Occasionally, DIC is the first presenting sign. Other life-threatening conditions, such as pulmonary embolism, sepsis, air embolism, eclampsia, and myocardial infarction, should be excluded. There will be radiological evidence of pulmonary edema with bilateral interstitial and alveolar infiltrates. Management is supportive and focuses on rapid maternal cardiopulmonary stabilization (as mentioned previously) and preventing subsequent end-organ damage.

XI. TRAUMA IN PREGNANCY

Treatment priorities for the pregnant patient with traumatic injury are the same as those for nonpregnant patients (**Chapter 9**). There are, however, unique changes that should be taken into account during clinical assessment. The gravid uterus complicates the initial abdominal assessment of the pregnant patient. The height of the uterus is roughly at the symphysis pubis at 12 weeks and the umbilicus at 20 weeks; then the height increases by 1 centimeter per week up to 36 to 40 weeks, when the uterus encompasses almost the entire abdomen. Late in pregnancy, a widened symphysis pubis and widened sacroiliac joints are possible. All pregnant patients with major traumatic injuries should be admitted to a facility with surgical obstetric capabilities. When evaluating mental status, be aware that neurologic symptoms of eclampsia may mimic head injury. Aortocaval compression can contribute to hypotension by restricting the return of blood to the heart. Whenever possible, the patient should be placed in the left lateral decubitus position; at a minimum, the right hip can be raised by 4 to 8 centimeters to displace the uterus off the inferior vena cava. If any question of spinal injury exists, spinal alignment is maintained and the patient is log-rolled.

The pregnant patient can lose up to 35% of blood volume before significant tachycardia, hypotension, and other signs of hypovolemia are seen. Therefore, the fetus may actually be in a state of hypoperfusion while the mother's condition seems stable. An assessment of the fetal heart rate is an essential part of the initial survey. This assessment can be accomplished easily with a fetoscope or a Doppler fetoscope. A conventional stethoscope can be used to auscultate the fetal heart rate in the third trimester, although it may be difficult to differentiate between maternal and fetal heart tones if the mother is tachycardic. If available, ultrasonography is very effective for documenting fetal cardiac activity and function. Late or persistent decelerations of the fetal heart rate are an ominous sign. If the fetus cannot be examined adequately at the facility, the patient should be stabilized and transported as soon as possible. A minimum of 4 hours of fetal monitoring is necessary after trauma.

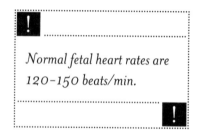

Normal fetal heart rates are 120–150 beats/min.

Secondary assessment should evaluate uterine irritability (spasms of the uterus), fetal heart rate, and fetal movement. A pelvic examination should be performed if necessary. If there is any question of blood from the vagina, a qualified, experienced person should do a sterile speculum examination. Preferably, a sonographic examination should be performed prior to the speculum examination to exclude placenta previa. A manual vaginal examination is contraindicated if placenta previa is a possibility.

Definitive care of the pregnant trauma patient includes adequate hemodynamic and respiratory resuscitation, stabilization of the mother, continued fetal monitoring, and radiographic studies as necessary in addition to obstetric care, critical care, and surgical consultation. If the mother is Rh-negative, $Rh_o(D)$ immune globulin (RhoGAM) should be given within 72 hours of injury, even when trauma is minimal. An assessment of the amount of fetal red blood cells in the maternal circulation by means of a Kleihauer-Betke stain is advised. Obstetrical consultation for appropriate dosage of $Rh_o(D)$ immune globulin is recommended.

XII. MECHANICAL VENTILATION DURING PREGNANCY

The indications for intubation and mechanical ventilation for pregnant patients are the same as those for nonpregnant patients. The maternal oxygen reserve is decreased and significant arterial desaturation occurs if the patient is hypoventilating or apneic for even a short time. Such episodes increase the hypoxic risk to the fetus as well. Mechanical ventilator parameters should be adjusted to maintain the $PaCO_2$ in the range of 30 to 32 mm Hg (4.0-4.3 kPa). Availability of data about permissive hypercapnic ventilation in the pregnant patient is limited, although chronic elevations of maternal PCO_2 up to 60 mm Hg (8.0 kPa) in patients with congenital heart diseases has not been shown to be detrimental to the fetus. Caution should be used when considering noninvasive ventilation due to the increased risk of aspiration during pregnancy.

Expeditious delivery is indicated only when evidence of placental abruption, DIC, chorio-amnionitis, or severe preeclampsia is seen. Delivery may also be indicated for patients with stiff, noncompliant lungs requiring high peak airway pressures or pressure control ventilation. Rapid delivery may improve diaphragmatic excursion and benefit the mother. Successful spontaneous delivery is possible during mechanical ventilation.

XIII. ADVANCED LIFE SUPPORT IN PREGNANCY

When cardiac arrest occurs in a pregnant woman, standard advanced life support resuscitative methods can and should be undertaken. A wedge should be placed under the right flank to displace the uterine contents to the left, improving venous return to the heart. Alternatively, the uterus can be displaced manually to the left. Chest compressions are performed slightly above the center of the sternum to account for elevation of the diaphragm. If initial attempts with standard ACLS resuscitative measures are unsuccessful and the fetal gestational age and size are estimated to be ≥24 weeks, then a decision to perform a perimortem cesarean section should be made rapidly so that delivery is accomplished within 4 to 5 minutes of arrest. This option is applicable only when the uterus is deemed large enough to impede life support efforts by significant aortocaval compression, which further worsens maternal hemodynamics. The principal reason for performing a perimortem cesarean section is to improve cardiac output by augmenting venous return to the heart with effective cardiac compressions. Standard medications for cardiopulmonary resuscitation should be used. Obstetric and neonatology assistance should be sought if at all possible.

XIV. PHARMACOTHERAPY

Choice of medications for the pregnant woman must take into account the potential for adverse effects on the fetus (**Table 14-2** and **Table 14-3**). Certain medications, such as warfarin, ACE inhibitors, diazepam, and phenytoin, have known or potential effects and should be avoided when acceptable alternatives are available. In general, the selection of any new medication for a critically ill or injured pregnant patient should include a review of its indications and pharmacodynamics as well as alternative approaches to management. A clinical pharmacist should be consulted to obtain information about fetal risk associated with drug therapy.

Table 14-2.	US Food and Drug Administration Categories of Fetal Drug Toxicities
Category	**Description**
A	Controlled studies in pregnant women have not demonstrated any risk to the fetus in the first trimester. These drugs are considered to be relatively safe for use during pregnancy.
B	No known specific risks are associated with the use of the drug in pregnancy, but controlled human studies are lacking. If adverse effects were shown in animal reproduction studies, these were not confirmed in controlled human trials.
C	Studies in women and animals are not available or studies in animals have revealed adverse effects on the fetus. Most new drugs fall into this category. These drugs should be given only if the potential benefit justifies the potential risk to the fetus.
D	These drugs have shown a definite fetal risk in controlled human trials. However, their use may be necessary during pregnancy, and a risk-benefit assessment needs to be performed before they are used.
X	These drugs have shown a definite risk to the fetus and their use is contraindicated because the potential risks to the fetus outweigh the potential benefits.

Table 14-3. Toxicity Categories for Selected Drugs During Pregnancy

Antiarrhythmics

Amiodarone	D
Lidocaine	C
Procainamide	C

Antibiotics

Acyclovir	C
Aminoglycosides	C
Azithromycin	B
Cefotetan (avoid)	B
Ceftriaxone (avoid)	B
Cephalosporins	B
Clindamycin	B
Gentamicin (safest)	C
Metronidazole (not in 1st trimester)	B
Penicillins	B
Quinolones	C
Sulfonamides	B
Trimethoprim	C
Vancomycin	C

Anticonvulsants

Carbamazepine	C
Magnesium sulfate	B
Phenobarbital	D
Phenytoin	D

Antihypertensives

ACE inhibitors	D
ß-Blockers	C
Clonidine	C
Hydralazine	C
Labetalol	C

Cardiovascular Medications

Amrinone/milrinone	C
Aspirin	D
Atropine	C
Digoxin	C
Dobutamine	C
Dopamine	C
Epinephrine	C
Nitroglycerin	C
Nitroprusside	C
Norepinephrine	D
Phenylephrine	C
Thrombolytics	C
Vasopressin	B
Verapamil	C

Diuretics

Furosemide	C
Spironolactone	C

Neuromuscular Blockers

Cisatracurium	B
Rocuronium	C
Succinylcholine	B
Vecuronium	C

Sedatives/Analgesics/Anxiolytics

Benzodiazepines	D
Codeine	C
Haloperidol	C
Morphine	B
Propofol	B

Steroids

Dexamethasone	C
Hydrocortisone	D
Prednisolone	B

Other

Aminophylline	C
H_2 blockers	B
Heparin	C
Insulin	B
Mannitol	C
Warfarins	X

Key Points

Critical Care in Pregnancy

■ A significant decrease in cardiac output may occur in the third trimester when the patient is placed in the supine position because the gravid uterus restricts venous return and aortic blood flow.

■ The diagnosis of preeclampsia is based on the development of pregnancy-induced hypertension with proteinuria, with or without edema, after 20 weeks of gestation. Eclampsia is defined as preeclampsia with generalized tonic-clonic seizures.

■ Magnesium sulfate (20% solution) is used in preeclampsia as seizure prophylaxis and as treatment for eclamptic seizures and requires close monitoring.

■ Lowering BP to normal levels is not necessary in the hypertensive states associated with pregnancy.

■ Anticoagulation with heparin (unfractionated or low-molecular-weight) is used in the treatment of pulmonary embolism in pregnancy. Warfarin is contraindicated in pregnancy, particularly in the first trimester.

■ Early and aggressive treatment with fluid and blood products is necessary in primary postpartum hemorrhage.

■ Treatment priorities for the resuscitation of the pregnant patient with trauma are the same as those for nonpregnant patients with trauma.

■ The pregnant patient can lose up to 35% of her blood volume before tachycardia, hypotension, and other signs of hypovolemia are seen. This can mask significant fetal compromise as well as ongoing maternal blood loss.

■ If the mother is Rh-negative, $Rh_o(D)$ immune globulin (RhoGAM) should be given, even after minimal trauma.

■ Indications for intubation and ventilation are the same for pregnant patients as for nonpregnant patients. Adjust mechanical ventilator settings to maintain the PCO_2 level in the range of 30 to 32 mm Hg (4.0-4.3 kPa).

■ A perimortem cesarean section should be considered within 4 to 5 minutes to improve maternal hemodynamics if initial resuscitative measures are ineffective.

■ When choosing medications for the pregnant woman, it is important to take into account their potential adverse effects on the fetus.

Suggested Readings

1. ACOG practice bulletin. Diagnosis and management of preeclampsia and eclampsia. *Int J Gynecol Obstet.* 2002;77:67.

2. Bates SM, Greer IA, Hirsch J, Ginsberg JS. Use of antithrombotic agents during pregnancy. *Chest.* 2004;126(suppl 3):S627.

3. Chan WS, Ray JG, Murray S, et al. Suspected pulmonary embolism in pregnancy, clinical presentation, results of lung scanning, and subsequent maternal and pediatric outcomes. *Arch Intern Med.* 2002;162:1170.

4. Gei AF, Vadhera RB, Hankins GDV. Embolism during pregnancy: thrombus, air, and amniotic fluid. *Anesthesiol Clin N Am.* 2003;21:165.

5. Guntupalli S, Stiengrub J. Hepatic disease in pregnancy: an overview of diagnosis and management. *Crit Care Med.* 2005;33(suppl):S332.

6. Hanania N, Belfort M. Acute asthma in pregnancy. *Crit Care Med.* 2005;33(suppl):S319.

7. Mallampalli A, Guy E. Cardiac arrest in pregnancy and somatic support after brain death. *Crit Care Med.* 2005;33(suppl):S325.

8. Montan S. Drugs used in hypertensive diseases in pregnancy. *Curr Opin Obstet Gynecol.* 2004;6:111.

9. Murali S, Baldisseri M. Peripartum cardiomyopathy. *Crit Care Med.* 2005:33(suppl):S340.

10. Naylor DF, Olson MM. Critical care obstetrics and gynecology. *Crit Care Clin.* 2003;19:127.

11. Pearson GD, Veille JC, Rahimtoola S, et al. Peripartum cardiomyopathy: National Heart, Lung, and Blood Institute and Office of Rare Diseases (National Institutes of Health) workshop recommendations and review. *JAMA.* 2000; 83:1183.

12. Shah AJ, Kilcline BA. Trauma in pregnancy. *Emerg Med Clin N Am.* 2003;21:615.

13. Stone S, Morris T. Pulmonary embolism during and after pregnancy. *Crit Care Med.* 2005;33(suppl):S294.

14. Whitty JE. Maternal cardiac arrest during pregnancy. *Clin Obstet Gynecol.* 2002;45:377.

Chapter 15:

ETHICS IN CRITICAL CARE MEDICINE

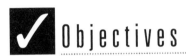

Objectives

- Review ethical principles.

- Discuss ethical dilemmas that involve triage, medical futility, do-not-attempt-resuscitation orders and withdrawal of life support in critically ill patients.

- Define types of advance directives used to guide care.

- Discuss examples that outline the decision making process used in medical ethics.

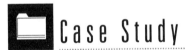

Case Study

A 68-year-old man, Mr. Hill, collapsed at home and sustained a cardiac arrest. Cardiopulmonary resuscitation was not initiated until paramedics arrived 6 minutes later. He was found in ventricular fibrillation, but he responded to intubation, defibrillation, and epinephrine. In the emergency department 30 minutes later, he is unresponsive to painful stimuli, pupils are dilated and fixed, and corneal reflexes are absent. He is breathing spontaneously and is hemodynamically stable. He is transferred to the ICU, but 3 days later he remains in a deep coma.

- Should further therapy be limited or withdrawn?

- What process should be utilized to address these issues?

- What potential dilemmas might arise in discussions with the patient's family?

I. INTRODUCTION

Medical ethics is at the heart of the patient-clinician relationship. However, ethics is also the foundation of laws, statutes, and regulations that govern the practice of medicine in many countries. Ethics in medicine impacts issues ranging from clinical research to bed utilization, from the interface between patients and their healthcare providers to healthcare policy formulation. Ethics is closely related to morality, culturally accepted norms regarding right and wrong, and duty, the principles guiding standards of behavior. Healthcare professionals have an obligation to act in their patients' best interests based upon the patient-clinician relationship, which is grounded in trust but complicated by an inequality of knowledge, information, and experience.

Three sets of circumstances typically bring patients at risk of dying in the hospital to the emergency department: (1) an acute event in an otherwise healthy person (such as trauma, stroke, myocardial infarction, or pneumonia); (2) a recurrent or relapsing decompensation in a patient with a chronic and progressive disease (such as respiratory failure in chronic lung disease, pneumonia complicating dementia, heart failure in cardiomyopathy); or (3) the reaching of a critical point by a patient with progressive, unrelenting decline (such as cancer or dementia). Many of these at-risk patients may be admitted to an ICU. Such patients may be unable to participate in decisions about their medical care and depend upon advance directives or surrogate decision makers to guide the healthcare team regarding treatment decisions.

The critical care team is involved in end-of-life care (EOLC) decision making in 3 key situations: triage, limitation of therapy and/or resuscitation, and withdrawal of life support. Therefore, the critical care team must be able to effectively communicate with patients and their families about prognosis and futility, reasonable goals of therapy, healthcare proxy stipulations and living wills, and options for limitation of resuscitation or removal of life support. Without formal discussions, patients' preferences are hard to predict; assumptions based upon quality of life, age, or functional status may be inaccurate; and physicians' choices may reflect their own preferences more than those of their patients.

Healthcare providers must be both cognitively and emotionally prepared to communicate among themselves and with patients and families regarding (1) realistic goals, (2) expectations for treatments and alternatives, (3) patients' expressed and implied desires regarding medical interventions and the implications of those desires, and (4) acceptable therapeutic options. Meaningful discussions of these issues are grounded in a thorough understanding of medical ethics, individual and collective cultural values, and pertinent legal principles. The competency of providers as communicators correlates directly with patients' and families' satisfaction with the medical care provided and also enhances the professional experience of the providers.

II. THE GUIDING ETHICAL PRINCIPLES OF HEALTHCARE

In healthcare, ethical principles protect patients against harm and focus action toward patient benefit. The guiding principles of healthcare are generally intended as a conceptual framework for providing patient-centered care (care that is appropriately respectful of patients) by identifying, analyzing, and contributing to the resolution of ethical problems that occur in the practice of medicine. The 4 guiding principles of healthcare are as follows:

■ Autonomy: This principle speaks to the right of an individual to be self-directing and to make decisions freely and independently; it recognizes the patient's sovereignty over his or her own body.

■ Beneficence: This principle refers to the obligation of physicians and healthcare providers to act in the best interest of their patients. Different value systems can lead to different concepts of what is best for an individual patient.

■ Nonmaleficence: This principle reflects the Latin tenet of primum non nocere, which translates as "above else, do no harm." Harm can be defined as the intentional or careless infliction of physical, psychological, or emotional distress through either acts of commission or acts of omission

■ Justice: This principle emphasizes the duty to treat all persons fairly and equitably.

III. ETHICAL DILEMMAS IN CRITICAL CARE

Many, if not all, ethical dilemmas can be handled professionally with utmost respect for patient needs when decisions involve consideration of the treatment situation, truthful exchange of information, thorough discussion of the patient's wishes and expectations, understanding of pertinent ethical principles, and coordination among members of the healthcare team. Uncertainty and ambiguity on the part of the physician, critical care team, patient, or family make meaningful discussion and decisions difficult. It is the responsibility of the team leaders to ensure that the healthcare environment is characterized by open communication, caring, and support. In situations where some members of the team have conflicting beliefs, emotional conflicts, or conflicts of interest that preclude open and objective communication and decision making, they may request to be excused and transfer patient-care responsibilities to a colleague. Patients and families can sense uncertainty and ambiguity, and are likely to react with suspicion and confusion. A consensus on the treatment plan and objectives also facilitates consistent communication and documentation and minimizes liability risks. In institutions where ethics consultation teams are available, their involvement has been regarded favorably by most participants.

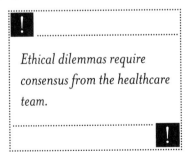

Ethical dilemmas require consensus from the healthcare team.

A. Triage

The ICU is characterized by resource-intensive medical care. Since the technology, physician presence, and staffing that characterize the ICU are costly and limited, triage decisions regarding the allocation of these physical and personnel resources are frequently necessary. Triage is most often necessary when demand for critical care beds exceeds their supply. Thus, patients may either be denied admission based on resource constraints; transferred from the ICU to another level of care based on severity of illness, prognosis, or wishes; or transferred to another institution. The minimum severity of illness required to meet ICU admission criteria is likely to fluctuate within an institution (such as during influenza season or disaster situations). Increasingly, however, patients who do not meet some minimum objective criteria for ICU admission are cared for on the wards regardless of the preference of patients, attending physicians, or staff. Critically ill patients who are not admitted to ICUs have significantly greater morbidity and mortality. Therefore, triage choices represent life-and-death decisions that must be based upon criteria that are as objective as possible and applied uniformly.

B. Medical Futility

Medical futility generally refers to therapeutic interventions that are highly unlikely to contribute to a meaningful outcome. The key problem associated with futility is that it is a fluid concept defined by the particular situation. Interventions perceived as futile in one institution by some providers at a certain point in time may not be perceived as such by others at a different time. Futility is also defined by the anticipated outcome based on probability of survival, values regarding minimally acceptable quality of life, and prognosis

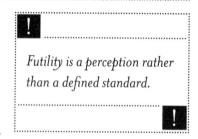

Futility is a perception rather than a defined standard.

or time frame for possible recovery. Thus, a determination of medical futility should be based on the predicted outcome, available medical evidence or experience, and patient expectations and wishes. Futility differs from cost-effectiveness, cost-utility, and cost-benefit analyses, which are based on principles of distributive justice rather than strict assessment of the probability of benefits derived from aggressive medical interventions. There is considerable ethical debate about whose views should prevail in decisions regarding discontinuation or limitation of care when providers and families disagree about the futility of care. Depending on the circumstances, a team of clinicians may declare a situation medically futile and limit medical treatment, an ethics team may evaluate the patient and make or concur with a determination of futility, or a legal process may make a determination of futility.

C. Advance Directives

In order to make binding decisions or enter into contracts such as informed consent, refusal of medical care, or limitation of resuscitation, a person must be legally able to do so. While competent patients are legally empowered to make decisions, unemancipated minors or mentally impaired individuals may not be competent for decision-making purposes. Capacity refers to the ability to make decisions in a specific circumstance; due to medications, injuries, or metabolic derangements that impair judgment, a patient may lack capacity. To give consent and to establish directives governing refusal or limitation of medical care, patients must have both competence and capacity, and their agreement must be obtained without fraud, duress, or coercion after full, reasonable disclosure. The basis, process, and outcome of all discussions leading to such decisions should be carefully documented to supplement any other required forms and clinician orders. Unlike informed consent, limitation or refusal of treatment is never implied.

An advance directive is an instructional statement that takes effect at some time in the future when specific conditions are met. A capable person can often leave verbal or written instructions directly for healthcare professionals or select a surrogate to guide medical decisions. If patients have left unambiguous and detailed instructions regarding their preferences for life-sustaining therapy in the event they become incapacitated, such instructions are usually binding and carried out. However, most patients' instructions are neither sufficiently detailed nor unambiguous for the circumstances of their illness. The role of the surrogate decision maker is to inform the healthcare team of what the patient's wishes would be under the circumstances; the wishes, therefore, are not those of the surrogate but of the patient in the form of a substituted judgment. Substituted judgments may be based on explicit instructions or direct and indirect communications regarding preferences and expectations. The following tools may be used to convey a patient's preferences:

- Living will: This document contains specific, substantive directives regarding medical procedures that the patient wants to receive or forgo in specific circumstances.

- Durable power of attorney for healthcare: A durable power of attorney (DPA) is a proxy directive that assigns one person authority to perform specified actions on behalf of the signer. The power is "durable" because, unlike the usual power of attorney, it continues to be in effect if the signer becomes incompetent.

- Healthcare proxy: A proxy is a person appointed by the patient specifically for the purpose of making healthcare decisions on the patient's behalf.

- Next of kin: Under some circumstances, in some countries or states, the next of kin are authorized by law to speak on behalf of an incapacitated patient. Surrogacy hierarchies that must be considered in healthcare decision making are usually defined by law.

The healthcare provider should be certain that the conditions for invoking an advance directive as intended by the patient have occurred before acting upon the directive. Similarly, acquiescing to requests made by surrogates occurs only after consideration of proper medical and ethical decision making principles.

D. Do-Not-Attempt-Resuscitation Orders

Do-not-attempt-resuscitation (DNAR) orders, also know as do-not-resuscitate (DNR) orders, are explicit physician orders restricting specific medical interventions in the event of a cardiopulmonary arrest. Such orders are usually based on a patient's expressed or written wishes or on such wishes as they are known to a proxy or surrogate decision maker. Do-not-attempt-resuscitation orders may include categorical specifications that limit blood transfusions, feeding

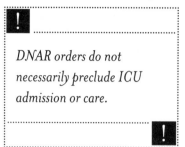

DNAR orders do not necessarily preclude ICU admission or care.

tubes, dialysis, intubation and mechanical ventilation, defibrillation, cardiopulmonary resuscitation in an already mechanically ventilated patient, or an escalation of existing ICU treatment. Factors that suggest a discriminatory intent must never form the basis for initiating DNAR discussions; these factors include gender, age, race, and economic or socioeconomic status. Suicidal ideation and depression must be excluded as reasons when a patient wishes to limit resuscitation or terminate life support.

E. End-Of-Life Care and Termination of Life Support

The goal of end-of-life care (EOLC) is to allow patients to die with dignity and respect and to exercise an element of control over their death. It is paramount that in all communications it is made clear that *care is not being withdrawn;* rather, it is life support that is withdrawn after the goals of treatment have changed. In many cases, the intensity of care may actually escalate following termination of life support as comfort needs are addressed. "Do not attempt resuscitation" never means "do not treat." Prior to the removal of life support, a proper DNAR order should be in effect based on local and institutional regulations. A plan for comfort measures should be developed by the healthcare team and must address anxiolysis and analgesia. Comfort care interventions are not intended to directly hasten death, which differentiates comfort care from euthanasia and physician-assisted suicide.

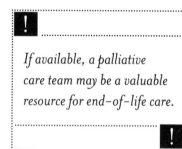

If available, a palliative care team may be a valuable resource for end-of-life care.

F. Organ Donation

After discussions regarding extent of care have been completed and a decision to withdraw life support has been made, organ-procurement representatives should be allowed to evaluate the patient and conduct discussions with the patient's family or surrogate decision maker about the potential for organ donation. Options include both conventional organ recovery after declaration of neurological death and potential organ donation after cardiac death. See **Appendix 11** for more information on brain death and organ donation.

IV. ETHICS AT THE BEDSIDE

When faced with an ethical dilemma, clinicians should incorporate one or more of the guiding principles of healthcare into a framework for resolution. As each principle is systematically addressed, specific components of conflict can be identified and their analysis can often be simplified. The clinician should always start with the medical facts of the patient's case and then proceed to related topics. Specific issues may include which persons are involved; whether time constraints apply; whether the chronology of events or decisions is important; what additional medical, legal, or social information is needed to facilitate decision making; what communication pathways will work best to resolve possible conflict; what values or rules are important to the patient, the family, and the institution; and what areas of consensus already exist among the participants. Any unsettled matters can often be organized into a series of steps within the process of resolution. Depending on the nature of the dilemma, other experts may be called upon for specific input. Some issues may need to be repeatedly examined to determine how to provide the highest level of biological and moral good for the patient. Some of the important elements of ethical decision making are summarized in **Table 15-1**.

Table 15-1. Key Elements of Ethical Decision Making
• Whenever possible, initiate discussions with patients regarding their preferences for life support before a medical crisis occurs and they lose capacity to make informed decisions.
• Utilize hospital and/or unit EOLC protocols. If such protocols are not in place, healthcare providers should work with appropriate legal and ethical advisers to develop them.
• Ensure that all decisions related to consent, refusal to consent, limitation of resuscitation, or termination of life support are clearly determined and documented according to policy and regulation.
• Make certain that all EOLC decisions are made with full disclosure of alternatives, implications, and potential conflicts of interest; are free of duress and coercion; and are made by persons who have competence and capacity.
• Ensure adherence to ethical principles and professional and legal standards of medical conduct.
• Communicate clearly and document extensively.
• Develop consensus and a plan with the care team and, when indicated, involve support services such as clergy, an ethics committee or consultant, social services, palliative care services, or hospital counsel.

Each patient's situation is unique and requires continual, caring communication and reassessment of needs and goals. Clinical judgment, practical wisdom, common sense, compassion, and empathy are the key attributes required by clinicians involved in any ethically complex problem.

V. CASE STUDIES

Case 1: Anoxic Encephalopathy Following Resuscitation
A 68-year-old man, Mr. Hill, collapsed at home and sustained a cardiac arrest. Cardiopulmonary resuscitation was not initiated until paramedics arrived 6 minutes later. He was found in ventricular fibrillation, but he responded to intubation, defibrillation, and epinephrine. In the emergency department 30 minutes later, he is unresponsive to painful stimuli, pupils are dilated and fixed, and corneal reflexes are absent. He is breathing spontaneously and is hemodynamically stable. He is transferred to the ICU, but 3 days later he remains in a deep coma.

Analysis
This scenario is not infrequent in critical care and often involves issues of limitation or withdrawal of care. The principles of autonomy, beneficence, nonmaleficence, and justice are presumed to apply in all clinical situations. Whenever possible, the members of the healthcare team should reach

a consensus before discussions are initiated with the family. However, early in the course of ICU care, there needs to be a determination of whether the patient had defined his wishes in advance, and/or who is authorized to speak and make decisions on the patient's behalf. The care team needs to convey a realistic attitude, using evidence-based data, accepted prognosis models, case studies, and anecdotal experience whenever possible, and acknowledging that all prognostication is highly subjective and everyone knows of someone who has survived as a "miracle." Communication is important, especially regarding reflexes and responses that the family witnesses and may place great hope in for eventual recovery. The patient's preferences and attitudes regarding acceptable minimum quality of life are essential here. The issues of feeding tubes, tracheostomy, gastrostomy tubes, and further resuscitation in the event of another cardiac arrest need to be explored. The ICU team should work closely with the patient's primary care physician, with whom the family is likely to have a close rapport. The early involvement of clergy or members of the ethics team may be beneficial. Further diagnostic data that may be more determinative should be considered if it may guide the surrogate decision maker. For example, if the cause of the initial event was a massive cerebrovascular accident, CT scan data is likely to result in a stronger prognostic stance. The help of a neurologist may be indicated to underscore estimates of recovery from anoxic brain injury. Documentation is important, and the elements of each conversation and the bases for prognosis should be clear. It is appropriate to discuss both possible ramifications of discontinuing life support and long-term-care issues. Finally, if the patient has left no advance directives and the surrogate cannot decide, it is not appropriate for providers to coerce a decision based on their personal values, the guilt of the surrogate, or resource constraints. Continued support and guidance are always appropriate and a decision may be forthcoming at a later date. However, when the patient is no longer critically ill and unstable, transfer to another unit is acceptable. The critical care team may then choose to continue in an advisory role, if appropriate.

Case 2: Triage

Six months pass and Mr. Hill develops urosepsis and becomes hemodynamically unstable on a chronic ventilator unit. He has not weaned from mechanical ventilatory support despite continued attempts. In addition, he has experienced repeated episodes of aspiration pneumonia for which he was successfully treated, has developed multiple decubitus ulcers, and is moderately malnourished. There has been no interval change in his mental status examination since ICU discharge. You receive a call from the pulmonary service requesting a transfer to your ICU. The ICU is presently full and there are no truly good candidates for discharge; you reasonably believe that all ICU patients have the potential to survive to discharge. The best potential candidate for transfer is a 35-year-old male with a closed head injury who was admitted 8 hours ago, is hemodynamically stable, and is not currently ventilated. He is in danger of developing worsening cerebral edema and may require intubation for airway protection—or then again, he may not.

Analysis

This is a triage/resource-allocation dilemma. The demand for ICU beds at the institution exceeds the supply, which requires a caring application of distributive justice. Defined hospital and ICU policies and protocols must be adhered to if they exist. The attending intensivist, as the leader of the critical care team, is responsible for determining how those resources will be allocated. The patient with the closed head injury is at high risk for acute decompensation outside the monitored setting of the ICU, and his long-term prognosis may not be better than that of Mr. Hill; however, his clinical course is indeterminate at this time. On the other hand, the course of events since Mr.

Hill's cardiac arrest suggests medical futility—meaningful outcomes may not be possible despite continued aggressive care. It is assumed that the family has continued to hope for recovery and has chosen not to limit resuscitation. It is appropriate to revisit the topic of limiting resuscitation, calmly and dispassionately; however, to avoid coercing the surrogate into a decision based on feelings of guilt, the triage considerations should not be a focus of the resumed discussion. There are 3 feasible alternatives: transfer Mr. Hill to the ICU in place of the patient with closed head injury; transfer Mr. Hill to another institution with available ICU beds, if possible; or deny Mr. Hill ICU admission at the present time.

Based on the immediate clinical situation, denial of ICU admission may be the most reasonable option. Autonomy must be respected. Beneficence toward the patient with closed head injury must be balanced with nonmaleficence to the older patient with anoxic injury. Supportive measures should begin to the extent possible on the wards. The family should be notified that he has taken a turn for the worse and that best efforts are under way. If there is continued deterioration without a response to therapy and an ICU bed remains unavailable, discussions with the family regarding futility may be appropriate. Careful documentation must accompany all treatment decisions and discussions. Clergy and the ethics committee may be notified if appropriate. Administrative notifications or advice of hospital counsel may also be needed.

Case 3: Advance Directive
Robert is a 17-year-old male patient with cystic fibrosis. He has written an advance directive. After much deliberation, Robert's parents and pediatrician have agreed to his wishes in writing. Robert has been getting progressively worse over the last 3 months, and in the last 24 hours he has had increasing respiratory distress. Robert developed respiratory failure at home while his parents were away, so a temporary caretaker called paramedics, who intubated him and placed him on mechanical ventilation, unaware of his advance directives. When Robert's parents arrive in the emergency department, they demand that he be extubated, that life support be withdrawn, and that he be made comfortable. Robert, who has been medicated with sedatives, is unable to participate in the discussions.

Analysis
Robert has a clear and unambiguous advance directive. Although he is legally a minor, his wishes have been endorsed by his parents. An advance directive written by a 17-year-old may not hold legal value, but it holds inherent value as a document that expresses the autonomy of the individual. The physician, when confronted with an advance directive, should always pursue, if possible, the true intent of the document and its validity. The paramedics, unaware of Robert's directive, appropriately initiated life support under the principle of beneficence and made a reasonable presumption of implied consent under the circumstances. However, given the information and documentation now available, it is important to consider discontinuation of life support to adhere to Robert's clearly stated wishes. Appropriate sedation and pain relief are indicated, and the ICU care team or palliative care services should be available to provide comfort care. It must be noted, however, that in some countries or institutions, laws and regulations may limit the ability of the care team to follow Robert's directive.

Key Points: Ethics in Critical Care Medicine

■ Healthcare professionals have an obligation to act in their patients' best interests based upon the ethical principles of autonomy, beneficence, nonmaleficence, and justice.

■ When faced with an ethical dilemma, consensus from the healthcare team on the treatment plan and objectives facilitates consistent communication and documentation and minimizes liability risks.

■ Specific components of conflict within an ethical dilemma can be identified and the analysis can often be simplified when each ethical principle is addressed systematically.

■ Life support may be withdrawn at the end of life, but care is never withdrawn.

 ## Suggested Readings

1. Annas GJ. The health care proxy and the living will. *N Engl J Med*. 1991;324:1210.

2. Cassell J, Buchman TG, Streat S, et al. Surgeons, intensivists, and the covenant of care: administrative models and values affecting care at the end of life. *Crit Care Med*. 2003;31:1263.

3. Consensus statement of the Society of Critical Care Medicine's Ethics Committee regarding futile and other possibly inadvisable treatments. *Crit Care Med*. 1997;25:887.

4. Davidson JE, Powers K, Hedayat KM, et al. Clinical practice guidelines for support of the family in the patient-centered intensive care unit: American College of Critical Care Medicine Task Force 2004-2005. *Crit Care Med*. 2007;35:605.

5. Giacomini M, Cook D, DeJean D, et al. Decision tools for life support: a review and policy analysis. *Crit Care Med*. 2006;34:864.

6. Prendergast TJ, Puntillo KA. Withdrawal of life support: intensive caring at the end of life. *JAMA*. 2002;288:2732.

7. Siegel MD. Alone at life's end: trying to protect the autonomy of patients without surrogates or decision-making capacity. *Crit Care Med*. 2006;34:2238.

8. Szalados, JE. Do-not-resuscitate and end-of-life care issues: clinical, ethical, and legal principles. *Curr Rev Clin Anesth*. 2003;24:47.

9. Truog RD, Cist AFM, Brackett SE, et al. Recommendations for end-of-life care in the intensive care unit: the Ethics Committee of the Society of Critical Care Medicine. *Crit Care Med*. 2001;29:2332.

10. White DB, Curtis JR, Lo B, et al. Decisions to limit life-sustaining treatment for critically ill patients who lack both decision-making capacity and surrogate decision-makers. *Crit Care Med.* 2006;34:2053.

11. Wueste, DE. A philosophical yet user-friendly framework for ethical decision making in critical care nursing. *Dimens Crit Care Nurs.* 2005;24:70.

Chapter 16:

CRITICAL CARE IN INFANTS AND CHILDREN: THE BASICS

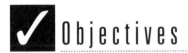 Objectives

- Review physiologic differences between pediatric and adult patients in terms of critical illness.

- Evaluate the differences in the incidence of conditions, consequences, and complications between the 2 groups.

- Identify general differences in therapy.

Case Study

A 3-month-old with a history of prematurity was brought to the emergency department by her father, who reported that for the past week she had nasal congestion, cough, wheezing, posttussive emesis, tachypnea, and fever. On arrival, the infant's vital signs were heart rate 182/min, respiratory rate 72/min, SpO$_2$ 87%, and temperature 101.7 °F (38.7°C). She was tachypneic, grunting, retracting intercostal muscles, and cyanotic, and was given nebulized albuterol with 100% oxygen by the staff. You have been asked to assist in her management.

– What is the most important initial intervention?

– What are the most immediate treatment strategies?

I. INTRODUCTION

The preceding chapters in the FCCS program have emphasized principles of critical care and specific management of a variety of conditions in adult patients. This chapter extends those principles to the treatment of pediatric patients. Due to issues related to maturation, habitus, anatomy, and physiology, the manifestations of critical illness in infants and children may differ from those in adults and may lead to different interventions.

II. GENERAL EXAMINATION

Because young children are unable to verbalize specific complaints, evaluation by the healthcare provider depends upon general and specific features of examination in addition to information obtained from a parent or guardian. Although many of the early signs of distress are subtle, their recognition can increase the likelihood that interventions will be successful and prevent more serious progression. If healthcare providers miss these elusive signs of illness, they sometimes assume that a child's condition has suddenly deteriorated when in fact the seemingly abrupt change reflects an advanced point along a continuum of physiologic compromise. Important factors to be considered in the general examination of a pediatric patient are listed in **Table 16-1.** See **Appendix 16** for age-appropriate normal values for vital signs and blood volume.

Table 16-1.	Important Aspects of the Physical Examination

Skin perfusion: Check for loss of normal pink mucosa and nail beds, mottling that has replaced the usually uniform skin color over the trunk and extremities, skin that has lost its warmth, and the slowing of capillary refill. To prevent an erroneous assessment, capillary refill should be determined with the extremity above the level of the patient's heart.

Degree of hydration: A dehydrated infant may have a sunken fontanelle in addition to signs that may be seen in older children, such as absent tears, sunken eyes, skin tenting, and dry mucous membranes.

Level of spontaneous reactivity and responsiveness: An ill child may initially have increased irritability, but this may be followed by decreasing responsiveness and increasing flaccidity. In most infants, alertness can be evaluated by observing the ability to fixate on objects, particularly a parent's face. The infant should turn toward sound and should follow an object horizontally and, within 1 month of age, vertically. Older children should exhibit stranger anxiety and show clear recognition of parents.

Position spontaneously assumed for comfort: Illness may be marked by the inability to find a position of comfort or to find more that a single position of comfort. Patients should not be forced to assume another position, as this could potentially compromise a tenuous airway.

(Continued on next page)

Table 16-1. Important Aspects of the Physical Examination

Tachypnea: Very rapid breathing is an important sign of illness in infants and young children. Etiologies include respiratory disease, hypovolemia, hyperviscosity syndromes, hyperglycemia, heart failure, adverse drug effect, metabolic acidosis, fever, pain, and anxiety.

Bradypnea: This ominous sign may be due to hypothermia, central nervous system injury, drug-induced depression, neuromuscular disease, severe shock, or some metabolic disorders.

Grunting during exhalation: Such grunting is ominous and occurs as part of respiratory distress, pain, or intra-abdominal disorders.

Nasal pathway: The nasal pathway is the primary route for normal breathing in an infant. Total airway resistance and the potential for compromised breathing are increased significantly in infants with nasal congestion or increased secretions, or by the presence of a nasogastric tube. Nasal flaring is a sensitive indicator of respiratory distress in the infant.

Early hypovolemic shock: The most reliable indicators of early, but compensated, hypovolemic shock in children are persistent tachycardia, cutaneous vasoconstriction, and diminution of the pulse pressure. The best clinical evidence of decreased tissue perfusion is the combination of skin mottling, prolonged capillary refill, and cool extremities. Systemic arterial blood pressure is frequently normal at this stage because of a compensatory increase in systemic vascular resistance. The neurologic status is normal or only minimally impaired. It remains important to measure blood pressure, as an abnormally low value suggests a decompensated state and requires immediate intervention.

Seizures: In infants seizures may be characterized by decreased alertness (the infant does not regard parents or track an object across the visual field), autonomic changes (tachycardia, elevated blood pressure, and dilated pupils), apnea, and subcortical muscle activity (bicycling movements of the legs, swimming movements of the arms, sucking, or tongue-thrusting movements). Tonic-clonic muscle motion may not occur during seizures in infants because neurons and their connections have not fully developed.

Infection: Fever should always suggest the possibility of serious bacterial disease. In the neonate, infections usually involve the bloodstream, although respiratory distress, temperature instability (including hypothermia), and gastrointestinal signs are frequent clinical findings of sepsis.

III. EVALUATION BY ORGAN SYSTEM

The healthcare provider who responds to a seriously ill pediatric patient must be able to promptly recognize respiratory, cardiovascular, metabolic, immunologic, and neurologic problems that affect children. Important differences between children and adults and basic treatment strategies are summarized below.

A. Respiratory System/Airway

Respiratory failure is particularly common in infants because of variable maturation in 3 areas:

■ The central nervous system receptor and effector mechanisms for the respiratory drive

■ Chest wall stability and respiratory muscular strength

■ Conducting airways and the alveolar-capillary complex

The respiratory response to hypoxemia in neonates may be biphasic (ie, hyperpnea initially, followed by hypopnea and hypoventilation). This response occurs despite apparently normal central and peripheral chemoreceptors to oxygen and CO_2.

1. Anatomic and Physiologic Considerations

The thorax is more cartilaginous in infants and young children and is, therefore, more compliant. Increased intrathoracic pressure during respiratory distress is less efficient in augmenting tidal volume because the chest retracts inward, reducing tidal ventilation and indirectly increasing the work of breathing. Soft-tissue retractions similarly reduce thoracic volume during vigorous respiratory efforts. In addition, the fact that the infant's ribs are aligned in a more horizontal plane decreases the inspiratory displacement of the thorax in the anteroposterior plane, further decreasing the efficiency of the bellows effect of the thorax.

The points of muscular insertion of the diaphragm on the thorax are more horizontal in the infant, as they are in the adult with obstructive lung disease and a flattened diaphragm. Therefore, the lower thorax may be drawn inward during inspiration, causing reduced inspiratory volume. Immature intercostal muscles cannot assist active ventilation for several years after birth; thus more dependency is placed upon diaphragmatic function and excursion. Compromise of diaphragmatic excursion by gastric distention, abdominal distension and surgery may quickly in turn compromise respiratory function.

Alveolar size and number increase substantially during childhood, and lung compliance also increases. Tidal volume remains fairly constant through childhood at 6 to 7 mL/kg body weight, but the fact that this small volume must also be available quickly indicates a need for high intrinsic or externally supplied airflow rates. Smaller anatomic conducting airways may produce high resistance if further narrowed by inflammation, edema, mucus, bronchospasm and bronchiolitis. Such high peripheral airway resistance may also alter exhalation and induce dynamic closure of the airways and auto-PEEP.

These factors combine to produce less respiratory reserve in the pediatric patient. Therefore, the etiology of cardiopulmonary arrest in pediatric patients is most commonly a primary respiratory disorder. The majority of deaths in children (especially those under 1 year of age) involve respiratory disorders resulting from infection, poisonings, trauma, submersion or suffocation, and sudden infant death syndrome. Airway obstruction, aspiration, and apnea are also among the major hazards to respiratory function. Thus, assuring a patent airway is the important first

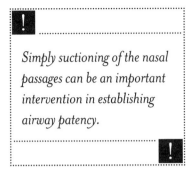

Simply suctioning of the nasal passages can be an important intervention in establishing airway patency.

step in care of the child with respiratory compromise. Neonates and young infants are dependent on their nasal airways (obligate nasal breathing). In young children, common causes of airway obstruction are congenital, infectious (viral croup, bacterial tracheitis, or, less commonly, epiglottitis), or related to ingestion of a foreign body. Clinical examination may help identify the site of obstruction. Airway obstruction above the thoracic inlet tends to cause stridor (inspiratory noise), whereas intrathoracic obstruction tends to cause wheezing (expiratory noise).

2. Airway Management

The first consideration in airway management is head position. A child who is obtunded or otherwise unable to maintain a position of comfort should be placed in the sniffing position to minimize upper airway obstruction from soft tissues. The sniffing position is accomplished by placing the child on a hard surface and rotating the head back so that the child's face is directed upward. A roll beneath the shoulders can work well to maintain the head position of an infant. In the child over 2 years of age, the sniffing position may be accomplished by placing a folded towel or sheet under the child's occiput. It must again be emphasized that, if able, children should be allowed to choose their position of comfort. After trauma involving a possible cervical spine injury, gentle in-line stabilization in the neutral position is used, and further manipulation is restricted to the jaw-thrust maneuver or insertion of an oropharyngeal or endotracheal airway.

Oxygen consumption by an infant is 2 to 3 times that of an adult. Residual oxygen reserves in the lung are rapidly depleted if oxygen availability is compromised and this situation quickly leads to hypoxemia and its consequences. Because children have less hemoglobin than adults and because cyanosis occurs only when a critical level of unsaturated hemoglobin is present, blood oxygen content must fall to very low levels before cyanosis is evident. Therefore, 100% oxygen should be administered to all dyspneic children or those in whom respiratory compromise is suspected.

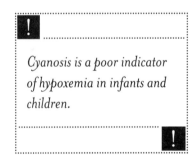

Cyanosis is a poor indicator of hypoxemia in infants and children.

Pulse oximetry is accurate and should be used to titrate the FiO_2. The mask used for oxygen supplementation may cause agitation in children, and several devices should be available for trial. Supplemental oxygen should be warmed and humidified to avoid heat and evaporative water loss from the airway. The nasopharynx in infants is large compared with the tidal volume and inspiratory flow so a nasal cannula will provide a much higher inspired oxygen concentration than in an adult. Issues relating to intubation are summarized in **Table 16-2.**

Table 16-2.	Factors That Affect Endotracheal Intubation in Children

- Positive pressure created during bag-mask ventilation may quickly cause gastric distension; a nasogastric tube may be needed. Gastric distension not only promotes vomiting and aspiration but also interferes with ventilation and leads to acceleration of hypoxemia during mask ventilation.

- Because the infant has a large occiput, the head flexes forward onto the chest when the infant is lying in supine position and the head is in the midline. In the absence of neck injury, the child's head should be placed in the sniffing position. Extreme neck extension, however, can obstruct the airway.

- The tongue in infants and children up to approximately 2 years of age occupies a relatively large portion of the oral cavity and may cause obstruction to spontaneous or assisted ventilation and intubation.

- The anterior and cephalad position of the larynx makes blind nasal intubation very difficult. In addition, the adenoidal tissue may be enlarged. Blind passage of a relatively rigid tube through this area can cause uncontrollable bleeding. This route is discouraged.

- The epiglottis often obscures the glottic opening because of its angle of attachment to the larynx and its relative lack of cartilage.

- Cricoid pressure may improve exposure of the glottis and reduce the risk of gastric distension, regurgitation, and aspiration by occluding the esophagus. The maneuver is accomplished by applying gentle pressure toward the spine at the level of the cricoid cartilage without displacing the larynx in the cephalad direction. Grasping the surface of the cricoid cartilage between the thumb and forefinger and pushing straight down will cause less lateral displacement than is sometimes seen when the tips of 1 or 2 fingers are used to push down on the trachea.

- The upper airway is narrowest at the cricoid ring. An oversized endotracheal tube may cause permanent injury to this area. In general, a properly sized tube is about the diameter of the child's small finger. In children over the age of 2 years, the following formula is used to determine the appropriate endotracheal tube size: [16 + (age in years)] /4. The use of cuffed endotracheal tubes is safe for infants beyond the newborn period and in children. Cuffed endotracheal tubes may be used in certain clinical conditions (poor lung compliance, large air leak or high airway resistance) as long as the tube size and position are correct and the cuff inflation pressure is monitored.

- A straight blade is most often used for children weighing <20 kg and should be long enough to reach the epiglottis.

- The trachea is short enough that special care must be taken to avoid bronchial placement of the endotracheal tube.

3. Respiratory Failure

Causes of respiratory failure in children can be usually be grouped by age (Table 16-3). The causes of respiratory failure in older children are similar to those found in adults.

Table 16-3.	Causes of Respiratory Failure
Premature neonates	Apnea of prematurity
	Infant respiratory distress syndrome (surfactant deficiency and ineffective chest bellows)
Term neonates	Bacterial pneumonia
	Sepsis
	Meconium aspiration
	Congenital airway abnormalities
Infants, toddlers	Pneumonia
	Bronchiolitis
	Asthma
	Foreign-body aspiration
	Upper-airway obstruction due to infection

Treatment of bronchiolitis includes supplemental oxygen administration and consideration of mechanical ventilation. Some infants respond to bronchodilators, and a trial of β-agonists may be useful. If there is no response to β-agonist trials, there is no defined advantage to corticosteroid therapy.

In asthma, treatment includes supplemental oxygen, inhaled β-agonist administration, and corticosteroids. β-Agonists may be administered intermittently or as continuous nebulization therapy. The suggested initial dosage for methylprednisolone is 1 mg/kg intravenously every 6 hours. Anticholinergic therapy such as ipratropium bromide may be beneficial. Patients with bronchiolitis or asthma with low oxygen concentration requirements may benefit from an oxygen-helium mixture (30% oxygen, 70% helium).

4. Mechanical Ventilation

The principle concepts of mechanical ventilation are similar in pediatric patients, but specific settings and adjustments may be different. The suggested initial mechanical ventilation settings for infants who weigh <5 kg are presented in **Table 16-4.**

Table 16-4.	Initial Mechanical Ventilator Settings: Infants Weighing <5 kg
Mode	Time-cycled, pressure-limited ventilation
Peak inspiratory pressure	Start at 18-20 cm H_2O and titrate to a pressure that provides adequate chest movement and tidal volume
Tidal volume	Approximately 8 mL/kg
Respiratory rate	20-30 breaths/min
PEEP	3-5 cm H_2O

Remember that tidal volumes measured at the ventilator also incorporate breathing circuit expansion and gas compression volumes, which can be a substantial portion of the total volume. Loss of ventilation can occur because the ventilator tubing is distended lengthwise and circumferentially by increases in peak airway pressure that create a back pressure. The amount of gas from the tidal inhalation that is trapped in the ventilator tubing is a function of the airway

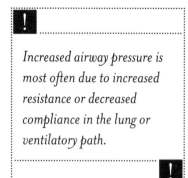

Increased airway pressure is most often due to increased resistance or decreased compliance in the lung or ventilatory path.

pressure and the distensibility (compliance) of the tubing. Soft plastic used in ventilator tubing distends more than hard plastic and the compliance volume of the tubing increases. As much as 3 to 4 milliliters of gas per centimeter H_2O airway pressure may be trapped in the tubing at end inspiration. This volume of gas remains in the tubing at peak inhalation without entering the lung and then exits the circuit through the exhalation valve as exhalation begins. This loss of alveolar ventilation is of less consequence in an adult with a tidal volume of 500 milliliters than it is in a child with a tidal volume of 150 milliliters.

Suggested initial ventilator settings for pediatric patients >5 kg are summarized in **Table 16-5.**

Table 16-5.	Initial Mechanical Ventilator Settings: Infants Weighing >5 kg
Mode	SIMV (volume or pressure-controlled)
Tidal volume	8-10 mL/kg for normal lungs or 6 mL/kg for acute lung injury/acute respiratory distress syndrome
Inspiratory time	Babies 0.5-0.6 sec Toddlers 0.6-0.8 sec School-age children/teens 0.8-1 sec
Respiratory rate	Adjust to maintain acceptable $PaCO_2$ levels; rates >18-20 are not usually necessary
Pressure support	5-10 cm H_2O to overcome resistance of endotracheal tube
PEEP	3-5 cm H_2O; higher levels in acute lung injury for alveolar recruitment

If volume-controlled ventilation is used, attention to the peak inflation pressure is required to prevent barotrauma. If pressure-controlled ventilation is used, attention to tidal volume is necessary to prevent hypoventilation or volutrauma. Always observe chest rise at initiation of mechanical ventilation and when tidal volume is adjusted. Sedation may be useful with increased respiratory rates and/or increased tidal volume.

B. Cardiovascular System

1. Anatomic and Physiologic Considerations

The circulating blood volume is higher per kilogram in children than in adults, but the absolute volume remains low because of the small body size. Therefore, small amounts of blood loss are less tolerated by children. Blood replacement is indicated when 5% to 10% of the circulating volume has been lost.

Cardiac output is high per kilogram of weight at birth, but the absolute amount is small (~600 mL/min) and largely depends on a rapid heart rate because the small heart size results in low stroke volume. In children, cardiac output remains dependent upon changes in heart rate. Bradycardia, therefore, may greatly limit systemic perfusion and is most often an ominous sign of significant hypoxemia or acidosis. Other arrhythmias usually do not produce significant changes in cardiac output unless sustained supraventricular tachycardia occurs. Ventricular arrhythmias are uncommon but, when present, may signify congenital heart disease, myocarditis, cardiomyopathy, electrolyte abnormalities, or asphyxia.

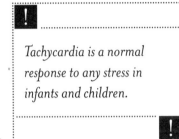

Tachycardia is a normal response to any stress in infants and children.

Myocardial maturation influences the heart's response to volume challenges intended to increase preload. Prior to the age of 8 weeks, infants may not respond to a fluid bolus by increasing cardiac output, but thereafter the response is similar to that of adults. The central venous pressure, however, does not necessarily reflect circulatory blood volume or left ventricular efficiency. Left and right heart function may be disparate, and each side may fail independently. Therefore, pulmonary artery catheters and expert consultation may occasionally be required to monitor left and right heart filling pressures.

Pulmonary vascular resistance falls quickly after birth, reaching normal adult levels by 8 weeks of life. However, the pulmonary vasculature may remain very reactive to hypoxia, hypercapnia, hypothermia, or acidosis, thereby increasing afterload to the right ventricle. Myocardial anatomy changes in such a way that after birth, the larger right ventricle decreases its mass and the left ventricle increases in size and mass. Similarly, neonatal response to catecholamines is limited until sympathetic nervous system innervation and β_1-receptors increase over several weeks. The physiologic effects of exogenous catecholamine administration, therefore, may be quite variable, and careful titration to the individual child's response is essential.

2. Shock

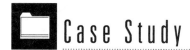 Case Study

A 4-month-old who was born prematurely is brought to the emergency department with a 3 day history of vomiting, diarrhea, and failure to thrive. He had been fed water and herbal tea for the previous 48 hours. On arrival he is found to be unresponsive and to have tonic-clonic activity, cool distal extremities, heart rate 165/min, temperature 97.2°F (36.2°C), blood pressure 68/47 mm Hg, and respiratory rate 56/min.

> – What is the possible diagnosis?
>
> – What interventions are appropriate?
>
> – What diagnostic modalities are indicated?

Pediatric patients are particularly susceptible to shock states. Shock in pediatric patients is defined and categorized as in adults (**Chapter 7**), but the etiologies may differ. Timely recognition of the shock state and aggressive intervention are essential to obtaining an optimal outcome. As soon as the diagnosis of shock is considered, early cardiopulmonary monitoring, vascular access, and treatment must be implemented. Fluid resuscitation is the initial therapy for most forms of shock. Rapid restitution of circulating intravascular volume is critical to restore tissue oxygenation and perfusion and avoid end-organ damage. Initial volume expansion with isotonic crystalloid solutions (normal saline or Ringer's lactate) at 20 mL/kg is recommended, repeated up to a total of 60 mL/kg in the first 15 minutes. Smaller volumes of 5 to 10 mL/kg should be used in patients with suspected myocardial dysfunction. Although hepatomegaly can be a sign of fluid overload in the pediatric patient, it must be viewed with caution. Disease processes common to children (eg, asthma, respiratory syncytial virus, pneumonitis) can cause lung hyperinflation and displacement of the liver. Other signs of volume overload should also be considered in the evaluation of these patients. If a child with an enlarged liver fails to respond to initial fluid administration, radiologic examination of the chest may help to evaluate heart size. In children, crackles may occur late in the process of developing heart failure, and a gallop may be difficult to discern in infants due to their rapid heart rate.

    a. Hypovolemic Shock

    The most common cause of shock in the pediatric patient is acute hypovolemia resulting from increased fluid and electrolyte losses (gastrointestinal disorders) or blood loss resulting from severe trauma. Hypovolemia can also result from capillary leak due to intestinal ischemia caused by volvulus, intussusception, or necrotizing enterocolitis. A detailed medical history should be obtained from the patient's caregiver and/or referring institution. A history of increased fluid losses (vomiting and diarrhea), lethargy, and decreased urine output is usually found in infants with hypovolemic shock. Blood pressure is maintained longer in hypovolemic children than in adults. Capillary refill and extremity temperature are much more reliable indicators of hypovolemia since they may become abnormal much earlier than blood pressure in the child with shock. Children with hypovolemic shock may require 40 to 60 mL/kg of isotonic fluids (normal saline or Ringer's lactate). Hypotonic or dextrose-containing fluids are not indicated during the initial treatment phase. A transfusion of packed red blood cells (10-15 mL/kg) should be considered in patients with hemorrhagic shock when signs of shock persist despite adequate isotonic fluid resuscitation. Inotrope/vasopressor support should be considered for patients who do not respond to isotonic fluids. Patients with concurrent adrenocortical problems can be refractory to fluids and inotropes and will respond only to glucocorticoid replacement.

b. Distributive Shock

As in adults, the most common cause of distributive shock in pediatric patients is sepsis. Other etiologies are similar to those in adults with the addition of congenital adrenal hyperplasia. Septic shock is characterized by changes in mental status, fever or hypothermia, and perfusion abnormalities such as vasodilation (warm shock) or vasoconstriction (cold shock). The therapeutic goal in septic shock is to restore and maintain optimal organ perfusion and oxygenation. Acceptable goals include restoration of the patient's mental status and urine output (1 mL/kg/h). Children in septic shock are usually severely hypovolemic and will respond to aggressive fluid resuscitation. Initial rapid fluid resuscitation with isotonic fluids (20 mL/kg) is suggested. Typical fluid requirements range from 40 to 200 mL/kg during the initial phase of resuscitation. Fluid choices are crystalloids (normal saline, Ringer's lactate) and colloids (5% albumin, dextran, gelatin). Vasopressor support with dopamine (5 to 10 µg/kg/min) is recommended as the first choice in patients with fluid-refractory vasodilated shock. Norepinephrine (0.05 µg/kg/min) or epinephrine (0.05 µg/kg/min) may be considered in patients unresponsive to dopamine. Dobutamine may be administered to patients with low cardiac output and elevated systemic vascular resistance states (vasoconstricted) after fluid resuscitation. Use of corticosteroids is indicated in patients with vasopressor-resistant shock, purpura fulminans, or suspected adrenocortical problems (chronic steroid use in immunodeficiency, malignant disease, collagen vascular disorders). The initial recommended dose is 50 mg/m²/24h of hydrocortisone. Early transfer to a pediatric intensive care unit for inotropic support and invasive cardiopulmonary monitoring is indicated in patients not responding to fluid resuscitation. Infants with sepsis are often profoundly hypoglycemic on presentation and glucose determinations should be performed on all infants with suspected sepsis.

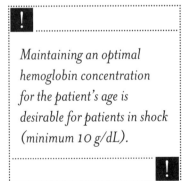

Maintaining an optimal hemoglobin concentration for the patient's age is desirable for patients in shock (minimum 10 g/dL).

c. Cardiogenic Shock

Congestive heart failure is the most common presentation of congenital heart anomalies in children and often precedes cardiogenic shock. Congestive heart failure can often be the result of acute or chronic changes in the heart's preload, afterload, contractility, or heart rate and rhythm. Signs and symptoms vary depending on the type of lesion. Infants with ductal-dependent lesions (coarctation of the aorta, transposition of the great vessels, tricuspid atresia, etc) will typically present in profound shock with a history of poor feeding, tachypnea, lethargy, cyanosis, thready or absent femoral pulses, and poor or absent urine output (obstructive shock). These patients will require prompt initiation of prostaglandin (PGE_1) and inotropes in addition to isotonic fluids. Patients with non-ductal dependent lesions can present with a history of tachycardia, gallop rhythm, heart murmur, tachypnea, hepatomegaly, and failure to thrive. These patients will often respond to diuresis with a loop diuretic (furosemide 0.5-1 mg/kg/ dose) rather than fluid resuscitation and to inotropic support (milrinone 0.5-1 µg/kg/ min or dobutamine 5-10 µg/kg/min) and/or afterload reduction. Fluid resuscitation must be titrated cautiously. Early transfer to a pediatric intensive care unit for further monitoring, inotropic support, and a complete evaluation by a pediatric cardiologist is recommended. Other common etiologies of cardiogenic shock include hypoxic-ischemic episodes after acute life-threatening events, near drowning, or strangulation.

d. Obstructive Shock

Congenital lesions that interfere with outflow from the left ventricle, such as coarctation of the aorta or interrupted aortic arch, commonly cause obstructive shock in infants. These infants develop signs of shock when the ductus arteriosus closes, thus interfering with the delivery of cardiac output to the distal aorta. A history of poor feeding, lethargy, decreased or absent urine output, decreased or absent femoral pulses, and metabolic acidosis is frequent. When treating hypotension in a child with non-hypovolemic shock, initial titrated boluses of 10 to 20 mL/kg crystalloid up to 40 mL/kg may not be effective. Inotropic support with dobutamine 5 to 10 µg/kg/min and a prostaglandin (PGE_1) infusion should be initiated rapidly to reopen the ductus arteriosus and restore perfusion to the distal aorta in infants and children with suspected left heart lesions. The usual dose is PGE_1 0.05 to 0.1 µg/kg/min as a continuous infusion. The side effects of PGE_1 infusion include periodic breathing, apnea, and peripheral vasodilatation, so the clinician must be prepared to support the patient's airway, provide ventilation, and administer additional fluids. Once the ductus arteriosus has reopened, it is critical to avoid hyperventilation and hyperoxia. Both of these conditions will lead to preferential pulmonary blood flow through the ductus and will worsen systemic shock and distal perfusion.

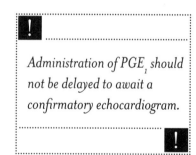

Administration of PGE_1 should not be delayed to await a confirmatory echocardiogram.

C. Metabolism/Temperature

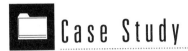

Case Study

A 6-month-old is brought by ambulance to the emergency department from his grandmother's house. He has been sick with diarrhea for 6 days. He refused to drink fluids except for water, rice water, and some juice. His grandmother found him unresponsive. En route to the hospital he develops tonic-clonic seizure activity and receives diazepam 5 mg per rectum. On arrival to the emergency department the patient is unresponsive, cyanotic, and apneic.

- What is the possible diagnosis?

- What interventions are appropriate?

- What diagnostic modalities are indicated?

Pediatric patients are particularly susceptible to abnormalities of water and temperature regulation as well as electrolyte abnormalities. The more common issues that can result in critical illness are discussed below.

1. Water/Temperature

Insensible water loss is higher in children than in adults because children have a higher ratio of surface area to body mass. This higher evaporative fluid loss, when combined with a higher metabolic rate, emphasizes that dehydration may occur quickly. Therefore, children require a greater amount of fluid per kilogram than adults do, but this volume is still a low absolute amount because of a child's small size. Titration of these small volumes usually requires infusion pumps for administration and frequent adjustment of intake to assure replacement of fluids lost from all sites. There are several approaches to fluid (**Table 16-6**) and electrolyte replacement that will help the clinician estimate the actual requirements.

Table 16-6. Estimating Fluid Requirements	
Body Weight in Kilograms	**Milliliters per Day**
<10 kg	100 mL/kg/day
11-20 kg	1000 mL + 50 mL/kg for each kg above 10 kg
>20 kg	1500 mL + 20 mL/kg for each kg above 20 kg

The method most widely used relates caloric expenditure to body weight for a resting patient. For every 100 calories expended 100 mL of water is lost (65% urine + 35% insensible water) plus 2 to 4 mEq of Na and K. Thus, a child weighing 25 kilograms would receive 1,600 milliliters of water per day (1,500 mL + 100 mL), 50 to 100 mmol/day of Na, and 25 to 50 mmol of K. The amount of dextrose required will depend on the patient's age and metabolic needs. Children who weigh <10 kg should receive a solution of 10% dextrose or higher. Children who weigh >10 kg will typically require a 5% dextrose-containing solution. Dextrose solutions should be withheld in hyperglycemic patients (glucose >180 mg/dL [9.9 mmol/L]). The recommended solution for the previously mentioned patient weighing 25 kilograms would then be 5% dextrose with 75 mmol of Na and 20 mmol of K in each 1,000 mL to run at 66 mL/h (1,600 mL/24h).

Under normal conditions, maintenance fluid needs are derived from normal urine, stool, and insensible water losses. Stool water losses are usually negligible in patients without gastrointestinal pathology. Minimally acceptable urine output is ~2 mL/kg/h for a well-hydrated infant and 1 mL/kg/h for a child.

The higher ratio of surface area to body mass and the decreased subcutaneous fat reserves in infants and young children allow greater heat loss through evaporation and radiation. Maintenance of body temperature is also limited in infants because they do not shiver to generate heat. The compensatory process of metabolizing brown adipose tissue to generate heat is harmful because it results in metabolic acidosis. It is important, therefore, to maintain an appropriate, neutral environment temperature to assure a rectal temperature of 98.6°F (37°C) for the neonate.

2. Glucose

Low glycogen stores and an increased metabolic rate make hypoglycemia more common in infants during stress. A continuous infusion of glucose (5 mg/kg/min) is often necessary. If glucose-containing fluids are withheld, blood glucose should be monitored very frequently (at least every 1-2 hours) to avoid hypoglycemia (glucose <65 mg/dL [3.6 mmol/L]). Glucose boluses of 0.5 to 1 g/kg with 10% glucose (5-10 mL/kg) in neonates and 25% glucose (2-4 mL/kg) in children will generally correct hypoglycemia.

3. Sodium

Hyponatremia (sodium <135 mmol/L) occurs during diarrhea or with diuretic use, especially when fluids are replenished with sodium-poor solutions, such as water or fruit juices. Children with cystic fibrosis, adrenal insufficiency, syndrome of inappropriate antidiuretic hormone (SIADH), and obstructive uropathy are also at risk for hyponatremia. In children with hyponatremia-induced seizures, 3% hypertonic saline can be titrated until seizures resolve. The usual 3% NaCl (0.513 mmol/mL) dose range is 3 mL/kg (2.5 mmol/kg). In patients with less severe acute hyponatremia (Na 120-130 mmol/L), a slow correction over 12 to 24 hours to Na levels of about 130 mmol/L is recommended. The patient's hydration status must be taken into consideration when treating hyponatremia. Hypovolemic patients must be hydrated with normal saline. In euvolemic or hypervolemic patients with mild hyponatremia, fluid restriction and loop diuretics in addition to the hyponatremia correction might be indicated. Early consultation with a pediatric intensivist and transfer to a pediatric intensive care unit for further monitoring are indicated in symptomatic patients.

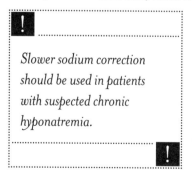

Slower sodium correction should be used in patients with suspected chronic hyponatremia.

Hypernatremia (sodium >145 mmol/L) results from excessive free-water losses in gastroenteritis, inadequate amounts of free-water intake, withholding of water, or nephrogenic or central diabetes insipidus. Infants are more susceptible to hypernatremia. Infants with hypernatremic dehydration can present with signs such as irritability, high-pitched cry, changes in mental status, hypertonia, and seizures. Isotonic fluids (normal saline) are recommended in these patients during the initial resuscitation phase to correct hypovolemia or shock. In children, the free-water deficit can be calculated as 4 mL/kg for every 1 mmol/L sodium >145 mmol/L. The serum sodium should be lowered no faster than 0.5 mmol/L/h over a period of 48 to 72 hours. Five percent dextrose half-strength normal saline (D5 ½ normal saline) can be used in patients whose serum sodium is <165 mmol/L, allowing for Na to drop no faster than 1 mmol/L/h. A more conservative approach should be considered in patients with serum Na >165 mmol/L. In these situations, the solution of choice may be D5 normal saline, provided an adequate hydration state was achieved. Central diabetes insipidus should be suspected in patients with brisk urine output after severe head injury or recent intracranial surgery. Early consultation with a pediatric neurosurgeon and or pediatric intensivist is advised.

4. Potassium

Hypokalemia (potassium <3.5 mmol/L) is usually the consequence of renal losses (diuretic therapy), renal tubular disorder resulting from chemotherapy, gastrointestinal losses (vomiting, fistulas), or decreased intake. In children with life-threatening hypokalemia (arrhythmia, paralysis), potassium chloride can be administered intravenously at a rate of ≤1 mmol/kg/h (maximum 20 mmol/h) with continuous ECG monitoring. The usual replacement rate of potassium is 0.2 to 0.3 mmol/kg/h. Serum potassium levels must be monitored at frequent intervals during the replacement phase.

Hyperkalemia (potassium >5.5 mmol/L) is most often the result of decreased losses, increased intake, or kidney dysfunction. Recommended treatment for hyperkalemia in children is listed in **Table 16-7.**

Table 16-7. Treatment of Hyperkalemia

If significant ECG abnormalities are present (peaked T waves, QRS widening, P-R interval prolongation)
- Administer calcium gluconate (10%) 50 mg/kg intravenously OR
- Administer calcium chloride (10%) 10 mg/kg intravenously

For redistribution of potassium
- Administer sodium bicarbonate 1 mmol/kg intravenously AND/OR
- Administer 25% dextrose 2-3 mL/kg (0.5-1 g/kg) + 0.1 unit regular insulin/kg intravenously (1 unit insulin for each 5 g dextrose)
- Administer inhaled ß₂-agonists (albuterol 2.5-5 mg/dose has been used successfully)

To remove potassium
- Administer loop diuretic: furosemide 0.5-1 mg/kg
- Administer sodium polystyrene sulfonate 1 g/kg/dose oral/rectal every 6 hours
- Administer dialysis

5. Calcium

Critically ill newborns are susceptible to hypocalcemia (total calcium <8.5 mg/dL [2.2 mmol/L], ionized calcium <1 mmol/L) because they experience a sudden withdrawal from the high rate of calcium intake associated with normal maternal-to-fetal transfer of calcium during gestation. In neonates with congenital heart disease, hypocalcemia may be the presenting sign for DiGeorge syndrome (22q11 microdeletion). Children with hypocalcemia may present with tetany, carpopedal spasm, laryngeal stridor, apnea, convulsions, hypotension, and congestive heart failure.

To correct life-threatening hypocalcemia in children, calcium gluconate 100 mg/kg/dose should be injected through a small needle into a large vein at a rate of approximately 1.5 mL/min if central venous access is not available. Calcium chloride 20 mg/kg per dose may be administered instead of calcium gluconate only if central venous access is available. Maintenance doses of calcium gluconate or calcium chloride may be delivered every 6 hours intravenously or by mouth (calcium gluconate 200-500 mg/kg/day) in cases of persistent hypocalcemia.

Hypercalcemia (total calcium >11 mg/dL [>2.75 mmol/L], ionized calcium >1.3 mmol/L) is rare in the pediatric population. Treatment is similar to that for adults: normal saline infusion 10 to 20 mL/kg followed by furosemide 1 to 2 mg/kg every 6 to 12 hours.

6. Magnesium

Hypomagnesemia (magnesium <1.8 mg/dL or 1.5 mEq/dL [0.75 mmol/L]) is commonly associated with malnutrition or malabsorption syndromes in children and with poor gut function in critically ill infants receiving prolonged intravenous fluid administration. It can be seen in patients with a renal tubular disorder resulting from chemotherapy for the treatment of bone tumors. Clinical manifestations of hypomagnesemia overlap those of hypokalemia and hypocalcemia. Life-threatening hypomagnesemia may be treated with magnesium sulfate 25 to 50 mg/kg intravenously over 5 to 15 minutes.

7. Phosphorus

Hypophosphatemia (phosphate <2.5 mg/dL [0.81 mmol/L]) is relatively uncommon in children and is usually associated with malnutrition, malabsorption syndromes, or renal tubular defects. Life-threatening hypophosphatemia, which may be signaled by muscle weakness, respiratory failure, coma, and seizures, can be treated with sodium phosphate or potassium phosphate 0.4 mmol/kg/dose infused over 6 hours (maximum 21 mmol).

D. Immune System

The following factors increase the risk of infection in neonatal patients:

- Decreased polymorphonuclear white cell function and storage reservoir

- Poor ability for antibody synthesis

■ Reduced delivery of phagocytes to inflammatory sites

■ Passive maternal immunity that is depleted by 2 to 5 months after birth, and amounts of immunoglobulins comparable to adult levels are not reached until 4 to 7 years of age

Because of their incompletely developed immune systems, children are treated with empiric antibiotic therapy more frequently than are adults. For the same reason, antibiotics are considered an emergency drug, particularly for febrile infants under 2 months of age. Under the age of 3 years, the risk of occult bacteremia is increased if temperature is >40°C (>104°F) or white blood cell count is <500 cells/mm^3 or >15000 cells/mm^3. Absolute neutrophil count <1,000 cells/mm^3 or significant bands of 25% to 30% are also markers of severe bacterial infection in children. In such situations, a full workup is recommended that should include blood culture, urine culture, and lumbar puncture, if clinically indicated. The stages of physiologic compromise due to infection in pediatric patients are similar to adult stages of sepsis, with some modifications. The systemic manifestations of sepsis are age adjusted for heart rate, blood pressure, and leukocyte count. Criteria for severe sepsis include cardiovascular dysfunction or acute respiratory distress syndrome or ≥2 other organ dysfunctions. Septic shock is defined by the presence of cardiovascular dysfunction.

In neonates, group B streptococci, such as *Escherichia coli,* Listeria, and Enterococcus, often cause life-threatening bacterial infections. The following organisms should be considered in children ages 2 months to 2 years: *Streptococcus pneumoniae, Haemophilus influenzae, Neisseria meningitidis,* and Salmonella. The organisms associated with serious infections in children and the suggested treatments are summarized in **Table 16-8.**

Table 16-8 Most Common Serious Infections in Infants and Children

Site	Organism	Treatment[a]
Neonates		
Bacterial meningitis	Group B streptococci, *Escherichia coli* (and other enteric Gram-negative organisms)	Cefotaxime 50 mg/kg/dose
	Listeria and Enterococcus	Ampicillin 50 mg/kg/dose
Viral meningitis	Neonatal Herpes simplex virus (HSV) and HSV encephalitis	Acyclovir 15 mg/kg/dose
Children		
Bacterial meningitis	*Haemophilus influenzae, Streptococcus pneumoniae, Neisseria meningitidis,* Salmonella	Cefotaxime 50 mg/kg/dose OR Ceftriaxone 50 mg/kg/dose Dexamethasone 0.15 mg/kg/dose for *H influenzae* and *S pneumoniae*
Viral meningitis	HSV encephalitis	Acyclovir 15 mg/kg/dose
Epiglottitis	*H influenzae*	Cefotaxime 50 mg/kg/dose OR Ceftriaxone 50 mg/kg/dose

Table 16-8	Most Common Serious Infections in Infants and Children	

Children (Continued)

Bacterial tracheitis	Staphylococcus Streptococcus *Moraxella catarrhalis*	Nafcillin 50 mg/kg/dose OR Clindamycin 10 mg/kg/dose and cefotaxime 50 mg/kg/dose
Retropharyngeal abscess	*Staphylococcus aureus* Group A streptococci (may be mixed infection) Gram-negative enteric organisms Anaerobes	Nafcillin 50 mg/kg/dose OR Clindamycin 10 mg/kg/dose and gentamicin 2.5 mg/kg/ dose OR Ampicillin/sulbactam 50-100 mg/kg/dose (based on ampicillin) and gentamicin 2.5 mg/kg/dose
Croup	Parainfluenza Influenza	Supportive care
Peritonitis	Gram-negative organisms *Escherichia coli*, Klebsiella Gram-positive organisms: Pneumococcus, Staphylococcus, α- hemolytic Streptococcus, Enterococcus Anaerobes: Bacteroides	Cefotaxime 50 mg/kg/dose, clindamycin 10 mg/kg/dose, and ampicillin 50 mg/kg/ dose OR Ampicillin 50 mg/kg/dose, gentamicin 2.5 mg/kg/dose, and clindamycin or metronidazole 7.5 mg/kg/ dose
Immunocompromised patients	Gram-positive organisms: Coagulase-negative Staphylococcus, α- hemolytic Streptococcus, Enterococcus, Coryneform bacteria	Vancomycin 10-15 mg/kg/ dose
	Gram-negative organisms: Klebsiella, Bacillus, Pseudomonas, *E coli*	Cefepime 50 mg/kg/dose OR Ceftazidime 50 mg/kg/dose
	Fungi: candida, aspergillus	Fluconazole: Loading dose 10 mg/kg; maximum loading dose 400 mg Amphotericin B: 0.25-1 mg/kg/day OR Caspofungin: 50 mg/m^2/dose Q 24h. Maximum dose 50 mg/dose.

[a] These recommendations are general guidelines only. Specific antibiotic choices should be individualized, taking into consideration clinical circumstances (renal function, liver function), patient age, immunization status, and local microbial virulence, sensitivities, and patterns of resistance. The antibiotic closing interval and frequency should be discussed with a pediatric intensivist or pediatric infectious disease expert.

E. Nervous System

The Glasgow Coma Scale (GCS) is difficult to apply in children, even when it is adapted for age as shown in **Table 16-9** (see **Chapter 8** for adult GCS). When assessing the need for further intervention, careful attention should be paid to the patient's ability to maintain the airway, the pupillary responses, the motor score, and, in infants, the fontanelle status. Any young child with a depressed level of consciousness, seizures, and/or coma should be evaluated for the possibility of occult trauma (eg, child abuse, especially shaken baby syndrome), even if there are no outward signs of injury. Infectious, metabolic, or toxic etiologies should also be considered. Boluses of 10% glucose in neonates and 25% glucose in children will generally correct hypoglycemia-induced coma and/or seizures (see above). Hyponatremia should be considered as a cause of seizures in small children. Diazepam may be administered rectally to children with ongoing seizure activity and no intravenous access (0.5 mg/kg/dose [use injectable or gel preparation]). Midazolam, diazepam, or lorazepam can be used in the initial treatment of seizures at a dose of 0.05 to 0.1 mg/kg given intravenously. Subsequently, a full intravenous loading dose of phenytoin or fosphenytoin 15 to 20 mg/kg should be administered if a second dose of benzodiazepine is ineffective. If the patient is already on phenytoin or the loading dose was ineffective, phenobarbital 15 to 20 mg/kg/dose should be considered. The physician caring for these patients should be aware of the cumulative respiratory depression potential of these medications and the resulting need for early airway support. General anesthesia should be considered in the event that seizures persist despite adequate treatment. Neuromuscular blocking agents are used only to facilitate endotracheal intubation. Early consultation with a pediatric neurologist and pediatric intensivist is recommended.

Table 16-9	Glasgow Coma Scale Modified for Infants and Children		
Clinical Parameter	**Infants (Ages 0-12 Months)**	**Children (Ages 1-5 Years)**	**Points[a]**
Eye opening	Spontaneous	Spontaneous	4
	Response to speech	Response to speech	3
	Response to pain	Response to pain	2
	No response	No response	1
Verbal response	Coos/babbles	Appropriate words	5
	Irritable cries	Inappropriate words	4
	Cries	Persistent cry	3
	Moans	Grunts	2
	No response	No response	1
Best motor response	Normal	Spontaneous	6
	Withdraws to touch	Localized pain	5
	Withdraws from pain	Withdraws from pain	4
	Flexor response	Flexor response	3
	Extensor response	Extensor response	2
	No response	No response	1

[a] Total Glasgow Coma Scale score = eye + verbal + motor points; best possible score = 15; worst possible score = 3

The unique features in the care of infants and children presented in this chapter highlight the very small margin for error in treating critically ill or injured pediatric patients. Specialty consultation should, therefore, be requested early.

Critical Care in Infants and Children: The Basics

■ Irritability is an early sign of changes in mental status in the young child.

■ In children, early signs of respiratory distress include tachypnea, grunting, and nasal flaring.

■ Ensuring a patent airway is the most important first step in treating a child with respiratory compromise.

■ Important anatomic differences between the airway of a child and the airway of an adult must be considered when intubating an infant or child.

■ Suggested initial ventilator settings for children are V$_T$ 8 to 10 mL/kg in normal lungs and 6 mL/kg if there is acute lung injury or acute respiratory distress syndrome. Respiratory rates in children may need to be higher than rates in adults to maintain acceptable PaCO$_2$ levels.

■ The perfusion status in children is best assessed initially by capillary refill and temperature of extremities. Hypotension is a late finding in shock.

■ Children with hypovolemic shock may require 40 to 60 mL/kg of isotonic fluids (normal saline, Ringer's lactate).

■ Vasopressor support with dopamine or norepinephrine is indicated in patients with fluid-refractory vasodilated shock. Epinephrine is indicated in patients with low cardiac output (vasoconstricted shock) after adequate fluid resuscitation is delivered.

■ Obstructive shock in infants is commonly caused by congenital lesions that interfere with outflow from the left ventricle, such as coarctation of the aorta or interrupted aortic arch.

■ Intracranial hemorrhage in the young infant can cause hemodynamically significant blood loss.

■ Hypoglycemia is common in infants during stress and must be corrected promptly.

■ Infants do not maintain body temperature well, and care must be taken to avoid hypothermia.

■ Young infants are at increased risk of infection due to their immature immune systems. Empiric antibiotics are considered an emergency drug for febrile infants <2 months of age.

■ Diazepam may be administered rectally to children with ongoing seizure activity and no intravenous access.

Suggested Readings

1. Carcillo JA, Fields AI, et al. Clinical practice parameters for hemodynamic support of pediatric and neonatal patients in septic shock. *Crit Care Med.* 2002;30:1365.

2. Goldstein B, Giroir B, Randolph A; and International Consensus Conference on Pediatric Sepsis. Definitions for sepsis and organ dysfunction in pediatrics. *Pediatr Crit Care Med.* 2005;6:2.

3. Smith L, Hernan L. Shock states. In: Fuhrman BP, Zimmerman JJ, eds. *Pediatric Critical Care.* 3rd ed. St. Louis, MO: Mosby; 2006:394.

4. Thompson AE. Pediatric airway management. In: Fuhrman BP, Zimmerman JJ, eds. *Pediatric Critical Care.* 3rd ed. St. Louis, MO: Mosby; 2006:485.

5. Wood EG, Lynch RE. Electrolyte management in pediatric critical illness. In: Fuhrman BP, Zimmerman JJ, eds. *Pediatric Critical Care.* 3rd ed. St. Louis, MO: Mosby; 2006:939.

MEDICAL EMERGENCY TEAMS

I. INTRODUCTION

Medical Emergency Teams (METs) have emerged as important resources that focus on the hospitalized patient at risk for unexpected or unrecognized events such as a sudden deterioration in condition or a reaction to medication. Typically, crisis teams are activated only after a significant event, like cardiac arrest, occurs. Until recently, there was no organized approach to identifying the at-risk hospitalized patient in order to prevent an untoward event. Most patients who have a cardiac arrest while in the hospital demonstrated identifiable signs of deterioration during the previous 8 hours. Patients with unexpected cardiac arrest or unplanned admission to intensive care often have deterioration in circulatory or respiratory systems for at least 1 hour. These serious events are neither sudden nor unpredictable. Early recognition of deterioration and timely intervention can reduce the incidence of cardiac arrest or need for intensive care and can improve patient outcomes.

Unfortunately, the early indicators of clinical deterioration can be difficult to identify. It is challenging to assess a patient's physiologic reserve. METs brings additional experienced providers with advanced monitoring tools to the patient's bedside. If needed, more advanced monitoring and therapy can be initiated immediately, and a decision can be made about the most appropriate care level. The most important action in the process is the call for help.

The MET model can be divided into three limbs, each of which plays an integral role in the success of the team.

Detection, or Afferent, Limb

- Early detection of signs and symptoms of clinical deterioration
- Predefined activation criteria

Intervention, or Efferent, Limb

- Concise plan for rapid assessment and intervention
- Effective communication of the assessment and recommendations to the responsible clinician
- Transfer to a higher level of care based on the rapid assessment and intervention

Oversight, or Administrative, Limb

- Clinical resource to the MET in management of individual patients
- Leads quality improvement efforts through data collection and analysis of MET activity
- Acts as program steward across the institution

II. BUILDING A MEDICAL EMERGENCY TEAM

A. Composition of a Medical Emergency Team

From hospital to hospital, METs may be called by various names, such as Rapid Response or ICU Outreach, and their composition may differ. While there is no one perfect team composition, the most successful METs have been developed by leveraging existing hospital resources and targeting them at a particular at-risk patient population. Multidisciplinary, physician-led teams are prevalent in academic centers with training programs. Nurse-led or nurse–respiratory therapist teams with physician backup (or medical control similar to the Emergency Medical Services model) are more often found in community hospitals without training programs. Regardless of the team composition, effective teamwork skills are essential to the success of the program. The implementation of standardized protocols or standing orders will allow the team to use evidence-based best practices to address commonly identified clinical issues, especially in circumstances where there is difficulty contacting the responsible physician. The MET administrative leadership should develop these protocols and standing orders in accordance with institutional policies and procedures. Possible members of a MET are identified in **Table A1-1**.

Table A1-1. Possible Members of a Medical Emergency Team	
Physicians Attending, fellow resident	Intensivist, hospitalist, emergency department physician, anesthesiologist, pulmonologist, surgeon, internist, physician assistant
Nurses Staff, advanced practice, clinical nurse specialist	Intensive care unit nurse, postanesthesia care unit nurse, emergency department nurse, telemetry unit nurse, certified registered nurse anesthetist, nursing supervisor
Other providers	Respiratory therapist, electrocardiography technician, emergency medical technician-paramedic

For example, at an academic hospital, METs may be composed of one of the following combinations of staff:

- Intensive care unit (ICU) fellow, ICU nurse, respiratory therapist

- Medicine resident, ICU nurse, respiratory therapist

- ICU nurse, respiratory therapist, physician (backup)

At a community hospital, a MET may consist of one of the following combinations:

- Emergency department physician, ICU nurse, respiratory therapist

- Emergency department nurse, ICU nurse, respiratory therapist

- Postanesthesia care unit nurse, respiratory therapist, physician (backup)

Typically, physician members are trained (or are training) in critical care or emergency medicine. They bring their knowledge of critical illness and skills in the management of life-threatening problems to the patient's bedside. Nurse members usually have many years of bedside experience and most often have extensive critical care training. Team members from other disciplines add value to the MET with their knowledge of such factors as airway and respiratory management, drug therapies, traumatic injury management, and critical care transport.

Team members usually are expected to maintain current provider status in basic and advanced cardiac life support, pediatric advanced life support (where applicable), and fundamental critical care. Periodic teamwork exercises in mock events or medical simulation centers can hone members' evaluation and management skills. Treatment protocols and standing orders should be reviewed and amended based on feedback from MET calls and quality improvement data.

B. Medical Emergency Team Equipment

The use of advanced physiologic monitors and equipment by appropriately trained MET members can provide crucial support to the at-risk patient. This can greatly enhance the team's ability to evaluate and manage signs and symptoms of clinical deterioration. Clearly, the earlier clinical abnormalities are identified and addressed, the greater the potential for a positive outcome and, often, the simpler the needed intervention. The MET first should evaluate the resources that are readily available in the areas it will support and then create a list of additional needed equipment. The MET must have access to cardiac, respiratory, and simple hemodynamic monitors. Other equipment and medications should be based on the patient populations served, the team composition, and local regulations and policies. Since the MET is expected to respond quickly, any additional needed equipment and supplies should be organized in appropriate bags or carts that can be readily transported to the patient. See **Table A1-2.**

III. ACTIVATING THE MEDICAL EMERGENCY TEAM

A. Activation Criteria and Triggers

The most important activation criterion is the bedside staff's concern that something is wrong, even if other indicators are within acceptable limits. This clinical intuition is often quite sensitive and warrants additional assessment. The fact that an intuition or a gut feeling is not very specific should not discourage activation of the MET.

Table A1-2.	Medical Emergency Team Equipment List*

Physiologic Monitors
Monitor/defibrillator with external pacing capability
Noninvasive blood pressure device
Pulse oximetry
Portable capnography (if available)

Respiratory Equipment
Portable oxygen tank
Portable suction device
High-flow oxygen reservoir face mask
Bag-mask device
Ventimask®, nasal cannula and simple face mask
Nebulizer mask
Oropharyngeal/nasopharyngeal airways
Laryngeal mask airways
Laryngoscopes and blades
Endotracheal tubes with stylets
Cricothyrotomy catheter kit
Stethoscope

Cardiovascular Equipment
Manual blood pressure device
IV administration kits
IV catheters

Miscellaneous
Personal protective equipment
Sterile gloves
Dressings and bandages
Antiseptics

Drug Bag (as appropriate for scope of practice)
Vasopressors
Inotropes
Vasodilators
Sedatives and analgesics
Bronchodilators
Crystalloid and colloid IV fluid
Aspirin

*Needed equipment and supplies should be available on the patient unit or carried by the MET

The distribution of a predefined set of MET activation criteria may help to focus attention on important early indicators and empower the bedside staff to call for help early. The criteria may be based on the detection of acute changes in physiology, organ system–specific signs and symptoms, and event triggers. Acute changes in physiology may include changes in vital signs that exceed predefined limits, like tachycardia, tachypnea, hypotension, and oliguria. The detection of one or more indicators of organ system dysfunction may trigger activation of the MET. Such pattern recognition may be more effective in detecting clinical deterioration when there is a more gradual change in physiologic variables.

Event triggers help emphasize that some patient incidents or interventions warrant further evaluation. The event may be a sign or a result of a larger issue that could be an ongoing threat to the patient's safety. For example, any administration of naloxone is an indicator that one or more undesirable side effects of opiates may be present. Although naloxone may temporarily reverse these side effects, they can recur as the antagonist effects wane. A more focused evaluation by the MET may avoid the undesirable consequences of these events. Models of activation criteria and event triggers are presented in **Table A1-3.**

Table A1-3	Models of Activation Criteria

Acute Physiologic Criteria

Acute change in heart rate to <40 or >130 beats/min
Acute change in systolic blood pressure to <90 mm Hg
Acute change in urine output to <50 mL in 4 hours
Acute change in respiratory rate <8 or >30 breaths/min
Acute change in pulse oximetry to <90% despite oxygen administration
Acute change in consciousness
Qualitative deterioration in clinical status

Organ System–Specific Criteria

Airway
   Respiratory distress
   Threatened airway

Breathing
   Respiratory rate >30 breaths/min
   Respiratory rate <6 breaths/min
   SpO_2 <90% on oxygen
   Difficulty speaking

Circulation
   Blood pressure <90 mm Hg despite treatment
   Pulse rate >130 beats/min

Neurology
   Any unexplained decrease in consciousness
   New agitation or delirium
   Repeated or prolonged seizures

Other
   Concern about the patient
   Uncontrolled pain
   Failure to respond to treatment
   Inability to obtain prompt assistance

Event Trigger

Unscheduled naloxone dose administered
Increase in oxygen requirement
  Any change to a 100% reservoir face mask
  Any change in FiO_2 delivery by ≥20%
After 3 unanswered pages to medical/surgical team for any patient in a shift
Response time to medical/surgical team page >30 min
Family concern about patient status
Any falls or traumatic injuries
Pain score ≥4 of 10 more than 30 min after highest ordered dose of analgesic
Persistent nausea/vomiting more than 30 min after highest dose of antiemetic
Any newly noted abnormal pulse

B. Medical Emergency Team Scoring Systems

The use of a scoring system in evaluating the at-risk patient can provide a graded assessment of clinical status and help to determine the level of response needed. An overall score is calculated based on the aggregate of points assigned to various symptoms, vital signs, and laboratory studies. Additional points are assigned to results that vary more greatly from normal. The Modified Early Warning Score (**Table A1-4**), which evaluates vital signs and mental status, has been validated in hospitalized medical patients. A score of 5 or greater has been associated with an increased mortality rate and increased admission to the ICU.

Individual MET programs may choose to define absolute value or trend thresholds that trigger a move to a higher level of care or mobilization of additional clinical resources. Collection and analysis of aggregate scores in patients receiving MET services can be used for quality improvement efforts, such as evaluation of standing orders, event cluster identification, and resource utilization.

Table A1-4.	Modified Early Warning Score						
				Points			
Indicator	**3**	**2**	**1**	**0**	**1**	**2**	**3**
Systolic blood pressure (mm Hg)	<70	71-80	81-100	101-199		≥ 200	
Heart rate (beats/min)		<40	41-50	51-100	101-110	111-129	≥ 130
Respiratory rate (breaths/min)		<9		9-14	15-20	21-29	≥ 30
Temperature (C)		<35		35-38.4		≥ 38.5	
AVPU score				**A**lert	Reacting to **V**oice	Reacting to **P**ain	**U**nresponsive

Subbe CP, Kruger M, Rutherford P, Gemmel L. Validation of a modified Early Warning Score in medical admissions. *QJM.* 2001;94:521-526.

IV. MEDICAL EMERGENCY TEAM RESPONSE

A. Medical Emergency Team Interventions

Interventions by the team should be aimed at rapidly stabilizing the patient and preventing further deterioration or full arrest. Studies have shown that the 3 most common reasons for activating a MET are hypoxemia, hypotension, and altered mental status. METs should identify the primary activating events in their facilities and build protocols to address each rapidly. Respiratory distress is the leading physiologic cause of MET activation. The reasons for acute changes can be related to fluid status, medications such as narcotics, progression of underlying disease, or patient noncompliance with physician-ordered oxygen therapies. Initial treatment is stabilization of the airway and application of high-flow oxygen to relieve the patient's distress and improve oxygen saturation. Following improvement in patient status, the team can evaluate for potential reversible causes.

Hypotension is a frequent physiologic cause of MET activation and can be related to volume status (both overall volume and blood volume); medications, including narcotics and antihypertensives; and the potential for sepsis. Initial treatment is administration of fluids to raise systolic pressure and/or immediate reversal of a known cause, such as narcotics.

Altered mental status, another common physiologic trigger of MET activation, is most often associated with hypoxemia, hypotension, or hypoglycemia. These should be evaluated and treated first. Altered mental status unrelated to those issues should be evaluated for either neurologic or medication causes, and treatment, including evaluation with CT scanning, should be guided accordingly.

METs should make every effort to involve the patient's primary physician and rounding team in decisions regarding disposition and care. The role of a MET is not to take the place of the primary team but to act for them at the bedside in an emergency.

B. Medical Emergency Team Communications

In the complex hospital environment, the use of a structured communication tool and a common critical language fosters the open communication between caregivers that is essential to the prompt evaluation and management of the at-risk patient. Incorporating the Situation, Background, Assessment, and Recommendation (SBAR) tool into MET documentation can facilitate effective communication by gathering all pertinent data in one place for any discussions to follow. This tool has proven to be most valuable in the effective communication of critical information.

SBAR Communication Tool

Situation: *What is happening with the patient?*

Background: *What is the clinical background or context?*

Assessment: *What do I think is the problem?*

Recommendation/interventions: *What would I do to evaluate and correct it?*

C. Medical Emergency Team Education

One of the primary goals of METs is education. The detection limb of the MET model relies heavily on the early recognition of signs and symptoms of clinical deterioration. Regularly scheduled staff in-services and mock-event drills are effective in maintaining competencies in identifying the at-risk patient. Public posting and discussion of activation criteria can further enhance the use of MET services and reduce patient clinical crises. Review of aggregate quality improvement data from MET activity also can reinforce education. Post hoc review of a patient event with the entire ward staff after a MET call serves to raise the entire group's collective knowledge and skill. This may help reduce the likelihood of subsequent problems and increase the likelihood that signs and symptoms of clinical deterioration will be detected at the earliest indication in future patients. Topic-of-the-week presentations, MET case reviews, and SBAR practice sessions are examples of targeted educational activities.

V. SUMMARY

Hospitalized patients can be at risk for clinical deterioration in part due to the complex nature of healthcare delivery systems. The goal of the MET model is to identify and manage signs and symptoms of clinical deterioration in at-risk patients through detection strategies at the bedside and mobilization of appropriate resources. Important factors in the successful implementation of MET include: (1) appropriate team composition; (2) activation criteria based on bedside staff concern, acute changes in physiology, or the use of scoring systems to identify at-risk patients; (3) interventions aimed at rapidly stabilizing the patient; (4) effective communication strategies like SBAR; (5) ongoing education to enhance detection and management of potential clinical crises; (6) availability of appropriate advanced clinical monitors, equipment, and medications to conduct MET activities; and (7) evaluation and correction of processes and causes that may put patients at risk.

Suggested Readings

1. Bellomo R, Goldsmith D, Uchino S, et al. A prospective before-and-after trial of a medical emergency team. *Med J Aust.* 2003;179:283-287.

2. Bristow PJ, Hillman KM, Chey T, et al. Rates of in-hospital arrests, deaths and intensive care admissions: the effects of a medical emergency team. *Med J Aust.* 2000;173:236-240.

3. Buist MD, Moore GE, Bernard SA, Waxman BP, Anderson JN, Nguyen TV. Effects of a medical emergency team on reduction of incidence of and mortality from unexpected cardiac arrests in hospital: preliminary study. *BMJ.* 2002;324:387-390.

4. DeVita MA, Bellomo R, Hillman K, et al. Findings of the First Consensus Conference on Medical Emergency Teams. *Crit Care Med.* 2006;9:2463-2478.

5. DeVita MA, Hillman K, Bellomo R, eds. *Medical Emergency Teams: Implementation and Outcome Measurement.* New York, NY: Springer Science + Business Media Inc; 2006.

6. Leonard M, Graham S, Bonacum D. The human factor: the critical importance of effective teamwork and communication in providing safe care. *Qual Saf Health Care.* 2004;13(suppl 1):i85-i90.

7. Subbe CP, Kruger M, Rutherford P, Gemmel L. Validation of a modified Early Warning Score in medical admissions. *QJM.* 2001;94:521-526.

 Web Sites

1. http://www.metconference.com. International Conference on Medical Emergency Team Response. Downloadable files from the conference presentations.

2. http://www.IHI.org/IHI/Programs/Campaign. Information regarding the IHI 5 Million Lives Campaign to Improve Patient Safety that includes creation of a MET team.

ENDOTRACHEAL INTUBATION

I. INDICATIONS, PATIENT EVALUATION, MANUAL MASK VENTILATION, PATIENT PREPARATION

See Chapter 2

II. EQUIPMENT

A. Bag-mask resuscitation unit with oxygen supplementation (with positive end-expiratory pressure valve if indicated)
B. Topical anesthetic spray
C. Medications as selected for analgesia/anesthesia, amnesia, and neuromuscular blockade
D. Towel roll or pad for occipital elevation
E. Pulse oximeter
F. Electrocardiography monitor
G. Automatic blood pressure device or frequent manual blood pressure monitoring
H. Gloves, mask, eye protection
I. Laryngoscope handle and blade(s): usually sizes #3 and #4 curved, #2 and #3 straight
J. Endotracheal tubes: usually 7.0- or 7.5-mm for adult women and 8.0-mm for adult men
K. Malleable stylet
L. Yankauer and tracheal suction catheters, suction device
M. Magill forceps
N. 10-mL syringe to inflate cuff
O. Water-soluble lubricant
P. Qualitative CO_2 detector, CO_2 monitor, or esophageal detector device
Q. Tape or tracheal tube stabilization device
R. Resuscitation cart

III. ROUTE OF INTUBATION

A. Orotracheal intubation via direct laryngoscopy

This route is generally favored in most circumstances, including when cervical spine injury is suspected.

B. Blind nasotracheal intubation

The nasotracheal route using a blind approach can only be attempted in a spontaneously breathing patient and may be favored by experienced operators in selected patients and situations. This technique has the advantage of allowing continued spontaneous ventilation and generally requires less sedation than direct laryngoscopy. It is more time-consuming than direct laryngoscopy and therefore is less useful in emergent intubation. Endotracheal tubes used for nasotracheal intubation have smaller diameters than those used for orotracheal intubation. Nasotracheal intubation should be avoided if basilar skull fracture is suspected and in the presence of coagulopathy. Nasotracheal intubation is discouraged in infants and small children due to anatomic differences from adults.

IV. OROTRACHEAL INTUBATION

A. Preparation

1. Don gloves, mask, and eye protection for universal precautions.
2. Explain the procedure, if patient is conscious.
3. Assure patent airway and optimal oxygenation and ventilation (**Chapter 2**).
4. Assure intravenous access.
5. Apply pulse oximeter, electrocardiography and blood pressure devices.
6. Assemble all equipment and ensure proper working order.
7. Prepare the endotracheal tube.
    a. Check cuff integrity by inflating and fully deflating.
    b. Insert stylet into endotracheal tube, bend to predicted configuration to assist glottic entry. Ensure the distal tip of the stylet does not protrude past the end of the endotracheal tube.
    c. Apply water-soluble lubricant to the cuff end of the tube.
8. Connect laryngoscope blade to handle.
    a. Select blade type (operator's choice).
        1. Straight blade — used to elevate the epiglottis anteriorly
        2. Curved blade — inserted into the vallecula
    b. Select blade length — #3 blade is proper unless patient's neck is very long.
    c. Assure that light is sufficiently bright.
9. Place pad or towel under occiput if cervical spine injury is not suspected.
10. Use topical anesthetic on the patient's oropharynx.
11. Preoxygenate with 100% oxygen for 2 to 3 minutes if time permits.
12. As necessary, proceed with sedation and neuromuscular blockade (**Chapter 2**).

B. Technique
    1. The operator stands at the head of the bed, and the bed is raised to a position of comfort for the operator. The head of the bed may be flat or raised slightly per operator preference.
    2. When no cervical injury is suspected, a small pad is placed under the occiput (the "sniffing" position) and the neck is gently extended (**Figure A2-1**). When cervical spine injury is possible, these steps are omitted, the neck is stabilized by an assistant (as described in **Chapter 2**), and the anterior portion of the cervical collar is removed.

Figure A2-1. Positioning for Orotracheal Intubation

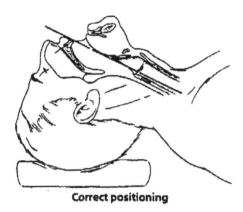

Correct positioning

To visualize the trachea, the axial planes of the oral, pharyngeal, and tracheal axes must be aligned. This alignment can be accomplished by flexing the neck at the level of the cervical spine and extending the head at the atlanto-occipital joint. Illustration © by Robert Margulies and reproduced with permission from the artist and *The Journal of Critical Illness.*

    3. Regardless of the operator's dominant hand in other contexts, the laryngoscope is always held in the left hand.
    4. Cricoid pressure should be gently but firmly applied by an assistant as soon as consciousness is lost and should be sustained until endotracheal tube placement is confirmed and the cuff inflated.
    5. Mouth opening in the sedated/relaxed patient may be assisted by a cross-finger technique wherein the thumb of the right hand is placed on the front lower teeth of the mandible and the first finger on the front upper teeth (maxilla). The mouth is gently opened by a "reverse scissor" movement of the fingers and the laryngoscope is introduced into the mouth.
    6. The tip of laryngoscope blade is inserted into the right side of the patient's mouth (**Figure A2-2**); the blade is advanced to the base of the tongue.
    7. The tongue should be swept to the left; proper tongue control is key to laryngeal visualization.
    8. The blade is gently advanced further to its proper position. A straight blade is placed beneath the epiglottis; a curved blade is placed into the vallecula above the epiglottis.
    9. Caution! Traction should be applied only along the long axis of the laryngoscope handle as the laryngoscope lifts the tongue upward away from the larynx, revealing the glottic opening. A rocking or rotating motion of the blade and handle may damage teeth, gingiva, or lips. The base of the laryngoscope blade should never contact the upper teeth!
    10. The vocal cords and glottic opening should be visualized.

Figure A2-2. Insertion of Laryngoscope

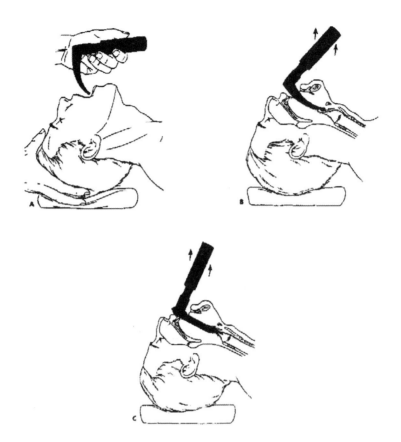

(A) The blade of the laryngoscope is inserted into the patient's mouth and pushes the tongue to the left. (B) The straight blade is inserted beneath the epiglottis, and (C) the curved blade follows the base of the tongue and is inserted into the vallecula. Illustration © by Robert Margulies and reproduced with permission from the artist and *The Journal of Critical Illness.*

11. If the vocal cords and glottis cannot be visualized, it may be helpful for an assistant to grasp the thyroid cartilage between the thumb and index finger and exert pressure in the following sequence: Pressure is applied backward against the cervical vertebrae and then in an upward direction to shift the larynx superiorly. Additional pressure is applied to shift the thyroid cartilage no more than 2 cm to the right side of the patient's neck. This procedure can be remembered by the acronym "BURP" (backward, upward, and rightward pressure on the thyroid cartilage).

12. The endotracheal tube is inserted gently through the vocal cords (**Figure A2-3**), holding the tube/stylet with the right hand. The stylet, if angled, may interfere with passage of the tube into the trachea. If resistance is encountered as the tube is advanced, consider having an assistant remove the stylet while the operator holds the endotracheal tube firmly in the glottic opening.

13. The stylet and laryngoscope should be removed carefully (**Figure A2-3**). The operator must continue to firmly hold the endotracheal tube and position it such that the external centimeter length markers on the tube show 21 cm (female) or 23 cm (male) adjacent to the front teeth.

14. The cuff is inflated.

Figure A2-3. Placement of Endotracheal Tube

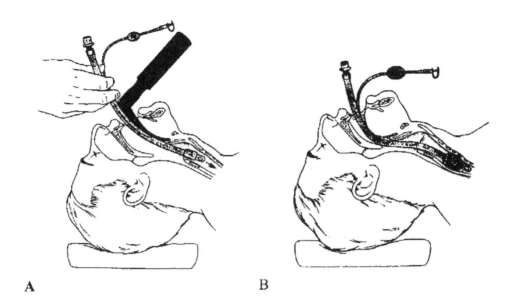

A   **B**

(A) The endotracheal tube is inserted through the vocal cords until the distal end rests approximately 2 to 3 cm above the carina. (B) Once the endotracheal tube is in proper position, the laryngoscope and stylet are removed and the cuff is inflated. Illustration © by Robert Margulies and reproduced with permission from the artist and *The Journal of Critical Illness.*

15. To ensure proper position of the tube:
    a. Auscultate the epigastrium; inspect and auscultate chest to assure equal bilateral gas entry.
    b. Use qualitative CO_2 detector or monitor or esophageal detector device. Lack of color change with a qualitative CO_2 detector or low exhaled CO_2 measurement may occur with a correctly placed tracheal tube in the patient with poor pulmonary perfusion such as during cardiac arrest or profound hypotension.
    c. Observe for condensation in the endotracheal tube during exhalation,
    d. Listen for breath sounds through the endotracheal tube as the patient is breathing spontaneously,
    e. Obtain chest radiograph (tube tip 2 to 3 cm above carina),
16. Secure endotracheal tube with tape or endotracheal tube stabilization device.

V. BLIND NASOTRACHEAL INTUBATION

A. Preparation

    1. See IV A, preparation for orotracheal intubation, steps 1-8.

    2. Position the patient's head on a small towel with the neck in a slightly extended position.

    3. Preoxygenate with 100% oxygen for 2 to 3 minutes if time permits.

    4. Use topical anesthetic on the nasal passages and pharynx and lubricate the nasal passages.

B. Technique

    1. The operator stands at the head of the bed, and the bed is raised to a position of comfort for the operator. The head of the bed may be flat or raised slightly per operator preference. The patient should have spontaneous ventilation and an adequate tidal volume.

    2. The larger naris should be used if there is significant deviation of the nasal septum.

    3. A well-lubricated endotracheal tube without a stylet is inserted gently through the nasal passage into the posterior oropharynx.

    4. Oxygen may be administered by face mask/blowby or by intermittently connecting the oxygen source to the endotracheal tube.

    5. The oropharynx should be inspected to assure that the endotracheal tube is in the midline.

    6. The amount of air movement at the endotracheal tube connector is assessed by either listening to air movement through the tube, using a specially designed "whistle," or using an exhaled CO_2 monitor.

    7. The endotracheal tube is advanced slowly while feeling and listening for air movement at the connector end of the endotracheal tube. Advancement continues if air movement increases through the tube. If air movement decreases, the endotracheal tube should be withdrawn until air movement resumes, re-advancing after repositioning the head.

    8. Advancing the tube through the glottis is usually easier during inspiration.

    9. The operator must continue to firmly hold the endotracheal tube and position it such that the external centimeter length markers on the tube show approximately 24 cm (female) or 26 cm (male) adjacent to the naris.

    10. The cuff is inflated.

    11. To ensure proper position of the tube:

        a. Auscultate epigastrium; inspect and auscultate chest to assure equal bilateral gas entry.

        b. Use qualitative CO_2 detector or monitor or esophageal detector device. Lack of color change with a qualitative CO_2 detector or low exhaled CO_2 measurement may occur with a correctly placed endotracheal tube in the patient with poor pulmonary perfusion.

        c. Observe for condensation in the endotracheal tube during exhalation.

        d. Listen for breath sounds through the endotracheal tube as the patient is breathing spontaneously.

        e. Obtain chest radiograph (tube tip 2 to 3 cm above carina).

    12. The endotracheal tube is secured with tape or endotracheal tube stabilization device.

VI. PEDIATRIC CONSIDERATIONS

A. Anatomic differences between adults and children
> 1. The larynx is more cephalad in infants than in adults, making it appear more anterior and resulting in a more difficult visualization during laryngoscopy.
> 2. Cricoid pressure is valuable during laryngoscopy because of the position of the larynx and assists in preventing aspiration.
> 3. In young children, the narrowest part of the airway is at the level of the cricoid cartilage, not at the larynx, making an anatomic "cuff" below the vocal cords.
> 4. In general, the diameter of the small finger approximates the properly sized endotracheal tube. A full-term neonate can accept a tube with 3.5-mm internal diameter.
> 5. Cuffed tubes therefore are usually limited to use in children >8 years old (endotracheal tube size >6.0-mm internal diameter); uncuffed tubes are generally used in younger children.

B. Technique differences between adults and children
> 1. Head position: a towel roll under the head is often needed in adults to achieve the sniffing position; a shoulder roll is usually needed to achieve this position in infants.
> 2. Laryngoscope blade selection: operator may choose a straight or curved blade; however, most clinicians do not use curved blades in infants. A common mistake in intubating a child is choosing a blade that is too small. The blade must be long enough to reach the epiglottis.
> 3. Proper depth of insertion in centimeters can be estimated by multiplying the internal diameter of the endotracheal tube by 3 (eg, internal diameter = 4.0; depth of insertion = $4.0 \times 3 = 12.0$ cm).
> 4. Appropriately sized equipment (eg, face mask, laryngoscope, endotracheal tube, suction catheter) should be used.

VII. PRECAUTIONS/COMPLICATIONS

A. Hypoxia, hypercapnia during procedure
B. Cardiovascular compromise during and immediately after procedure
C. Damaged teeth, lips, gingiva
D. Malpositioned tube (esophagus, right main-stem bronchus)
E. Pharyngeal, laryngeal, tracheal damage
F. Gastric distension and aspiration of gastric contents
G. Bronchospasm
H. Pneumothorax

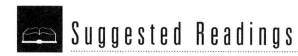 Suggested Readings

1. Balk RA. The technique of orotracheal intubation. *J Crit Ill.* 1997;12:316-323.

2. Knill RL. Difficult laryngoscopy made easy with a "BURP." *Can J Anaesth.* 1993;40:279-282.

3. Popovich MJ, Hoffman WD. Endotracheal intubation. In: Parrillo JE, ed. *Current Therapy in Critical Care Medicine.* St. Louis, MO: CV Mosby; 1997:8.

4. Thompson AE. Pediatric airway management. In: Fuhrman BP, Zimmerman JJ, eds. *Pediatric Critical Care.* 3rd ed. St. Louis, MO: CV Mosby; 2006:485.

AIRWAY ADJUNCTS

I. LARYNGEAL MASK AIRWAY (LMA)

A. Indications

    1. Provide an airway and ventilation when bag-mask ventilation is difficult

    2. Provide a temporizing airway when endotracheal intubation is unsuccessful

B. Equipment

    1. Bag-mask resuscitation unit with oxygen supplementation

    2. Pulse oximeter

    3. Electrocardiographic monitor

    4. Blood pressure monitoring

    5. Gloves, mask, eye protection

    6. Laryngeal mask airway of appropriate size (**Table A3-1**)

    7. Syringe for cuff inflation

    8. Water-soluble lubricant

    9. Qualitative CO_2 detector or CO_2 monitor

    10. Resuscitation cart

Table A3-1. Laryngeal Mask Airway Size and Cuff Inflation

LMA Size	Patient Size	Maximum Cuff Volume	Largest ETT ID (mm)*
1	Neonate/infant to 5 kg	Up to 4 mL	3.5
1.5	5-10 kg	Up to 7 mL	4.0
2	10-20 kg	Up to 10 mL	4.5
2.5	20-30 kg	Up to 14 mL	5.0
3	>30 kg/small adult	Up to 20 mL	6.0 cuffed
4	Average adult	Up to 30 mL	6.0 cuffed
5	Large adult	Up to 40 mL	7.0 cuffed

* Largest endotracheal tube size (ETT ID) that will fit through LMA tube lumen.

C. Preparation for insertion
    1. Don gloves, mask, eye protection
    2. Assure patent airway and optimal oxygenation and ventilation
    3. Assure IV access
    4. Apply pulse oximeter, electrocardiographic and blood pressure monitor
    5. Select appropriate size LMA
    6. Check cuff integrity by inflating and fully deflating
    7. Lubricate only the posterior aspect of the deflated mask with a water-based lubricant
    8. Preoxygenate with 100% oxygen for 2 to 3 minutes if time permits

D. Technique (**Figure A3-1**)
    1. The cuff is deflated completely so that it forms a spoon shape and there are no folds in the mask.
    2. The operator stands behind the head of the bed, and the bed is raised to a position of comfort for the operator.
    3. The patient is placed in the sniffing position (ie, head extended, neck flexed), unless potential or definite cervical spine injury prevents neck extension.
    4. Cricoid pressure is not recommended during placement of the LMA because it may interfere with correct placement.
    5. The mask is positioned with the bowl facing anteriorly. Hold the device like a pencil, with the index finger of the dominant hand at the junction of the bowl and tube, pressing against the palate and pharyngeal wall with the index finger.
    6. The cuff is inserted into the hypopharynx until definite resistance is felt.
    7. Without the operator holding the device, the cuff is inflated with enough air to obtain a seal around the laryngeal inlet. This step results in an outward movement of the tube.
    8. The cuff is inflated with enough air to obtain a seal (intracuff pressure of approximately 60 cm H_2O. Maximum volumes are listed in **Table A3-1**, but lesser volume may provide an adequate seal.
    9. A manual ventilation device is attached, and chest movement and breath sounds are verified in both lung fields. Correct position should be confirmed with a qualitative or quantitative end-tidal CO_2 detector.
    10. If chest movement is inadequate, or if a large air leak is present, the device should be removed and reinserted.
    11. When the LMA is positioned appropriately, the tube is secured with tape.

Figure A3-1. Insertion technique for laryngeal mask airway

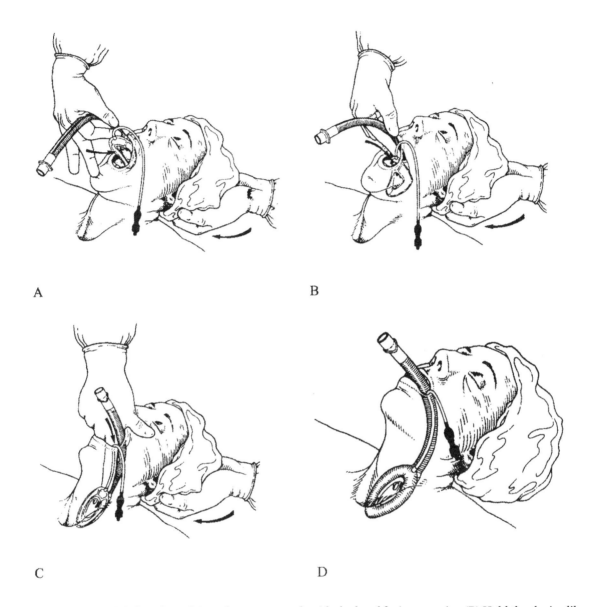

A

B

C

D

A) Insert lubricated and deflated mask into the open mouth with the bowl facing anterior. (B) Hold the device like a pencil, pressing against the palate and pharyngeal wall with the index finger. (C) Continue inserting the cuff behind the tongue into the hypopharynx until finite resistance is felt. (D) Without holding the device, inflate cuff with enough air to obtain a seal. Attach manual ventilation device and ensure chest movement. Adapted from Brain AIJ. *The Intravent Laryngeal Mask Instruction Manual.* Berkshire, UK: Brain Medical, 1992.

II. ESOPHAGEAL-TRACHEAL DOUBLE-LUMEN AIRWAY DEVICE

A. Indications
    1. Cardiorespiratory arrest and inability to provide an airway by other means

B. Equipment
    1. Bag-mask resuscitation unit with oxygen supplementation
    2. Pulse oximeter
    3. Electrocardiographic monitor
    4. Blood pressure monitoring
    5. Gloves, mask, eye protection
    6. Esophageal-tracheal double-lumen device
    7. Syringe for cuff inflation
    8. Water-soluble lubricant
    9. Qualitative CO_2 detector or CO_2 monitor
    10. Resuscitation cart

C. Preparation for insertion
    1. Don gloves, mask, eye protection
    2. Assure patent airway and optimal oxygenation and ventilation
    3. Assure IV access
    4. Apply pulse oximeter, electrocardiographic and blood pressure monitor
    5. Select appropriate size device
    6. Check integrity of both cuffs by inflating and fully deflating
    7. Preoxygenate with 100% oxygen for 2 to 3 minutes if time permits

D. Technique
    1. The cuffs should be deflated completely.
    2. The operator stands behind the head of the bed, and the bed is raised to a position of comfort for the operator.
    3. The patient is placed in a neutral or sniffing position (ie, head extended, neck flexed), unless potential or definite cervical spine injury prevents neck extension.
    4. The patient's tongue and jaw are grasped between the thumb and index finger, and the device is inserted blindly. It is advanced until the placement ring markers on the tube are positioned as indicated by the manufacturer. Do not force the tube if resistance is met. A laryngoscope can be used to assist with placement.
    5. The pharyngeal cuff is inflated first to seal the posterior pharynx.
    6. The distal cuff is then inflated.
    7. Ventilation should be attempted first through the pharyngeal lumen, and the chest should be auscultated for breath sounds and observed for movement. The tube enters the esophagus approximately 95% of the time.
    8. If breath sounds are absent, ventilation should be attempted through the tracheal lumen while auscultating for breath sounds.
    9. Use of the correct lumen for ventilation should be confirmed with a qualitative/ quantitative end-tidal CO_2 or esophageal detector device.
    10. When the device is positioned appropriately, the tube is secured with tape.

Suggested Readings

1. Danks RR, Danks B. Laryngeal mask airway: review of indications and use. *J Emerg Nurs.* 2004;30:30-35.

2. Krafft P, Schebesta K. Alternative management techniques for the difficult airway: esophageal-tracheal Combitube. *Curr Opin Anaesthesiol.* 2005;17:499-504.

3. Mace SE. The laryngeal mask airway: guidelines for appropriate usage. *Resid Staff Physician.* 2001;47:30.

Appendix 4:

ADVANCED LIFE SUPPORT ALGORITHM

Figure A4-1. Pulseless Arrest Algorithm

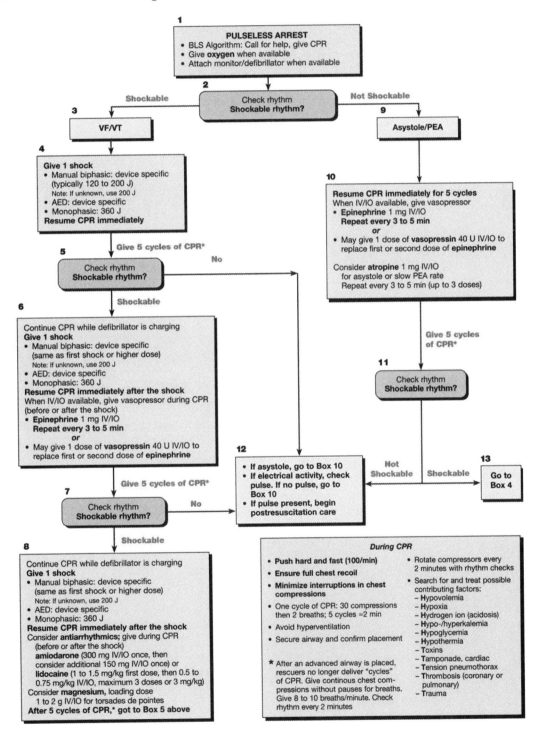

Reproduced with permission from The American Heart Association in Collaboration with the International Liaison Committee on Resuscitation (ILCOR): 2005 American Heart Association Guidelines for Cardiopulmonary Resuscitation and Emergency Cardiovascular Care. *Circulation* 2005;112:IV58-IV66.

Figure A4-2. Bradycardia Algorithm

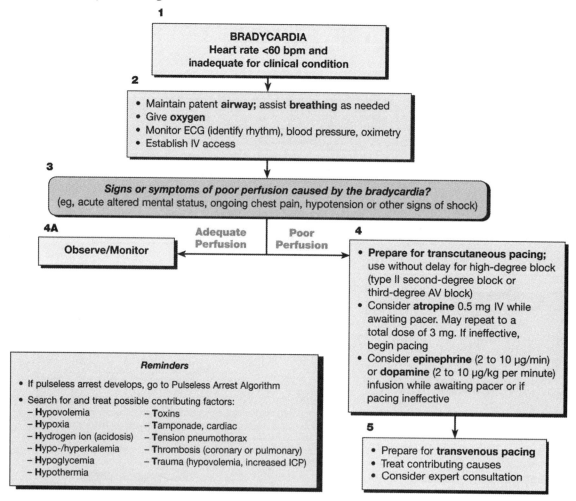

Reproduced with permission from The American Heart Association in Collaboration with the International Liaison Committee on Resuscitation (ILCOR): 2005 American Heart Association Guidelines for Cardiopulmonary Resuscitation and Emergency Cardiovascular Care. *Circulation* 2005;112:IV67-IV77.

Figure A4-3. Tachycardia Algorithm

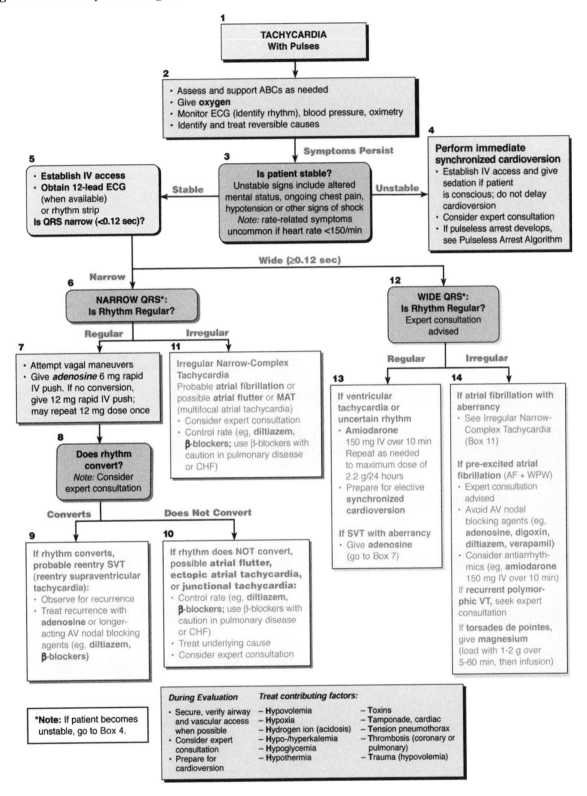

Reproduced with permission from The American Heart Association in Collaboration with the International Liaison Committee on Resuscitation (ILCOR): 2005 American Heart Association Guidelines for Cardiopulmonary Resuscitation and Emergency Cardiovascular Care. *Circulation* 2005;112:IV78-IV83.

Figure A4-4. Pediatric Pulseless Arrest Algorithm

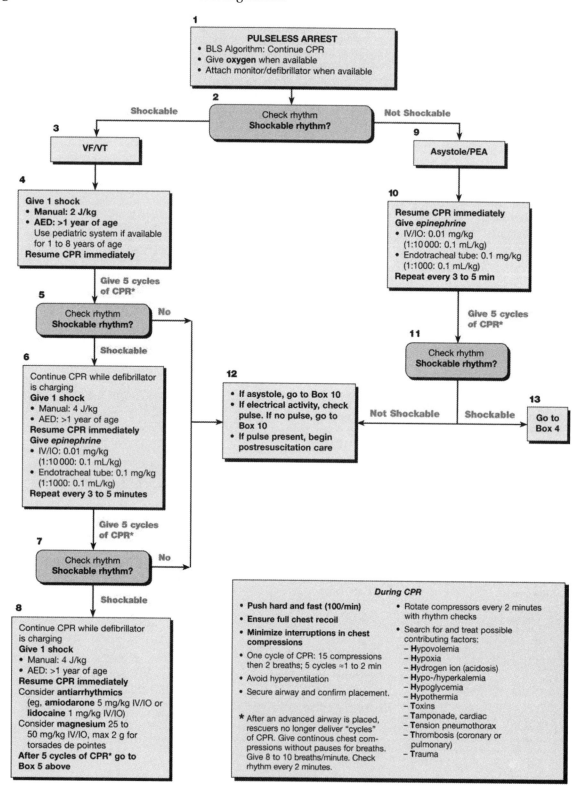

Reproduced with permission from The American Heart Association in Collaboration with the International Liaison Committee on Resuscitation (ILCOR): 2005 American Heart Association Guidelines for Cardiopulmonary Resuscitation and Emergency Cardiovascular Care. *Circulation* 2005;112: IV167-IV187.

Figure A4-5. Pediatric Bradycardia Algorithm

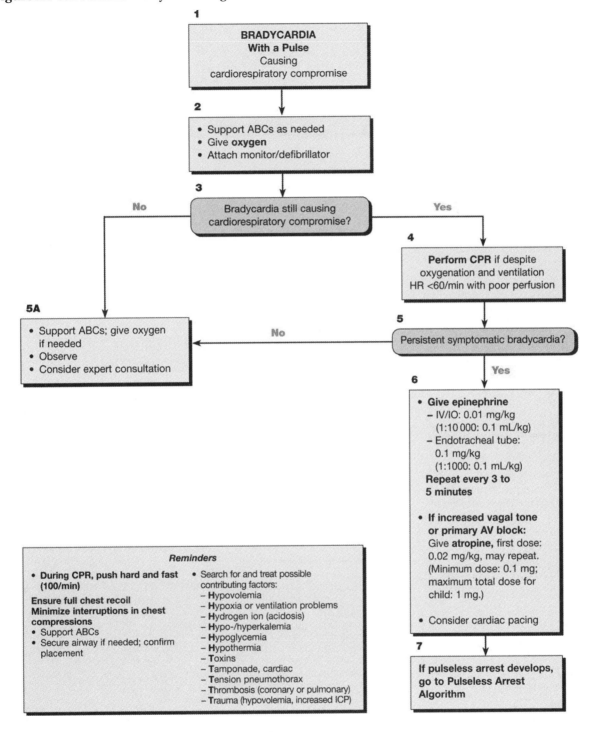

Figure A4-6. Pediatric Tachycardia Algorithm

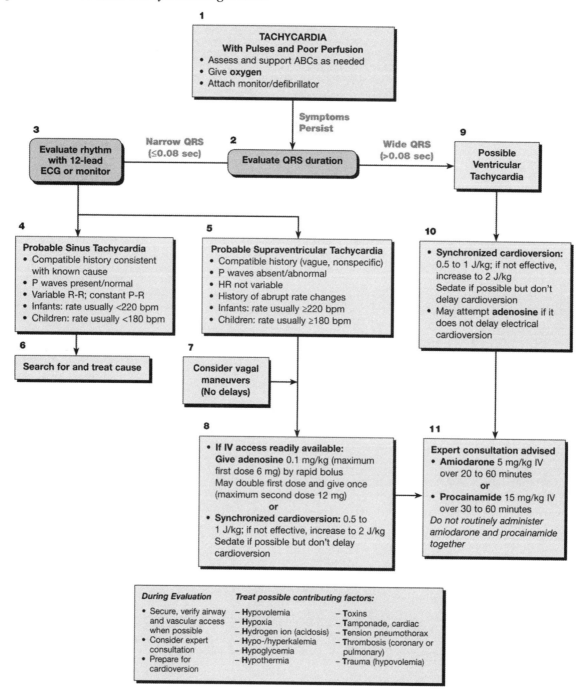

Reproduced with permission from The American Heart Association in Collaboration with the International Liaison Committee on Resuscitation (ILCOR): 2005 American Heart Association Guidelines for Cardiopulmonary Resuscitation and Emergency Cardiovascular Care. *Circulation* 2005;112: IV167-IV187.

DEFIBRILLATION/CARDIOVERSION

I. INDICATIONS

A. Defibrillation/unsynchronized cardioversion
1. Ventricular fibrillation
2. Pulseless ventricular tachycardia
3. Polymorphic ventricular tachycardia

B. Synchronized cardioversion
1. Unstable or stable ventricular tachycardia with a pulse
2. Unstable or stable supraventricular tachycardia, atrial fibrillation, or atrial flutter

II. EQUIPMENT

A. Conductive gel or self-adhesive defibrillation pads
B. Defibrillator/cardioverter
C. Connecting cable, leads, and electrodes
D. Medication for sedation
E. Supplemental oxygen with bag-mask oxygen delivery device
F. Emergency suction and intubation equipment
G. Pulse oximeter
H. Electrocardiography and blood pressure monitor
I. Intravenous catheter, infusion pump, tubing, fluids
J. Resuscitation cart

III. TECHNIQUE

A. Recognize cardiac rhythm, determine severity of its physiologic effect
B. In patients with unstable rhythms or adverse physiologic effects on systemic perfusion, begin immediate defibrillation/cardioversion, after initiation of cardiopulmonary resuscitation
C. Recognize that time delays under the above circumstances decrease the likelihood of conversion to a stable rhythm
D. Inform and prepare patient as clinical situation dictates; sedate if necessary
E. Assure intravenous access
F. Provide supplemental oxygen

G. Monitor pulse oximeter and electrocardiography

H. Turn on defibrillator/cardioverter

I. Attach monitoring electrodes (if needed)

J. Apply conductive gel to paddles or apply conductive pads to chest wall

    1. Male patients with a hirsute chest may require rapid shaving to ensure adequate contact

K. Paddle/electrode placement

    1. Anterolateral

        a. One paddle/electrode to right of upper sternum below clavicle

        b. One paddle/electrode to left of nipple with center in midaxillary line

    2. Anteroposterior

        a. One paddle/electrode anteriorly over left precordium, below clavicle

        b. One paddle/electrode posteriorly in left infrascapular location, left of thoracic spine

    3. Avoid placement over permanent pacer or implantable cardioverter-defibrillator

L. Paddle pressure (if used)

    1. Adult — approximately 25 lb of pressure to each paddle

    2. Pediatric — ensure good contact with chest wall

M. Activate appropriate switch for synchronized cardioversion or unsynchronized defibrillation

N. Set energy level of electrical discharge (in accordance with recommendations of the American Heart Association)

    1. Adult defibrillation

        a. Manual biphasic waveform device: energy level is device-specific (typically between 120 to 200 J). If unknown, use 200 J for initial shock. Subsequent shocks should be same or higher energy level as initial shock.

        b. Monophasic waveform device: 360 J, initial and subsequent shocks

    2. Adult cardioversion (synchronized)

        a. Ventricular tachycardia (stable): with monophasic device, 100 J for initial attempt and advance energy level as needed; with biphasic device, lower doses may be used (consult manufacturer).

        b. Polymorphic ventricular tachycardia: treat as ventricular fibrillation (see above).

        c. Atrial fibrillation: 100 J with monophasic device; 100 J to 120 J with biphasic device, or consult manufacturer. Escalate energy levels as needed for subsequent shocks.

        d. Atrial flutter: 50 J; if rhythm persists, advance energy levels as needed.

        e. Paroxysmal supraventricular tachycardia: 50 J; if rhythm persists, advance energy levels as needed.

        f. If delays in synchronization occur or conditions are critical, use immediate unsynchronized shocks (defibrillation mode).

O. Ensure electrical safety (all personnel clear of contact with the patient, bed, and equipment)

P. Charge capacitors through defibrillator/cardioverter

Q. Depress discharge button(s) on the device or simultaneously on the defibrillator/paddles (with synchronized cardioversion, the discharge buttons must remain depressed until the energy is released)

R. If defibrillation performed, immediately resume chest compressions; if cardioversion performed, assess patient (respiration, pulse, and rhythm)

S. If unsuccessful, repeat process, following standard Advanced Cardiovascular Life Support protocols

IV. PEDIATRIC CONSIDERATIONS

A. Manual Defibrillator
1. Appropriate paddle size is important; use the largest paddle size possible, assuring good chest contact over its entire area and good separation between the two paddles (about 3 cm)
    a. Infants (< 10 kg) — 4.5-cm paddles usually used
    b. Children (>10 kg) — 8.0- to 13-cm paddles usually used
2. Paddle placement is similar to that for adults
3. Be sure that the defibrillator/cardioverter provides a low-dose range for infants. Some defibrillators do not go below 10 joules and therefore should not be used for converting infants/children weight <20 kg (5 to 6 yrs of age)
4. Pediatric defibrillation
    a. 2 joules/kg (initial)
    b. Advance to 4 J/kg if rhythm persists
    c. Use adult energy levels in children ≥ 50 kg
5. Pediatric cardioversion
    a. Stable or unstable ventricular tachycardia: 0.5 to 1.0 J/kg
    b. Stable or unstable supraventricular tachycardia: 0.5 to 1.0 J/kg
    c. Advance to 2 J/kg if unsuccessful
B. AED (Automatic external defibrillator)
1. > 25 kg (8 years old): Use standard adult AED with adult pad-cable system
2. < 25 kg (>1 year old but < 8 years old): Use attenuated dose if a pediatric system is available. Use adult system if pediatric system is not available
3. < 1 year old. There is currently insufficient evidence to recommend for or against the use of an AED

V. PRECAUTIONS/COMPLICATIONS

A. During procedure
1. Skin burn may occur if insufficient gel or improper pads are used, poor contact with the chest wall occurs during discharge, or if the pads/paddles are too close to each other.
2. All metal objects should be removed from the patient to avoid skin burns.
3. Patient's environment and chest must be dry to avoid current traveling across water, resulting in a decreased amount of delivered energy.
4. Transdermal patches should be removed as they may impede transmission of current.
5. Medical personnel may sustain electrical shock or burn if safety precautions are not followed.
B. After procedure
1. Arterial embolization
2. Pulmonary edema
3. Postcardioversion arrhythmias; be prepared to institute cardiopulmonary resuscitation
4. Post-shock syndrome (myocardial damage)

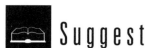 Suggested Readings

1. American Heart Association. *Advanced Cardiovascular Life Support: Provider Manual.* Dallas, TX: American Heart Association; 2006.

2. 2005 American Heart Association Guidelines for Cardiopulmonary Resuscitation and Emergency Cardiovascular Care. Electrical Therapies: Automated external defibrillators, defibrillation, cardioversion, and pacing. *Circulation.* 2005;112(suppl IV):IV-35-IV-46. Available at www.circulationaha.org

3. Wiegand D, Carlson, K. *AACN Procedure Manual for Critical Care.* 5th ed. St. Louis, MO: Elsevier Saunders; 2005.

INTRAOSSEOUS NEEDLE INSERTION

I. INDICATIONS

A. Emergency vascular access in children and adults if intravenous access is delayed

B. Any fluid or medication that can be given intravenously can be given by the intraosseous route in the same dosages

II. EQUIPMENT

A. Conductive gel or self-adhesive defibrillation pads
B. Sternal or iliac bone marrow aspiration needle (15- to 18-gauge) or disposable intraosseous needle
C. Sterile syringes and infiltrating needles
D. Sterile 4 × 4 gauze sponges
E. Medication for local anesthesia
F. Gloves, sterile drapes
G. Skin disinfectant
H. Supplemental oxygen
I. Pulse oximeter
J. Electrocardiography monitor
K. Intravenous tubing, T-connector, and fluid

III. SITE SELECTION

A. Young children
    1. In neonates, proximal tibia, just below the growth plate, distal to the tibial tubercle; in infants 6 to 12 months old, insert 1 cm distal to tibial tuberosity; in children > 1 year of age, insert 2 cm distal to the tibial tuberosity
B. Adults
    1. Sternum
    2. Distal tibia above the medial malleolus
    3. Lateral or medial malleolus
    4. Distal radius and distal ulna
    5. Distal femur
    6. Anterior-superior iliac spine

IV. TECHNIQUE (TIBIAL SITE)

A. Apply oxygen, monitor pulse oximeter and electrocardiography
B. Restrain leg with a small sandbag or intravenous fluid bag behind the knee for support
C. Create sterile field
D. Infiltrate local anesthetic if clinical situation permits
E. Use proximal anterior tibia, midpoint of the medial flat surface, 1 to 3 cm below the tibial tuberosity (**Figure A6-1**)
F. Insert the needle at 60° to 90° to the skin away from the growth plate; advance with a screwing motion
G. Use the distal tibia only if the proximal tibia is impenetrable (just proximal to the medial malleolus and posterior to the saphenous vein)

Figure A6-1. Intraosseus Needle Insertion

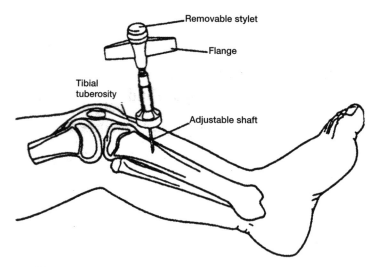

Approach to puncture of the proximal anterior tibia. Reprinted with permission from Fiser HD. Intraosseous infusion.. *N Engl J Med* 1990; 322:1579-1581.

H. Confirm entry into the marrow space by noting a lack of resistance after the needle has passed through the cortex

I. Aspirate marrow into the syringe; this should be accomplished easily, but failure to do so does not necessarily indicate improper placement

J. Infuse fluids; fluids should flow freely

K. Secure needle by taping flanges to the skin (may require support of external portion of the needle)

L. Consider flushing with heparin-saline solution

M. Infuse intravenous fluids

N. Observe for infiltration of fluids

O. Continue attempts to place intravenous catheter(s)

P. Discontinue intraosseous infusion and withdraw needle after intravenous access is established (preferably within 1 to 2 hours)

Q. Apply pressure to puncture site for approximately 5 minutes

R. Apply sterile dressing

V. PRECAUTIONS/COMPLICATIONS

A. Inability to place needle (approximately 20% of patients)

B. Subcutaneous and/or subperiosteal infiltration of fluid

C. Tibial fracture

D. Compartment syndrome

E. Clotting of marrow within the needle

F. Cellulitis, subcutaneous abscess

G. Osteomyelitis (0.6%)

H. Pain (usually minor))

 Suggested Readings

1. 2005 American Heart Association Guidelines for Cardiopulmonary Resuscitation and Emergency Cardiovascular Care: Pediatric advanced life support. *Circulation*. 2005;112: IV-167--IV187. Available at www.circulationaha.org.

2. Fiser HD. Intraosseous infusion. *N Engl J Med*. 1990;322:1579-1581.

3. Fiorito BA, Mirza F, Doran TM, et al. Intraosseous access in the setting of pediatric critical care transport. *Pediatr Crit Care Med*. 2005;6:50-53..

4. The International Liaison Committee on Resuscitation (ILCOR) consensus on science with treatment recommendations for pediatric and neonatal patients: Pediatric basic and advanced Life support: *Pediatrics*. 2006;117:e955-e977.

Temporary Transcutaneous Cardiac Pacing

I. INDICATIONS/CONTRAINDICATIONS

A. Indications
  1. Symptomatic bradycardia (hypotension, chest pain, syncope, altered mental status, heart failure, etc) unresponsive to pharmacologic management
  2. Overdrive pacing of tachycardias, refractory to drug therapy or electrical cardioversion
B. Contraindications
  1. Severe hypothermia
  2. Not recommended for asystole

II. EQUIPMENT

A. Cardiac pacing electrode pads
B. Pulse generator
C. Connecting leads
D. Medication for sedation and/or analgesia, if necessary
E. Supplemental oxygen (cannula, mask, other as necessary)
F. Pulse oximeter
G. Electrocardiography monitor
H. Intravenous catheter, tubing, fluids
I. Resuscitation cart

III. TECHNIQUE

A. Recognize cardiac rhythm, determine severity
B. Prepare patient
C. Obtain intravenous access if not done previously
D. Apply oxygen; monitor pulse oximeter and electrocardiogram
E. Attempt pharmacologic management, including atropine, epinephrine, and/or dopamine when appropriate (follow Advanced Cardiovascular Life Support guidelines)
F. Assemble equipment

G. Apply electrode pads

    1. Anteroposterior

        a. One electrode anteriorly over left precordium as close as possible to maximal cardiac impulse, below clavicle

        b. One electrode posteriorly in left infrascapular location directly behind anterior electrode, left of thoracic spine

    2. Anterolateral

        a. One electrode to right of upper sternum below clavicle

        b. One electrode to left of nipple with center in midaxillary line

    3. Shaving of excessive body hair may be required to ensure good contact

H. Administer sedation or analgesia as necessary and tolerated by patient

I. Connect leads to pulse generator

J. Turn on pulse generator and monitor

K. Set rate at 60 to 100 beats/min; adjust as needed, based on clinical response

L. Adjust pulse generator output (mA) upward until electrical and mechanical ventricular capture (threshold) occurs (usually 20 to 60 mA). Set output 2 mA above threshold to allow for safety margin. In the setting of severe symptoms or bradyasystolic arrest, it may be appropriate to start at the maximal output and then decrease if capture is achieved.

M. Criteria for proper electrical capture

    1. Pacer spike followed by a ventricular complex 100% of the time

    2. Wide QRS complex

    3. T-wave in an opposite deflection from baseline as the QRS complex

N. Assess efficacy of mechanical capture — obtain blood pressure and palpate pulse. Palpate pulse distal to carotid site as electrical stimulation from the pacemaker may mimic a carotid pulse.

O. Arrange for temporary or permanent transvenous pacemaker as necessary

IV. PEDIATRIC CONSIDERATIONS

A. Bradycardia in children is most often secondary to hypoxemia

B. Pacing for bradycardic rhythms secondary to hypoxemic insult may be considered after airway management, oxygenation, ventilation, chest compressions, epinephrine bolus (0.01 mg/kg, 1:1,000 concentration) and infusion, and possibly atropine bolus (0.02 mg/kg, may repeat; minimum dose 0.1 mg and maximum total dose for child 1 mg) have been accomplished

C. The effectiveness of cardiac pacing in this setting is unproven

D. Even if electrical capture of the heart is accomplished, contractility and myocardial blood flow may not improve without mechanical capture

E. It is recommended to use the largest available paddles or self-adhering electrode pads that will fit on the chest wall without touching (allow at least 3 cm between paddles or pads).

    1. For children > 10 kg (> 1 year of age) use large adult paddles.

    2. For children < 10 kg (< 1 year of age) use small infant paddles (4.5 cm)

V. PRECAUTIONS/COMPLICATIONS

A. Inability to capture (~20% of patients), usually related to delay in attempting to pace

B. Painful skeletal muscle contraction

C. Skin or tissue damage

D. Temporizing measure only, prior to transvenous pacing

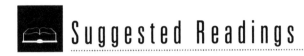 Suggested Readings

1. American Heart Association. *Advanced Cardiovascular Life Support: Provider manual.* Dallas, TX: American Heart Association; 2006.

2. Hazinski MF, Nadkarni VM, Hickey RW, O'Connor R, Becker LB, Zaritsky A. Major changes in the 2005 AHA Guidelines for CPR and ECC: reaching the tipping point for change. *Circulation.* 2005;112(24 suppl):IV206-IV211.

3. Wiegand D, Carlson K. *AACN Procedure Manual for Critical Care.* 5th ed. St. Louis, MO: Elsevier Saunders; 2005.

THORACOSTOMY

I. INDICATIONS/CONTRAINDICATIONS

A. Indications
  1. Tension pneumothorax
  2. Large simple pneumothorax
  3. Penetrating thoracic wound with concurrent need for positive-pressure ventilation
  4. Hemothorax
  5. Symptomatic pleural effusion (recurrent, following thoracentesis)
  6. Empyema
  7. Chylothorax
B. Contraindications
  1. Coagulopathy
    a. Correct prior to nonemergent thoracostomy.
    b. Risk of hemorrhage must be accepted with tension pneumothorax.
  2. Inability to aspirate fluid or air to confirm a patent pleural space
    a. This dictum holds in all circumstances except a penetrating thoracic wound with need for positive-pressure ventilation.
    b. Attempted tube placement in the presence of an obliterated pleural space risks pulmonary injury and potentially fatal hemorrhage.
    c. Aspiration is performed most conveniently through the thoracostomy incisional wound immediately before tube placement.
    d. Aspiration is most important when an apparent effusion presents as "whiteout" on chest radiograph, and its free-flowing nature cannot be confirmed radiographically. Such an apparent effusion in reality may be solid tumor; blunt dissection into such tumor may have devastating hemorrhagic consequences.

II. EQUIPMENT

A. Needle thoracostomy
  1. 14- to 16-gauge catheter over needle
  2. 23-gauge butterfly needle (infants)
B. Tube thoracostomy
  1. Sterile gloves, gown, eye protection, mask, cap, and drapes
  2. Intravenous catheter, tubing, and fluid
  3. Supplemental oxygen
  4. Monitors (echocardiographic, pulse oximeter)
  5. Skin disinfectant
  6. Sterile syringes and infiltrating needles
  7. Local anesthetic
  8. Scalpel with #10 or #15 blade
  9. Forceps
  10. Curved clamp
  11. 24- to 40-French thoracostomy tube
      a. 32- to 40-French thoracostomy tubes are placed in trauma settings to evacuate an acute hemothorax that potentially contains clots. The largest diameter tube accommodated by the intercostal space is used in this circumstance.
      b. For infants and children, see **Table A8-1.**
  12. Water-seal drainage system
  13. Needle holder
  14. 0-silk or 0-polypropylene suture on cutting needle
  15. Suture scissors
  16. 1/4-inch-wide adhesive tape strips or "cable ties" with applicator
  17. Sterile 4 × 4 gauze sponges
  18. Petroleum jelly gauze
  19. Antiseptic ointment
  20. 4-inch-wide impervious tape strips
  21. 1-inch-wide adhesive tape
  22. Resuscitation cart

Table A8-1. Approximate Sizes for Pediatric Thoracostomy Tubes by Age and Weight*		
Age	**Approximate Weight (kg)**	**Tube Size (French)**
Newborn to 9 months	3.5-8	12-18
10 to 17 months	10	14-20
18 months to 3 years	12-15	14-24
4 to 7 years	17-22	20-32
8 years	28	28-32
≥9 years	≥35	28-38

* Needle thoracostomy can usually be accomplished on infants with a 23-guage butterfly needle.

III. TECHNIQUE

A. Analgesia/Sedation

    1. Tube thoracostomy is a painful procedure. In nonemergent and semiurgent circumstances, intravenous narcotic analgesia and a benzodiazepine should be titrated to effect as hemodynamic and respiratory status allow. Local anesthetic should be infiltrated generously throughout the tube thoracostomy tract.

B. Preliminary needle thoracostomy (**Figure A8-1**)

    1. Indication: before tube thoracostomy for rapid temporizing treatment of tension pneumothorax.

    2. Site

        a. Midclavicular line at the second intercostal space; necessitates that the pectoralis major muscle and possibly breast tissue be penetrated before the intercostal space.

        b. Midaxillary line at the fifth intercostal space; placed in the auscultatory triangle posterior to the pectoralis and anterior to latissimus dorsi muscles where only the thin serratus anterior muscle need be penetrated prior to the intercostal space.

    3. Don cap, mask, eye protection and sterile gloves.

    4. Quickly prepare the access site with povidone-iodine solution.

    5. Advance 14-gauge catheter over needle with attached syringe immediately over the superior aspect of the rib while aspirating.

    6. When air is aspirated, advance catheter completely, and withdraw needle and syringe. Withdraw catheter following completion of tube thoracostomy.

    7. Note: 1 mL of saline in the aspirating syringe allows access of intrapleural air to be recognized as bubbles.

Figure A8-1. Sites for needle thoracostomy

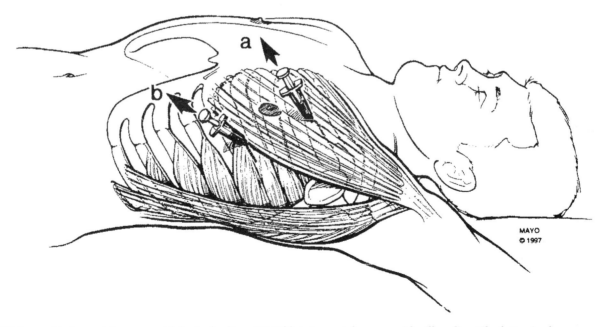

(A) Second intercostal space, midclavicular line. (B) Fifth intercostal space, midaxillary line. The latter is also the incision site for placement of a thoracostomy tube and necessitates transgression of much less chest wall musculature and no breast tissue. Reprinted with permission of the Mayo Foundation.

C. Preparation for tube thoracostomy
1. Provide supplemental oxygen.
2. In nonemergent circumstances, establish intravenous access, electrocardiographic monitoring, and pulse oximetry.
3. Assemble the following nonsterile materials: water-seal drainage system, 1/4-inch-wide strips of adhesive tape or cable ties to secure thoracostomy tube to drainage system, 4-inch-wide impervious tape strips to secure dressing.
4. Ensure adequate lighting.
5. Place patient in supine position with ipsilateral arm extended.
6. Don cap, mask, eye protection, and sterile gloves.
7. Paint patient's anterior and lateral chest wall with antiseptic solution. Remove gloves.
8. Don sterile gown and gloves.
9. On a sterile work space, lay out, from left to right, the following sterile instruments and materials in sequence: syringe with infiltrating needle loaded with local anesthetic, scalpel with blade, forceps, curved clamp, thoracostomy tube, needle holder loaded with suture, suture scissor, dressing comprised of gauze 4 × 4 sponges, petroleum jelly gauze, and antiseptic ointment. These instruments and materials will be used in this sequence.

D. Insertion

Instrument	Maneuver
1. Syringe and needle with local anesthetic	a. Raise cutaneous wheal at incision site. b. Deeply infiltrate underlying subcutaneous tissue.
2. Scalpel	a. 3-cm incision at position *B* in **Figure A8-1** through the skin and subcutaneous tissue of the fifth intercostal space. b. Deepen incision to level of chest wall musculature. Note: The skin incision parallels the intercostal space. It should be placed one interspace below the intended level of pleural entry so that a tract deep to subcutaneous tissue can be created for the tube. This tract closes spontaneously upon tube removal.
3. Syringe and needle with local anesthetic	a. Through wound, infiltrate subcutaneous tissue cephalad to incision.
4. Forceps	a. Using left hand, retract subcutaneous tissue cephalad away from chest wall to create tension at junction of subcutaneous tissue and chest wall musculature (**Figure A8-2**).
5. Curved clamp	a. Continue to apply above traction with forceps. b. With curved clamp in right hand, spread at junction of subcutaneous tissue and chest wall musculature to open this plane (**Figure A8-2**).
6. Syringe and needle with local anesthetic	a. Through incisional wound, infiltrate musculature and pleura of fourth intercostal space. b. Advance needle into pleural space while aspirating syringe. c. Confirm presence of air or fluid in the pleural space.

7. Curved clamp

    a. With curved clamp in right hand, hold tips against superior aspect of fifth rib with concavity of clamp facing pleural space.

    b. Intercostal dissection must be performed immediately superior to a rib to avoid injury to the neurovascular bundle that lies inferior to each rib.

    c. Advance curved clamp through musculature (serratus anterior and intercostal muscles) and pleura into the pleural space (**Figure A8-3**). Note: This maneuver may need to be forceful but must always be restrained. A dramatic loss of resistance will signal entry into the pleural space and will be followed by egress of fluid and/or air.

    d. Ensuring that the tips of the clamp remain on the superior aspect of the fifth rib, widely separate the jaws of the clamp to create a generous opening through the serratus anterior muscle, intercostal muscles, and pleura.

    e. Insert the left index finger into the pleural space as the clamp is withdrawn. Palpation of the smooth pleura confirms the intrapleural location. Sweep the finger through 360° to ensure the absence of adhesions between parietal and visceral pleura. Such adhesions and obliteration of the pleural space would predispose to pulmonary injury during tube insertion.

8. Thoracostomy tube

    a. Keep the left index finger in the pleural space.

    b. With the right hand, advance the thoracostomy tube over the tip of the left index finger into the pleural space (**Figure A8-4**). Passage of the tube over the tip of the intrapleural index finger ensures intrapleural placement of the tube.

    c. Advance the tube until resistance is encountered (approximately 15 to 25 cm). The last side hole of the tube should reside 2 cm within the pleural cavity. Ideally, the tip of the tube lies at the pleural apex.

9. Water-seal drainage system

    a. Connect the thoracostomy tube to the drainage system.

10. Needle holder and suture

    a. Place a suture of 0-nonabsorbable material through the wound on either side of the thoracostomy tube.

    b. Tie each suture to close the wound.

    c. Tie each suture about the thoracostomy tube to secure it.

    d. Place additional sutures as necessary to close the wound.

11. 1/4-inch adhesive tape or cable ties

    a. Secure connection between chest tube and drainage system tubing (**Figure A8-5**).

    b. Tape should never be placed in such a manner as to obscure the connection from view. One must be able to see that the connections are intact at all times.

12. Dressing of gauze, 4 x 4 sponges, petroleum jelly gauze, antiseptic ointment, and impervious tape

    a. Place dressing over thoracostomy site.

    b. Secure dressing with impervious tape.

13. 1-inch adhesive tape

    a. Secure chest tube and drainage system tubing to patient's trunk.

Figure A8-2. Blunt Dissection for Thoracostomy

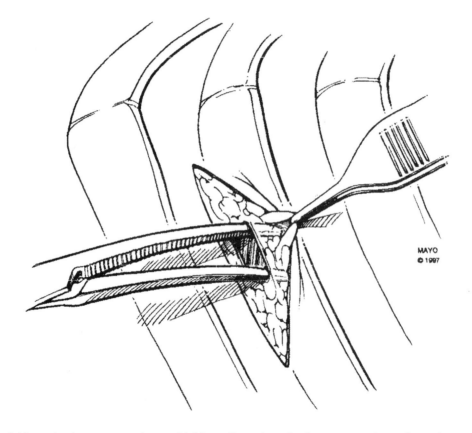

Retraction of skin and subcutaneous tissue with blunt dissection of subcutaneous tissue from chest wall musculature superior to incisional wound. Reprinted with permission of the Mayo Foundation.

Figure A8-3. Creation of Pleural Opening

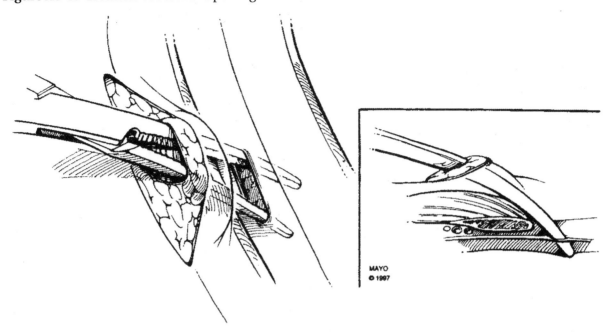

The curved clamp has been advanced into the superior aspect of the incisional wound and advanced through the intercostal musculature and pleura at the superior margin of the fifth rib. The jaws of the clamp are then spread to create a pleural opening. The opening should be generous enough to simultaneously admit a finger and the thoracostomy tube. Insert shows the path of the curved clamp in cross-section. Reprinted with permission of the Mayo Foundation.

Figure A8-4. Placement of Thoracostomy Tube

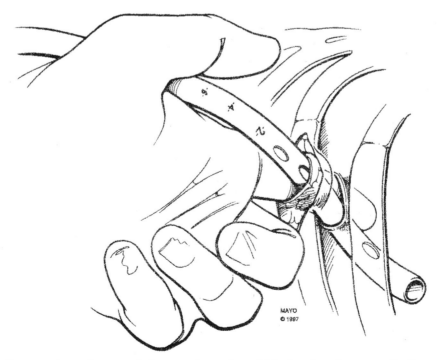

The left index finger replaces the curved clamp and remains within the pleural space as the thoracostomy tube is advanced over the tip of the finger, ensuring intrapleural location. Reprinted with permission of the Mayo Foundation.

Figure A8-5. Connection of Thoracostomy Tube

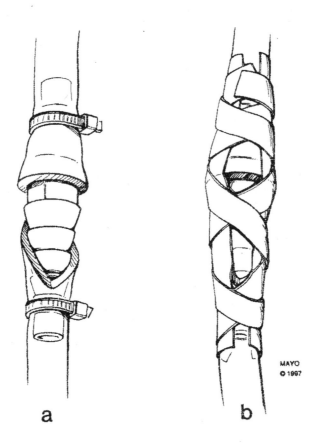

a   b

The thoracostomy tube and tubing from the draining system are secured about a conical connecting adaptor with "cable ties" (a) or strips of adhesive tape placed longitudinally and in a spiral fashion (b). Reprinted with permission of the Mayo Foundation.

E. Pleural decompression
  1. Adjust suction to 20 cm H_2O.
  2. Consider prophylactic antibiotic coverage.
F. Thoracostomy tube monitoring
  1. A thoracostomy tube should be monitored frequently with portable chest radiography to ensure appropriate tube placement and the absence of iatrogenic pneumothorax. The last side hole of the thoracostomy tube lies on a radiopaque line and thus is visible on the radiograph as a gap in this line; the gap should always appear well within the pleural space.
  2. Patency of the chest tube is assured by the presence of a to-and-fro movement of fluid with respiration (respiratory variation). This may be detected within the thoracostomy tube, the tubing of the collection device, or the water-seal chamber. As the pleural space is definitively decompressed, the thoracostomy tube will become loculated from the general pleural space by adhesion of visceral and parietal pleura around it; respiratory variation will then be lost.
  3. The character and volume of pleural drainage must be assessed frequently. The significance of diminished drainage volume can only be determined in light of concurrent chest radiographic findings. For example, diminishing sanguineous drainage

may mean cessation of bleeding or occlusion of the thoracostomy tube by clot; the chest radiograph will reveal increasing effusion/hemothorax in the latter circumstance, but not the former.

4. Air leaks are apparent as air bubbling through the water seal (not the suction regulator). Small air leaks will demonstrate bubbling only during spontaneous expiration or mechanical inspiration. Large air leaks will demonstrate bubbling through both phases of the respiratory cycle. These continuous air leaks may indicate a bronchopleural fistula or tracheobronchial laceration.

G. Thoracostomy tube removal

    1. General criteria for thoracostomy tube removal

        a Complete radiographic expansion of the lung

        b. Absence of air leak for 24 hours

        c. Drainage volume <100 mL over 24 hours

    2. Prepare a dressing of impervious tape, gauze 4 × 4 sponges, petroleum jelly gauze, and antiseptic ointment.

    3. With a sterile scissors, divide the sutures securing the thoracostomy tube.

    4. Instruct the patient to take a full inspiration, hold the breath, and perform a Valsalva maneuver. Practice this sequence several times.

    5. Repeat the above sequence, briskly withdraw the thoracostomy tube with the patient performing a Valsalva maneuver at full inspiration, and immediately apply the occlusive dressing to the thoracostomy wound.

    6. Do not close the thoracostomy site with suture or other material.

    7. Obtain an immediate portable chest radiograph to ensure the absence of pneumothorax.

IV. PEDIATRIC CONSIDERATIONS

A. Approximate sizes for pediatric thoracostomy tubes by age and weight are shown in **Table A8-1.**

V. PRECAUTIONS/COMPLICATIONS

A. Possible injury to intercostal artery, vein, or nerve

B. Extrapleural tube position

C. Subcutaneous emphysema

D. Break in water seal, resulting in pneumothorax

E. Chest wall hematoma/ecchymosis

F. Chest wall or intrapleural hemorrhage

G. Infection

    1. Insertion-site cellulitis

    2. Tract infection

    3. Empyema

H. Laceration of diaphragm or intrathoracic/intra-abdominal viscera

I. Recurrence of pneumothorax (upon removal, secondary to entrained room air or rupture of pulmonary bulla/bleb).

J. Clamping a chest tube in the presence of an air leak may result in life-threatening tension pneumothorax.

Suggested Readings

1. Etoch SW, Bar-Natan MF, Miller FB, Richardson JD. Tube thoracostomy. Factors related to complications. *Arch Surg.* 1995;130:521-525.

2. Martino K, Merrit S, Boyakye K, et al. Prospective randomized trial of thoracostomy removal algorithms. *J Trauma* 1999;46:369-371.

3. Richardson JD, Spain DA. Injury to the lung and pleura: In: Mattox KL, Feliciano DV, Moore EE, eds. *Trauma.* 4th ed. New York, NY: McGraw-Hill, 2000; 523-543.

4. Warren WH. Chest tube thoracostomy. In: Parrillo JE, Dellinger RP, eds. *Critical Care Medicine.* 2nd ed. St. Louis, MO: Mosby, Inc., 2001; 238-248.

ARTERIAL CATHETERIZATION

I. INDICATIONS

A. Continuous assessment of systolic, diastolic, and mean blood pressures
B. Frequent arterial blood sampling
C. Evaluation of cardiac output, stroke volume, and/or systolic pressure variation to evaluate volume responsiveness using special systems

II. EQUIPMENT

A. Catheter
    1. Diameter

Artery	Diameter (gauge)
Radial	20 or 22
Femoral#	20 or 18
Axillary#	20
Dorsalis pedis	20 or 22

    # Soft, flexible material is preferable to minimize vessel injury.

    2. Type
        a. Catheter over the needle
        b. Arterial catheterization kit with guidewire (preferred for femoral artery)
B. General
    1. Arterial catheter or kit (above)
    2. Tape
    3. Sterile 2 × 2 and 4 × 4 gauze sponges
    4. Medication for local anesthesia
    5. Medication for sedation, if necessary
    6. Sterile gloves, gown, mask, cap, drapes, eye protection for universal precautions
    7. Chlorhexidine 2%
    8. Pressure transducer, tubing, pressure monitor

III. TECHNIQUE

A. Radial artery
    1. Inform patient
    2. Assure intravenous access
    3. Position patient as shown in **Figure A9-1**
    4. Don mask, cap, and eye protection
    5. Wash hands and don sterile gloves
    6. Create sterile field and disinfect skin
    7. Identify anatomic landmarks
    8. Palpate radial artery at head of the radius
    9. Infiltrate anesthetic
    10. Insert needle over radial artery approximately 1 cm distal to radial head (**Figure A9-1**)
    11. Advance needle at approximately 20° to 45° angle
    12. Entry into artery will be signaled by appearance of pulsating arterial blood
    13. Once in artery, immobilize needle with free hand
    14. If using catheter over the needle, advance the catheter with a rotating motion to hub and remove needle (**Figure A9-1**)
    15. Modified Seldinger technique (**Figure A9-2**)
        a. Advance the guidewire
        b. Pass arterial catheter over the guidewire
        c. Remove needle and guidewire
    16. Connect tubing to pressure transducer
    17. Secure the catheter to the skin with suture and apply sterile dressing

Figure A9-1. Catheter-over-needle technique

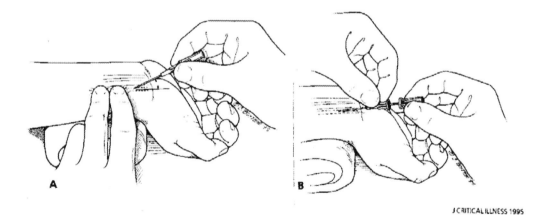

J CRITICAL ILLNESS 1995

(A) After extending and immobilizing the wrist, the radial artery is localized by palpation. The needle is inserted at a 20° to 45° angle. (B) After the artery is entered, the catheter is advanced over the needle and the needle is withdrawn. Illustration © by Charles H. Boyter and reproduced with permission from the artist and *The Journal of Critical Illness*.

Figure A9-2. Modified Seldinger technique

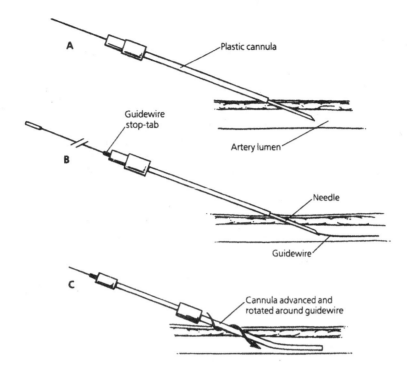

(A) The needle is inserted into the artery. (B) The guidewire is advanced until the stop-tab reaches the needle hub. (C) The catheter is advanced over the guidewire into the artery. Illustration © by Robert Margulies and reproduced with permission from the artist and *The Journal of Critical Illness*.

B. Femoral artery cannulation
- 1. Inform patient
- 2. Assure intravenous access
- 3. Position patient
- 4. Don mask, cap, and eye protection
- 5. Wash hands and don gown and sterile gloves
- 6. Create sterile field and disinfect skin
- 7. Identify anatomic landmarks
- 8. Palpate femoral artery below the inguinal ligament
- 9. Infiltrate anesthetic
- 10. Enter skin over femoral artery approximately 1 to 2 cm below the inguinal ligament
- 11. Advance needle at approximately 45° angle
- 12. Entry into the artery will be signaled by appearance of pulsating arterial blood
- 13. Once in artery, immobilize needle with free hand
- 14. Advance guidewire through needle
- 15. Remove needle, leaving guidewire in place
- 16. Use scalpel and make a small incision at insertion site
- 17. Dilate subcutaneous tissue and artery with dilator and remove
- 18. Pass arterial catheter over the guidewire
- 19. Remove guidewire
- 20. Connect tubing to pressure transducer
- 21. Secure the catheter with suture and apply sterile dressing

IV. VALIDATION OF MEASUREMENTS AND SYSTEM CHARACTERISTICS

A. Systolic return-to-flow blood pressure assessment (**Figure A9-3**)
    1. Observe arterial waveform
    2. Place a manual blood pressure cuff on the same extremity as the arterial catheter and inflate until the arterial waveform flattens
    3. Release pressure in cuff slowly until the first evidence of pulsatile waveform is again observed, and note pressure on sphygmomanometer
    4. Sphygmomanometer pressure is the "true" systolic blood pressure and should correlate with pressure measured through arterial catheter

B. Square wave test
    1. Use to test system characteristics of tubing (eg, length, stiffness, presence of bubbles)
    2. Rapidly flush the arterial line tubing (**Figure A9-4**)
    3. Observe waveform for underdamping or overdamping (**Figures A9-5, A9-6**)

C. Factors that may interfere with monitoring accuracy
    1. Connections of stopcocks and interface
    2. Constant pressure application (300 mm Hg)
    3. Elasticity alterations of the blood vessel wall
    4. Reflectance of the pulse wave from the walls or tubing
    5. Air bubbles in the fluid column throughout the system
    6. Thrombi around or in the catheter
    7. Stiffness and length of the plastic tubing

Figure A9-3. Instructions for obtaining systolic return-to-flow blood pressure

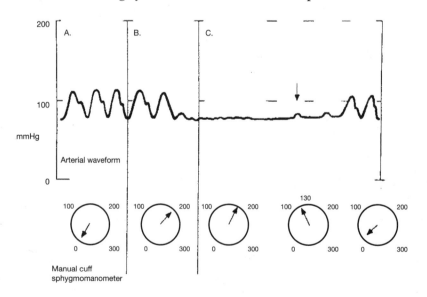

(A) Observe arterial waveform. (B) Place a manual blood pressure cuff on the same extremity as the radial or dorsalis pedis arterial catheter and inflate it. Arterial waveform flattens as the manual blood pressure cuff is inflated. (C) Release pressure in cuff slowly until the first evidence of pulsatile waveform is again observed, at which point the pressure on the sphygmomanometer is noted. This sphygmomanometer pressure is the return-to-flow or "true" systolic blood pressure. In this example, systolic pressure is 120 mm Hg.

Figure A9-4.

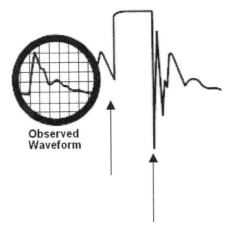

Application of a rapid in-line flush and the correlating evaluation of the monitoring system. First arrow indicates flush applied and second arrow indicates the rapid frequency response when released. Reprinted with permission from Edwards Lifesciences.

Figure A9-5.

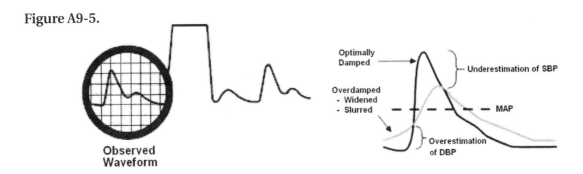

An overdamped signal indicates loss of signal related to loose connections, air bubbles in the system, and/or inadequate fluid and pressure applied. SBP, systolic blood pressure; MAP, mean arterial pressure; DBP, diastolic blood pressure. Reprinted with permission from Edwards Lifesciences.

Figure A9-6.

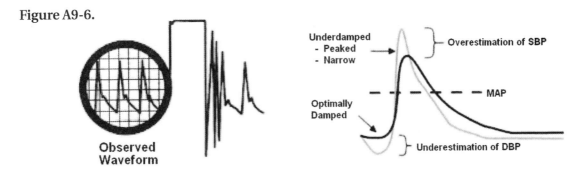

An underdamped signal indicates significant increase in frequency response and is in general related to loss of calibration of the transducer, requiring a transducer change. SBP, systolic blood pressure; MAP, mean arterial pressure; DBP, diastolic blood pressure. Reprinted with permission from Edwards Lifesciences.

V. PEDIATRIC CONSIDERATIONS

A. Both radial artery and femoral artery cannulation may be safely performed in children using the techniques described here.

B. Suggested catheter sizes are 22- and 24-gauge (radial) and 20-gauge (femoral)

VI. PRECAUTIONS/COMPLICATIONS

A. Contraindications
    1. Ischemia of the extremity
    2. Infection at the puncture site
    3. Raynaud disease
    4. Prior vascular surgery involving the artery to be punctured

B. Complications
    1. Digit, hand, leg, foot ischemia
    2. Hemorrhage
    3. Arterial air embolism
    4. Infection
    5. Arteriovenous fistula
    6. Arterial aneurysm

 Suggested Readings

1. Franklin C. The technique of radial artery cannulation. Tips for maximizing results while minimizing the risk of complications. *J Crit Illn.* 1995;10:424-432.

2. Jastremski MS. Vascular access: Arterial cannulation. In: Jastremski MS, ed. *Emergency Procedures.* Philadelphia, PA: WB Saunders; 1992:403.

Central Venous Catheter Insertion

I. INDICATIONS

A. Inability to cannulate peripheral veins
B. Administration of medications through a multilumen catheter
C. Administration of irritating, caustic, or hypertonic solutions
D. Hemodynamic monitoring, insertion of a transvenous cardiac pacing catheter
E. Rapid infusion of resuscitation fluids

II. EQUIPMENT

A. Single-lumen or multilumen central venous catheter or insertion kit
B. General supplies
    1. Sterile central venous catheter, guidewire, 18-gauge, thin-walled central venous needle
    2. Syringe, scalpel, dilators, suture, syringes, and infiltrating needles
    3. Tape
    4. Sterile 2 × 2 and 4 × 4 gauze sponges
    5. Medication for local anesthesia and sedation
    6. Sterile gloves, gown, goggles or face shield, mask, cap, and full-length drapes for universal precautions
    7. Chlorhexidine 2%
    8. Supplemental oxygen (cannula, mask, other as appropriate)
    9. Pulse oximeter
    10. Electrocardiographic monitor
    11. Intravenous tubing and fluid
    12. Ultrasound for vascular imaging, if available
    13. Resuscitation cart available

III. TECHNIQUE

A. Modified Seldinger technique
   1. Inform patient and obtain consent.
   2. Assure peripheral intravenous access, if possible.
   3. Apply oxygen, monitor pulse oximeter and electrocardiography as appropriate.
   4. Position patient (see specific site below).
   5. Don mask with face shield or goggles and cap.
   6. Wash hands.
   7. Don sterile gown and gloves.
   8. Create sterile field.
   9. Prepare site with chlorhexidine and drape.
   10. Identify anatomical landmarks; locate vessel with ultrasound if available.
   11. Establish the needle entry site and the angle/depth of insertion.
   12. Assemble equipment.
   13. For internal jugular and subclavian vein cannulations, estimate the length of central venous catheter needed by laying the catheter over the patient's chest. The tip of the catheter should rest just above the junction of the superior vena cava and right atrium (approximately at the second intercostal space).
   14. Infiltrate local anesthetic.
   15. Advance 18-gauge needle with the bevel up at the specific angle and direction to the predetermined depth while applying suction to the syringe.
   16. Verify entry into the vein, which will be signaled by rapid flush of venous blood into the barrel of the syringe.
   17. If a rapid flush of blood does not occur as the needle is advanced to the predetermined depth, continue to apply suction to the syringe and withdraw the needle slowly along the same pathway. Often, a flush of venous blood will occur during withdrawal, indicating that the needle collapsed the vein and perforated both anterior and posterior walls during advancement.
   18. If the vein is not encountered, do not change needle direction midcourse; rather, retract the needle tip slowly to a subcutaneous position and redirect the tip.
   19. Once in the central vein, rotate the syringe so that the bevel of the needle opens to the vessel lumen, then hold the needle steady with the free hand.
   20. Remove the syringe from the needle and cover the hub of the needle with the thumb of the hand holding the needle.
   21. Note: some needle/syringe units are made to insert the guidewire directly through the syringe and needle without disconnecting needle and syringe (see package insert of specific equipment in use)
   22. Advance guidewire through needle; minimal to no resistance should be met (**Figure A10-1**)
   23. Many guidewires are long enough to reach the heart and cause ectopy. It is not necessary to insert the guidewire more then 20 cm; monitor the electrocardiogram carefully during passage of the guidewire. When guidewire is in place, withdraw needle from the insertion site over the wire, leaving guidewire in place.
   24. Use scalpel to make a small incision at the incision site.
   25. Use dilator to dilate skin, subcutaneous tissue, and vein and then remove.

26. Using a rotating motion, advance catheter over the guidewire into the vein to predetermined depth.
27. Remove guidewire; aspirate free flow of venous blood through the catheter to confirm that catheter tip is within vessel lumen.
28. If the catheter is correctly positioned, blood should be aspirated easily from all ports of a multilumen catheter.
29. Apply caps to ends of the lumens. Flush each lumen and clamp until ready for use.
30. Secure the catheter with suture and apply sterile dressing.
31. Obtain a chest radiograph to confirm correct position for internal jugular and subclavian vein catheters.

Note: During subclavian and internal jugular line placement, aspiration of air into the venous circulation is possible while syringes, tubing, and guidewires are exchanged and connected. This is a particular risk in patients who are breathing spontaneously and are not receiving positive-pressure ventilation. Care should be taken to occlude intravascular catheters any time syringes and lines are being connected, so as to minimize the risk of air entrainment and embolization.

Figure A10-1. Modified Seldinger technique.

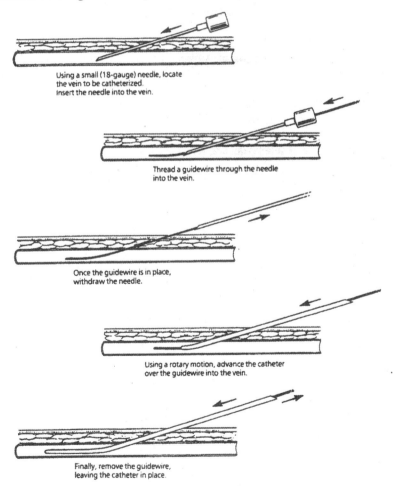

Using a small (18-gauge) needle, locate the vein to be catheterized. Insert the needle into the vein.

Thread a guidewire through the needle into the vein.

Once the guidewire is in place, withdraw the needle.

Using a rotary motion, advance the catheter over the guidewire into the vein.

Finally, remove the guidewire, leaving the catheter in place.

Illustration © by Robert Margulies and reproduced with permission from the artist and *The Journal of Critical Illness.*

B. Internal jugular vein (central approach)
1. Position patient in a 15° head-down (Trendelenburg) position to ensure filling of the internal jugular vein.
2. Stand at the head of the bed.
3. Turn patient's head away from the side to be cannulated.
4. Both right and left internal jugular veins can be cannulated; however, the right side has several advantages over the left:
    a. It offers a more direct route to the superior vena cava.
    b. The apex of the left lung is higher than that of the right; therefore, the possibility of pneumothorax is greater on the left.
    c. The thoracic duct is on the left; therefore, the possibility of thoracic duct injury is greater on the left.
5. The medial (sternal) and lateral (clavicular) bellies of the sternocleidomastoid muscle form a triangle with the clavicle at the base.
6. The internal jugular vein lies within the carotid sheath just beneath the apex of the triangle formed by the bellies of the sternocleidomastoid.
7. The carotid artery also lies within the carotid sheath just medial and deep to the internal jugular vein.
8. A smaller finder needle may be used (25-gauge, 1 1/4-inch needle) to locate the vein before using the 18-gauge insertion needle.
9. The skin is punctured at the apex of the triangle; the needle tip is directed caudally at a 45° to 60° angle to the frontal plane and laterally toward the ipsilateral nipple.
10. The needle is advanced to a depth of 3 to 5 cm, depending on the size of the patient.
11. If the vein is not entered, redirect the needle tip slightly more medially and repeat; do not direct the needle tip across the midline, as the carotid artery may be punctured.
12. When the vein is entered, proceed as above for passage of the guidewire and catheter.

C. Subclavian vein (infraclavicular approach)
1. Position patient in a 15° head-down (Trendelenburg) position to ensure filling of the subclavian vein.
2. Stand at the side of the bed.
3. Turn patient's head away from the side to be cannulated. A rolled towel placed vertically between the scapulae is advocated by some operators.
4. Both right and left subclavian veins can be cannulated.
5. The skin is punctured at the junction of the medial and middle thirds of the clavicle.
6. The needle is advanced beneath the clavicle parallel to the frontal (horizontal) plane and directed toward the sternal notch.
7. Care should be taken never to allow the needle tip to dip beneath the frontal plane, as the risk of pneumothorax increases significantly.
8. The needle is advanced to a depth of 3 to 5 cm, depending on the size of the patient.
9. When the vein is entered, proceed as above for guidewire and catheter insertion.

D. Femoral vein
    1. The patient is placed in supine position with the legs slightly abducted.
    2. Stand at the side of the bed.
    3. Both right and left femoral veins can be cannulated.
    4. Palpate the anterior superior iliac spine and the pubic tubercle. These bony landmarks delineate the course of the inguinal ligament. The abdominal compartment lies cephalad to the inguinal ligament, the leg caudal. Do not attempt venous access cephalad to the inguinal ligament.
    5. The femoral artery runs directly beneath the inguinal ligament. It should be identified by palpation of its pulse and its course determined.
    6. The femoral vein lies about 1 cm medial and parallel to the femoral artery.
    7. The skin is punctured 1 to 2 cm below the inguinal ligament.
    8. The needle is advanced at an angle of approximately 45° and directed cephalad.
    9. The needle is advanced until venous blood is freely aspirated.
    10. When the vein is entered, proceed as above for guidewire and catheter placement.

IV. PEDIATRIC CONSIDERATIONS

A. The intraosseous route may be used as a temporary route when other vascular sites are not immediately available in children (**Appendix 6**).
B. Central venous cannulation via the subclavian and internal jugular routes is possible even in babies, but these routes may be unwise for the operator inexperienced with catheterization of children; the femoral venous route may be preferable.
C. Pediatric catheter insertion kits use 4-French and 5-French catheters and 18- to 21-gauge introducer needles.

V. PRECAUTIONS/COMPLICATIONS

A. Pneumothorax, hemothorax, chylothorax (subclavian and internal jugular approaches)
B. Local subcutaneous tissue, nerve, artery, and vein damage. Note: If a large catheter is inadvertently placed in an artery, it should be left in place and expert consultation obtained.
C. Thrombophlebitis and deep vein thrombosis
D. Infection
E. Catheter, guidewire embolism
F. Cardiac arrhythmias
G. Hemorrhage
H. Air embolism

Suggested Readings

1. Bone RC. The technique of subclavian and femoral vein cannulation. *J Crit Illn.* 1988;3:61.

2. O'Grady NP, Alexander M, Dellinger EP et al. Guidelines for the prevention of intravascular catheter-related infections. *MMWR Recomm Rep.* 2002;51(RR-10):1-29.

BRAIN DEATH AND ORGAN DONATION

I. BRAIN DEATH (DEATH BY NEUROLOGIC CRITERIA)

Brain death is usually a clinical diagnosis based upon the total and irreversible cessation of all brain function, including that of the brain stem. Criteria and methods to diagnose/certify brain death may be established by national laws, state regulations, or hospital policy and often vary among countries and institutions. Major differences in requirements may include the number of observers, the specialty of the physician assessor, the duration of observation, and the use of confirmatory tests. However, common requirements are listed in **Table A11-1**. A mistaken diagnosis of brain death must never occur. Because variations in some physical examination features may exist, a physician experienced in brain-death certification, hospital policy, and state and national laws should always participate in this process.

Table A11-1. Clinical Criteria for Brain-Death Certification

1. Identifiable cause of coma

2. Exclusion of reversible CNS depression

   Absence of hypothermia (>34°C [>93.2°F])

   Absence of hypotension

   Absence of drugs (e.g., ethanol, barbiturates, sedative hypnotics, neuromuscular blocking agents)

   Absence of metabolic abnormalities that could potentiate CNS depression (e.g., abnormalities in electrolytes, osmolality, serum ammonia, hypercapnia, hypoxemia)

3. Absent cortical function

   Unresponsive to painful stimuli administered via cranial nerves (spinal cord reflexes may persist in brain death)

   No spontaneous muscular movements

   No posturing, shivering, or seizure activity

4. Absent brainstem function

   Pupils nonreactive

   No corneal reflexes

   No gag or cough reflexes

   No oculocephalic reflexes

   No oculovestibular reflexes

   No sucking or rooting reflexes (pediatric patients)

continued next page....

Table A11-1.	Clinical Criteria for Brain-Death Certification

5. Documentation of apnea

  Absence of spontaneous breathing after a $PaCO_2$ >60 mm Hg (>8.0 kPa) or 20 mm Hg (2.7 kPa) above normal baseline values has been reached during apnea testing

6. Additional confirmatory studies (usually optional in adults but may be required in some countries)

  Cerebral blood flow study (4-vessel angiogram preferred/required in some countries or radionuclide imaging) – absent cerebral blood flow

  Transcranial Doppler ultrasonography – absence of diastolic or reverberating flow

  Electroencephalogram – no activity recorded at full gain (consult with a neurophysiologist)

CNS, central nervous system.

The interval between two evaluations and the use of confirmatory tests according to the patient's age are listed below.

Age	Interval	Confirmatory test(s)
Term to 2 months	48 hours	2
2 months to 1 year	24 hours	1
1 year to < 18 years	12 hours	Optional
≥ 18 years	Optional	Optional

II. ORGAN DONATION

A. Brain Death

Transplantation of organs and tissues is possible from donors who fulfill brain-death criteria. This process is facilitated by a local organ procurement organization representative, the procurement transplant coordinator. This representative can provide information about criteria for accepting specific organs or tissue and can assist in or conduct the process of requesting donation from the family.

Care of the brain-dead organ donor awaiting organ procurement is challenging. Homeostasis must be maintained to assure perfusion of donor organs before removal. Somatic physiology is disrupted during brainstem destruction and may result in hypotension, cardiac dysfunction, hypothermia, and electrolyte and endocrinologic abnormalities. Bradyarrhythmias do not respond to atropine because the vagal nuclei are not functional after brain death, and treatment with primary cardiac chronotropic agents (e.g., isoproterenol or dopamine) may be needed. Diabetes insipidus is common and often requires treatment with aggressive hypotonic fluid replacement or desmopressin. Table **A11-2** lists physiologic goals useful in maintaining optimal organ/tissue function.

Table A11-2.	Suggested Parameters for Optimal Donor Organ Function Before Procurement

Systolic blood pressure >90 mm Hg or mean arterial pressure >60 to 65 mm Hg (adults)

Dopamine or dobutamine ≤10 μg/kg per minute

Central venous pressure 4 to 10 mm Hg

Urine output 100 to 200 mL/h, or 2 to 3 mL/kg per hour

Arterial oxygen saturation (SaO_2) >95% or PaO_2 >100 mm Hg (13.3 kPa)

Hematocrit >30%

Temperature 36.5 to 37.5°C (97.7 to 99.5°F)

Normal electrolytes

Serum glucose 120 to 180 mg/dL (6.6 to 9.9 mmol/L)

Eyelids taped shut/eye drops

B. Cardiac Death

Organs may be procured from donors after cardiac death. Once futility has been determined and the decision has been made to withdraw care, families may be approached regarding the possibility of organ donation after cardiac death. In this instance, care is withdrawn in a controlled environment and the patient is formally declared dead after 5 minutes of cardiac asystole. At that time, procurement of organs such as kidneys, pancreas, liver, and lungs may be undertaken. In addition to solid organ procurement, cornea, heart valves, bones and skin may similarly be procured with consent. The process for organ donation is greatly facilitated by the involvement of the local organ procurement organization.

 # Suggested Readings

1. Haupt WF, Rudolf J. European brain death codes: a comparison of national guidelines. *J Neurol.* 1999;246:432-437.

2. The Quality Standards Subcommittee of the American Academy of Neurology. Practice parameters for determining brain death in adults (summary statement). *Neurology.* 1995;45:1012-1014.

3. Shemie SD, Doig C, Dickens B, et al. Brain arrest: the neurological determination of death and organ donor management in Canada. *CMAJ.* 2006;174:S1-S30.

4. Shemie SD, Ross H, Pagliarello J, et al. Organ donor management in Canada: recommendations of the Forum on Medical Management to Optimize Donor Organ Potential. *CMAJ.* 2006;174:S13-S32.

5. Task Force for the Determination of Brain Death in Children. Guidelines for determination of brain death in children. *Arch Neurol.* 1987;44:587-588.

6. Van Norman GA. A matter of life and death: what every anesthesiologist should know about the medical, legal, and ethical aspects of declaring brain death. *Anesthesiology.* 1999;91:275-287.

7. Wijdicks EFM. The diagnosis of brain death. *N Engl J Med.* 2001;344:1215-1221.

8. Wood KE, Becker BN, McCartney JG, D'Alessandro AM, Coursin DB. Care of the potential organ donor. *N Engl J Med.* 2004;351:2730-2739.

💻 Web Sites

1. United Network for Organ Sharing. http://www.unos.org/resources/ donorManagement.asp?index=1. Contains check list for management of the organ donor.

2. UK Transplant. http://www.uktransplant.org.uk/ukt/about_transplants/donor_care/ donor_care.jsp. Contains chapter on organ donor management from the Intensive Care Society guidelines for adult organ and tissue donation.

TETANUS IMMUNOPROPHYLAXIS
FOR THE INJURED PATIENT

Patients who have completed a 3-dose primary tetanus vaccination series and have received a tetanus toxoid-containing vaccine <5 years before the injury do not require a tetanus toxoid-containing vaccine for wound management.

Table A12-1. Summary of Tetanus Prophylaxis in Routine Wound Management for Patients Between the Ages of 11 and 64 Years

HISTORY OF ADSORBED TETANUS TOXOID (Doses)	CLEAN. MINOR WOUNDS (Not Prone to Tetanus)		ALL OTHER (Tetanus-Prone) WOUNDS	
	Tdap or Td[a]	TIG	Tdap or Td[a]	TIG
Unknown or <3	Yes	No	Yes	Yes
≥3	No[b]	No	No[c]	No

Tdap, tetanus toxoid, reduced diphtheria toxoid, acellular pertussis vaccine; Td, tetanus toxoid and reduced diphtheria toxoid — for adult use (dose = 0.5 mL); TIG, tetanus immune globulin — human (dose = 250 IU).

[a] *Tdap is preferred to Td for adults vaccinated ≥5 years earlier and adolescents who have never received Tdap. Td is preferred to tetanus toxoid (TT) for patients who received Tdap previously or when Tdap is not available. If TT and TIG are both used, tetanus toxoid adsorbed rather than tetanus toxoid for booster use only (fluid vaccine) should be used.*

[b] *Yes, if≥10 years since the last tetanus toxoid-containing dose.*

[c] *Yes, if≥5 years since the last tetanus toxoid-containing dose.*

Table A12-2. Summary of Tetanus Prophylaxis in Routine Wound Management for Children and Adolescents

HISTORY OF ADSORBED TETANUS TOXOID (Doses)	CLEAN, MINOR WOUNDS		ALL OTHER WOUNDS[1]	
	Td or Tdap[2]	TIG[3]	Td or Tdap[2]	TIG[3]
Unknown or <3	Yes	No	Yes	Yes
≥3[4]	No[5]	No	No[6]	No

Td, adult type diphtheria and tetanus toxoid vaccines; TIG, tetanus immune globulin (human); Tdap, booster tetanus toxoid, reduced diphtheria toxoid, acellular pertussis.

¹ *Such as, but not limited to, wounds contaminated with dirt, feces, soil, and saliva; puncture wounds; avulsions; and wounds resulting from missiles, crushing, burns, and frostbite.*

² *Tdap is preferred to Td for adolescents who never have received Tdap. Td is preferred to tetanus toxoid (TT) for adolescents who received Tdap previously or when Tdap is not available.*

³ *Intravenous immune globulin should be used when TIG is not available.*

⁴ *If only 3 doses of fluid toxoid have been received, a fourth dose of toxoid, preferably an adsorbed toxoid, should be given. Although licensed, fluid TT rarely is used.*

⁵ *Yes, if ≥10 years since the last tetanus-containing vaccine dose.*

⁶ *Yes, if ≥5 years since the last tetanus-containing vaccine dose. More frequent boosters are not needed and can accentuate adverse effects.*

From American Academy of Pediatrics. Tetanus. In: Pickering, LK, Baker, CJ, Long, SS, McMillan JA, eds. *Red Book: 2006 Report of the Committee on Infectious Diseases.* 27th ed. Elk Grove Village, IL: American Academy of Pediatrics; 2006: 648-653

Suggested Readings

1. Broder KR, Cortese MM, Iskander JK, et al. Preventing tetanus, diphtheria, and pertussis among adolescents: use of tetanus toxoid, reduced diphtheria toxoid and acellular pertussis vaccines recommendations of the Advisory Committee on Immunization Practices (ACIP). *MMWR Recomm Rep.* 2006;55(RR-3):1-34.

2. Kretsinger K, Broder KR, Cortese MM, et al. Preventing tetanus, diphtheria, and pertussis among adults: use of tetanus toxoid, reduced diphtheria toxoid and acellular pertussis vaccine recommendations of the Advisory Committee on Immunization Practices (ACIP) and recommendation of ACIP, supported by the Healthcare Infection Control Practices Advisory Committee (HICPAC), for use of Tdap among healthcare personnel. *MMWR Recomm Rep.* 2006; 55(RR-17):1-37.

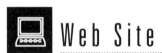

Web Site

Centers for Disease Control and Prevention. http://www.cdc.gov

UNFRACTIONATED HEPARIN ANTICOAGULATION

I. VENOUS THROMBOEMBOLISM

1. Make calculations using total body weight in kilograms.
2. Administer heparin, 80 U/kg, as an intravenous bolus.
3. Start intravenous heparin infusion, 18 U/kg per hour (20,000 U heparin in 500 mL of D5W = 40 U/mL).
4. Obtain stat activated partial thromboplastin time (APTT) 6 hours after heparin bolus.
5. Adjust heparin infusion based on sliding scale below.

APTT (s)	Dose Change
<35 (1.2 × control)	80 U/kg bolus, increase drip by 4 U/kg per hour
35-45 (1.2 to 1.5 × control)	40 U/kg bolus, increase drip by 2 U/kg per hour
46-70 (1.5 to 2.3 × control)	No change
71-90 (2.3 to 3 × control)	Reduce drip by 2 U/kg per hour
>90 (>3 × control)	Hold heparin for 1 hour, reduce drip by 3 U/kg per hou

6. Order APTT 6 hours after dosage change, adjusting heparin infusion based on the sliding scale until APTT is therapeutic. Problems with standardizing APTT monitoring suggest that the therapeutic range should be determined by calibrating reagent lots to APTT values that correlate with therapeutic heparin levels. When 2 consecutive APTT levels are therapeutic, order APTT (and readjust heparin drip as needed) every 24 hours.
7. Make changes as promptly as possible and round off doses to the nearest mL/h (nearest 40 U/h).

II. CORONARY ARTERY DISEASE

1. Unstable angina and non-ST-segment myocardial infarction
   a. Administer heparin as an initial bolus dose of 60 to 70 U/kg (maximum dose 5,000 U) is recommended.
   b. Start an intravenous heparin infusion of 12 to 15 U/kg per hour (maximum 1,000 U/h).
   c. Adjust heparin infusion to maintain a therapeutic APTT value.
2. ST-segment myocardial infarction with use of alteplase, reteplase or tenecteplase
   a. Administer heparin as an initial bolus dose of 60 U/kg (maximum dose 4,000 U)
   b. Start an intravenous heparin infusion of 12 U/kg per hour (maximum 1,000 U/h).
   c. Adjust heparin infusion to maintain a therapeutic APTT value.
3. Percutaneous coronary interventions with use of glycoprotein IIb/IIIa inhibitors
   a. Administer heparin as an initial bolus dose of 70 U/kg.
   b. Additional boluses are administered to keep the activated clotting time at > 200 seconds.

Suggested Readings

1. Antman EM, Anbe DT, Armstrong PW, et al. ACC/AHA guidelines for the management of patients with ST-elevation myocardial infarction: executive summary: a report of the American College of Cardiology/American Heart Association Task Force on Practice Guidelines (Committee to Revise the 1999 Guidelines on the Management of Patients With Acute Myocardial Infarction). *J Am Coll Cardiol.* 2004;44:671-719. Full text available at: http://www.acc.org/qualityandscience/clinical/guidelines/stemi/Guideline1/index.pdf.

2. Braunwald E, Antman EM, Beasley JW, et al. ACC/AHA 2002 guideline update for the management of patients with unstable angina and non–ST-segment elevation myocardial infarction: a report of the American College of Cardiology/American Heart Association Task Force on Practice Guidelines (Committee on Management of Patients with Unstable Angina). *J Am Coll Cardiol.* 2002;40:1366-1374. Full text available at: http://www.acc.org/qualityandscience/clinical/guidelines/unstable/unstable.pdf.

3. Hirsh J, Raschke R. Heparin and low-molecular-weight heparin: the Seventh ACCP Conference on Antithrombotic and Thrombolytic Therapy. *Chest.* 2004;126(Suppl):188S-203S.

4. Raschke RA, Reilly BM, Guidry JR, Fontana JR, Srinivas S. The weight-based heparin dosing nomogram compared with a "standard care" nomogram. A randomized controlled trial. *Ann Intern Med.* 1993;119:874-881.

Short ACTH Stimulation Test

1. Blood for serum cortisol is drawn at baseline.

2. For patients older than 2 years of age, synthetic 1-24 adrenocorticotropic hormone (ACTH; Cortrosyn®, cosyntropin), 250 μg, is administered intravenously or intramuscularly. For patients younger than 2 years of age, 125 μg synthetic 1-24 ACTH should be administered.

3. A serum cortisol level is drawn 30 or 60 minutes after cosyntropin administration.

4. A cortisol level >18 to 20 μg/dL (>500 to 550 nmol/L) at 30 or 60 minutes indicates adequate adrenal function.

5. Failure to attain adequate cortisol levels indicates the need for further testing and expert consultation.

6. Since cortisol levels may not be reported quickly, corticosteroids should be administered while awaiting results if the clinical situation is suggestive of acute adrenal insufficiency.

THROMBOPROPHYLAXIS FOR VENOUS THROMBOEMBOLISM

Table A15-1. Pharmacologic and Mechanical Interventions for VTE Prophylaxis

Clinical Situation	Intervention
General, vascular, and urologic surgery	
Low risk: minor surgery in patients <40 years with no additional risk factors, transurethral procedures, or low-risk urologic or vascular surgery without risk factors	Early, persistent mobilization
Moderate risk: minor surgery in patients with risk factors, major surgery in patients <40 years with no risk factors	Low-dose UFH twice daily or LMWH once daily
High risk: surgery in patients >60 years or >40 years with additional risk factors; major vascular surgery with risk factors; major, open urologic surgery	Low-dose UFH three times daily or LMWH
Highest risk: surgery in patients with multiple risk factors (>40 years, cancer, prior VTE); hip or knee arthroplasty, hip fracture surgery; major trauma, spinal cord injury	Low-dose UFH three times daily or LMWH with CS and/or IPC
Gynecologic surgery	
Brief procedures (<30 min) for benign disease	Early, persistent mobilization
Laparoscopic procedures with risk factors	Low-dose UFH, LMWH, CS, or IPC
Major gynecologic surgery for benign disease without risk factors	Low-dose UFH twice daily, or LMWH, or IPC started before surgery and used continuously while patient is nonambulatory
Extensive surgery for malignancy and additional VTE risk factors	Low-dose UFH three times daily, LMWH or IPC started before surgery and used continuously during hospital stay; or low-dose UFH or LMWH and CS or IPC
Laparoscopic surgery	
Laparoscopic surgery without risk factors	Early, persistent mobilization
Laparoscopic surgery with risk factors	Low-dose UFH, LMWH, IPC, or CS

continued next page...

Table A15-1. Pharmacologic and Mechanical Interventions for VTE Prophylaxis, continued

Orthopedic surgery

Elective hip arthroplasty	LMWH at high-risk dose, fondaparinux, or adjusted-dose VKA
Elective knee arthroplasty	LMWH at high-risk dose, fondaparinux, adjusted-dose VKA, or IPC (if pharmacologic prophylaxis is contraindicated)
Knee arthroscopy, elective spine surgery with no risk factors	Early, persistent mobilization
Arthroscopic knee surgery with risk factors	LMWH
Hip fracture surgery	Fondaparinux, LMWH at high-risk dose, adjusted-dose VKA, or low-dose UFH
Elective spine surgery with risk factors	Low-dose UFH, LMWH postoperatively, or perioperative IPC and/or CS
Elective spine surgery with multiple risk factors	Low-dose UFH or LMWH with CS and/or IPC

Neurosurgery

Intracranial neurosurgery	IPC ± CS or low-dose UFH or postoperative LMWH

Trauma, burns

	LMWH or low-dose UFH (if no contraindication), or IPC or CS alone (if LMWH is contraindicated)

Spinal cord injury

	LMWH, low-dose UFH or LMWH with IPC, or IPC ± CS when anticoagulant prophylaxis is contraindicated

Critical care

ICU patients or medical conditions with moderate risk and/or confined to bed	Low-dose UFH, LMWH, or CS and/or IPC if high risk of bleeding
ICU patients with higher risk	LMWH

Abbreviations: VKA, vitamin K antagonist; IPC, intermittent pneumatic compression; UFH, unfractionated heparin; LMWH, low-molecular-weight heparin; CS, graduated compression stockings; VTE, venous thromboembolism; ICU, intensive care unit.

Suggested Reading

Geerts WH, Pineo GF, Heit JA, et al. Prevention of venous thromboembolism: the Seventh ACCP Conference on Antithrombotic and Thrombolytic Therapy. *Chest.* 2004;126:338S-428S.

Appendix 16:

PEDIATRIC NORMAL VALUES

Table A16-1. Blood Volume in Children

Age Group	Weight (kg)	Blood Volume (mL/kg)	Total Volume (mL)
Newborn	2.5-4.0	90	290
Infant	4-12	75	600
2-4 years	10-20	75	1200
4-7 years	15-30	75	2000
7-12 years	20-50	75	2500
≥13 years	≥40	70	3000-5000

Table A16-2. Vital Signs in Children

Age Group	Heart Rate (beats/min)	Respiratory Rate (breaths/min)	Systolic Blood Pressure (mm Hg)	Diastolic Blood Pressure (mm Hg)
Newborn	100-180	30-60	50-70	25-50
Infant	80-180	30-40	85-100	50-60
2-4 years	70-140	20-30	87-105	53-66
4-7 years	60-110	20-30	95-105	53-66
7-12 years	60-100	16-20	97-112	57-71
≥13 years	50-90	12-16	112-128	66-80

SIMULATION IN FCCS

I. INTRODUCTION

Until recently, the approach to critical care knowledge, problem solving, and technical skills depended largely on written material and lecture-based learning followed by on-the-job practice. There are numerous disadvantages to these methods for both the learner and patient. Learning in a setting without close supervision and the inability to practice repeatedly also creates concerns about patient safety and medical error. Many situations in the critical care environment are rare and practitioners might not be exposed to them during training. Simulation permits repeatable experiential learning. The recent technological growth in medical simulation provides experiential learning for a growing number of critical care practitioners.

II. FUNDAMENTAL CONCEPTS

■ *What is simulation?*

Simulation is a science primarily developed over the past several decades in the military and aviation fields. Medical simulation is a relatively recent application of the science with commercial simulators becoming available in the mid 1990s. Simulation is a method for implementing a model over time or, perhaps more simply, the technique of imitating the behavior of a situation or process by means of an analogous situation or apparatus. For FCCS training, "simulation" refers to the use of a computer-controlled manikin in replicating clinical situations encountered in a critical care environment.

■ *When is simulation used?*

Simulation is typically used in the following situations:

- ■ Reality is dangerous

- ■ Events are uncommon

- ■ Errors are expensive

Consider the example of pilots being trained to respond to engine failure (a rare event). Deliberately causing an engine to fail in mid-flight would be dangerous and any error in the response could be expensive (i.e., loss of aircraft, loss of life). Of course, a similar case can be made when experiential learning is employed to teach the management of patients in the critical care environment. In FCCS, the application of simulation is useful in teaching the management of rapidly escalating, complex, and uncommon events. Examples include management of ventilator settings, septic shock, a difficult airway, or patients with multiple trauma.

A. Fidelity, Validity, and Reliability

For simulation to be effective for learning and assessment, three key aspects must be considered: fidelity, validity, and reliability.

1. **Fidelity** is defined as the accuracy of the representation when compared to the real world or the degree of exactness to which something is copied or reproduced (of reality).

> Equipment fidelity: Degree to which the simulator duplicates the appearance and feel of a real system.

> Environment fidelity: Extent to which the simulation duplicates motion cues, visual cues, and other sensory information from the task environment.

> Psychological fidelity: Degree to which the trainee perceives the simulation to be a believable surrogate for the trained task, or the match between the trainee's performance in the simulated environment and the real world.

Applied to simulation in critical care, equipment fidelity would refer to the human likeness of the computer-manikin interface and the reality of procedural interventions. Environment fidelity would refer to the replication of the critical care environment (eg, bed, ventilator, medications, infusion pump, procedure kits, clinical staff). Ultimately, however, the fidelity of the equipment and environment only need to be sufficient to establish the psychological fidelity in which the learner can suspend disbelief and "buy into" the simulation to maximally benefit from experiential learning,

2. **Validity** refers to the degree to which a model or simulation is an accurate representation of the real-world from the perspective of the intended uses of the model or simulation.

> **Face validity:** Simulation will have face validity if it "looks like" it is going to measure what it is supposed to measure (eg, does it seem as though it will work the way we would expect?).

> **Content validity:** Experts have performed a detailed examination of the contents of the simulation to determine if it is appropriate and situation-specific (eg, does it demonstrate or test all facets of a given concept?).

Construct validity: Experts perform better than novices and post-test scores would be better than pre-test scores after a teaching session.

Concurrent validity: Performance in the simulation corresponds to currently accepted measures, such as written or oral examinations.

Predictive validity: Those who perform well in the simulation go on to perform well in the real world.

A number of studies have validated clinical simulation for both individual and team performance of technical and nontechnical skills. Validation studies have demonstrated the interest and enthusiasm of students, high levels of realism, and both construct and content validity with full-scale simulation. To date, there has been only limited assessment of the transfer of training to the real environment and no assessment of effectiveness in reducing risk or improving patient outcomes.

3. **Reliability** of a simulation refers specifically to inter-rater reliability and test-retest reliability. Put simply, if two different evaluators (raters) come up with the same score for a learner's performance during a simulation, then a high inter-rater reliability is established. Likewise, if learners get an equivalent performance score during different sessions with the same simulation, then high test-retest reliability is established.

B. Categories of Simulation

Simulation can be grouped into three principal categories.

Case studies and role plays: Designed to be interactive, critical thinking exercises. Examples include oral examinations, verbal role playing, and standardized patients.

Part-task trainers: Focused on a specific skill or task. Examples include manikins for intubation and arterial or venous cannulation.

Full-mission (or full-scale) simulations: Designed to simulate a complex process, with all of the environmental complexities involved. Examples include aircraft flight simulators; haptics-based surgical simulators, and manikin-based human patient simulators.

As summarized in **Table A17-1**, fidelity (but not necessarily validity) varies depending upon the category of simulation. Choice of the appropriate category of simulation primarily depends on the learning domains to be addressed and cost (**Table A17-2**).

Table A17-1. Simulation Fidelity Comparison

CATEGORY	EQUIPMENT FIDELITY	ENVIRONMENT FIDELITY	PSYCHOLOGICAL FIFDELITY
Case Studies/Role Plays	Low	Low to Medium	Low to Medium
Part-Task Trainers	Medium	Low	Medium
Full-Mission Simulations	High	Medium to High	High

Table A17-2. Benefit-Cost Matrix

CATEGORY	COGNITIVE (Knowledge)	PSYCHOMOTOR (Skills)	AFFECTIVE (Attitudes)	RELATIVE COST
Case Studies/Role Plays	Moderate	Weak	Moderate	Low
Part-Task Trainers	Moderate	Moderate	Weak	Moderate
Full-Mission Simulations	Strong	Strong	Strong	High

III. PATIENT SIMULATION

Full-scale or patient simulation refers to a comprehensive simulation of the clinical management of a patient, including both the clinical environment (patient bed, and equipment) and representation of the patient. Briefly, a patient simulator is an anatomic and physiologic replica of a patient, composed of a computer-controlled manikin (**Table A17-3**) and models of physiology and pharmacology.

Table A17-3. Possible Features of a Human Patient Simulator

CLINICAL FEATURES	MONITORED PARAMETERS
• Voice and phonation	• Electrocardiogram
• Eye blinking, pupil dilation and constriction	• Invasive (arterial, central venous, pulmonary artery, and intracranial) pressures
• Infant anterior fontanelle	• Noninvasive blood pressure
• Breathing with chest rise and fall	• Thermodilution cardiac output
• O_2 and CO_2 exchange	• Pulse oximetry
• Normal and abnormal breath sounds	• Temperature
• Normal and abnormal heart sounds	• Capnography
• Palpable pulses	• Arterial and venous blood gases
• Laryngospasm, swollen tongue	• Pulmonary compliance, resistance; flow-volume loops
• Twitch, train-of-four monitoring	• Urine output

Under computer control, the patient simulator manikin exhibits clinical signs and monitored parameters comparable to a real patient. With less sophisticated, instructor-driven patient simulators, an instructor at the controls of the computer drives the behavior of the simulated patient, observes the student's clinical interventions, makes a clinical assessment about how a real patient would respond, and then commands the simulator manikin to exhibit the appropriate clinical signs and monitored parameters.

With more sophisticated, model-driven simulators, the "patient" behavior is determined by complex mathematical models of human physiology and pharmacology that are embedded in the computer control software. With these simulators, the student (for some parameters) or instructor inputs the intervention (e.g., give 100-mg bolus of succinylcholine, increase FiO_2 to 1.0, start norepinephrine at 0.1 µg/kg per minute, or perform needle aspiration of a tension pneumothorax) and the patient responses are displayed automatically.

Table A17-4 offers a brief comparison of instructor-driven and model-driven simulators.

Table A17-4. Comparison of Instructor and Model-Driven Simulators		
CAPABILITY	**INSTRUCTOR-DRIVEN SIMULATOR**	**MODEL-DRIVEN SIMULATOR**
Physiology	Subjectively controlled by instructor	Objectively controlled by computer
Fidelity	Limited by knowledge and capabilities of instructor	Limited by capabilities of computer software
Reliability	Varies by instructor	Does not vary
Validity	Requires validation of each instructor	Requires validation of computer software

IV. APPLICATION FOR CRITICAL CARE MEDICINE AND FCCS

A. Experiential Learning

Table A17-5 summarizes the levels of competency, with each level building on the foundation of the previous levels. Typically, lower levels of learning, such as knowledge acquisition and comprehension (the "Knows" and "Knows How" levels), are more easily taught in classrooms and assessed using written and oral examinations; however, there is a role for simulation even at this level. Because adult learners have varied learning styles, simply hearing a lecture or reading a chapter may not be enough to reinforce important information. For visual learners, even basic physiologic and pharmacologic responses can be taught using a simulator. In the FCCS lectures or skills stations, the cardiovascular response to a fluid challenge or the response to a pharmacologic therapy can be demonstrated.

Table A17-5. Levels of Competency	
Knows	Does the learner know the basic information?
Knows How	Can the learner describe how to apply the basic information?
Shows How	Can the learner demonstrate the application of cognitive, psychomotor, and affective skills?
Does	Does the learner perform in the real-world situation?

The application and analysis of learned rules (data integration and problem solving) lend themselves readily to simulation, and the "Shows How" level is where simulation-based learning stands out. Simulators become most effective when training involving data acquisition and motor skills (physical examination, airway management, etc.) is mixed with cognitive analysis and synthesis in a realistic distracting environment of alarms, monitors, and other personnel. Although simulation may not offer an exact replica of the critical care environment, it offers a close approximation while avoiding the problematic nature of learning on patients and goes far beyond the limitations of written and oral exams and testing using workplace assessments (e.g., patient consent, subjective evaluation, stochastic variables). Learners can practice physical examination skills, evaluate monitored and laboratory data, and integrate the information into a problem list and management plan in real time. They then can implement management strategies and practice serial reevaluation of the patient. If the response is incorrect, the simulated clinical experience can be restarted and a different strategy applied. Thus, pattern recognition and learning by experience is applied.

■ Full-scale simulation easily can be applied to many of the FCCS skill stations.

Mechanical ventilation skill stations: Many full-scale simulators allow independent adjustment of right and left lung compliance and resistance, and also permit demonstration of the hemodynamic consequences of auto-PEEP (positive end-expiratory pressure), pneumothorax, and initiation of positive pressure ventilation.

Airway skill station: Real-time scenarios of cannot intubate or cannot intubate/cannot ventilate can be demonstrated and practiced with the use of airway adjuncts (oro- and nasopharyngeal airways, laryngeal mask airways). Methods to assure correct placement of tracheal tubes can be taught better than with a part-task trainer, and the effects and complications of sedatives and neuromuscular blockers can be examined using a full-scale simulator.

Trauma skill station: This is the ideal venue to use full-scale simulation. The standard FCCS trauma scenarios, all requiring rapid evaluation and management of multiple trauma-related hypotension, intracranial hypertension, and thermal injury can be performed in a team setting with full-scale simulation.

B. Team Building/Crisis Management

A second application of simulation is team building and crisis management. Critical care practitioners must employ a large knowledge base, solve problems, and perform psychomotor skills rapidly, but they do not do so in a vacuum; they interact in concert with a number of other trained practitioners with a wide variety of complex interpersonal behaviors. Problems of human performance are recognized as major contributors to preventable errors and undesirable outcomes may relate to errors in technique, judgment, compliance, vigilance, or fixation as well as difficulties in communication. During simulator sessions, defining leaders and followers, assuring high-quality communication, stressing early request for help, utilizing all forms of resources, and avoiding errors of fixation can be emphasized.

When simulation is used for teaching or crisis management, some form of feedback or debriefing is desired. The goals of debriefing are verbal feedback and constructive criticism in a safe educational atmosphere. It is vital to encourage self-assessment and sponsor a change in culture if it is so required. The instructor must correct problem behaviors, attitudes, and actions that hamper individual and team performance. Video analysis of the session, along with other visual tools, can be used to improve the effectiveness of teaching points during debriefing. While not mandatory, video recording can provide examples of communication, leadership, critical thinking, and problem solving by individuals or teams. In the absence of video, students may refute or deny actions, behaviors, or comments.

C. Assessment

Beyond fundamental learning and team building, simulation also has an application in the assessment of competence, especially the "Shows How" level of learning. The development of simulation as a tool in assessment in critical care is evolving and there are numerous challenges in using simulation for high-stakes certification or credentialing. Problem-solving and decision-making skills can be tested in real time and in scenarios containing uncommon events where errors are not reversible. Consistent and reliable simulated clinical experiences and quality scoring systems must be developed, studied, and validated before simulation is used in credentialing. In testing using standardized patients, checklists alone may be used; however, in full-scale simulations, checklists are problematic. Actions must be weighted based on importance, and the timing and sequence of interventions are also significant, which makes scoring more complicated. A holistic global scoring system may be better than a checklist, but it tends to be subjective. Assessment with several simulations rather than one and use of multiple raters may assure that holistic scoring will be more objective. Patient simulators employing physiological models may address some assessment shortcomings, because patient outcome is determined by the quality and timeliness of the care. Lastly, whether simulation can be an indicator of how the student or team will do in the "Does" level of learning (real-world delivery of critical care) must be studied and validated. Inferring real-world behavior from simulation can be problematic because simulation includes inadvertent cueing, scenarios that are not open-ended, and differences in data gathering that may improve performance during testing compared to the critical care environment.

V. LIMITATIONS IN SIMULATION

Simulation in healthcare education and training appears to be gaining acceptance, but it has not yet reached the point of widespread adoption. A number of problems may be encountered with simulator training. Although the cost of full-scale simulators is decreasing, the costs are still high enough to keep this technology from being universally available. Early simulator systems were not easily moved, but the portability of newer systems has improved greatly. The manikins have well-described weaknesses in fidelity, including extraneous nonclinical noises due to valves, solenoids, and the movement of compressed gases within the manikin. There are also impediments to the physical examination, especially in skin (warmth, vasodilatation), abdominal examination (organ enlargement, bowel sounds, ascites), and neurologic evaluation (consciousness, abnormal movements, tendon reflexes).

Although the cost and technical problems may be a limiting factor, a more important shortcoming derives from the limited research into validation of the effectiveness, transfer of training to the clinical environment, and cost-effectiveness of this technology.

 Suggested Readings

1. Beaubien, JM, Baker DP. The use of simulation for training teamwork skills in health care: how low can you go? *Qual Saf Health Care.* 2004;13(suppl 1):51-56.

2. Department of Defense Manual 5000.59-M. Modeling and Simulation Glossary. Washington, DC: Department of Defense, January 1998. Available at: http://handle.dtic.mil/100.2/ADA349800

3. Dunn WF, ed. Simulators in Critical Care and Beyond. Des Plaines, IL: Society of Critical Care Medicine, 2004.

4. Maran, NJ, Glavin RJ. Low- to high-fidelity simulation—a continuum of medical education? *Med Educ.* 2003;37(suppl 1):22-28.

5. Schuwirth LWT, van der Vleuten CP. The use of clinical simulations in assessment. *Med Educ.* 2003;37(suppl 1):65-71.

6. Shapiro MJ, Morey JC, Small SD, et al. Simulation based teamwork training for emergency department staff: does it improve clinical team performance when added to an existing didactic teamwork curriculum? *Qual Saf Health Care.* 2004;13:417-421.

7. Steadman RH, Coates WC, Huang YM, et al. Simulation-based training is superior to problem-based learning for the acquisition of critical assessment and management skills. *Crit Care Med.* 2006;34:151-157.

INDEX